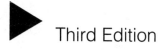

Third Edition

Communication for the Speechless

Franklin H. Silverman
Marquette University
Medical College of Wisconsin

Allyn and Bacon

Boston • London • Toronto • Sydney • Tokyo • Singapore

Series Editor: Kris Farnsworth
Editorial Assistant: Christine M. Shaw
Production Administrator: Joe Sweeney
Editorial-Production Service: Walsh Associates
Cover Administrator: Suzanne Harbison
Composition Buyer: Linda Cox
Manufacturing Buyer: Louise Richardson

Library of Congress Cataloging-in-Publication Data

Silverman, Franklin H.
    Communication for the speechless / Franklin H. Silverman.—3rd ed.
      p.   cm.
    Includes bibliographical references and index.
    ISBN 0-01-318487-4
    1. Speech disorders.   2. Communication devices for the disabled.
  3. Handicapped—Means of communication.   I. Title.
    [DNLM: 1. Speech Disorders—rehabilitation.   2. Manual Communication.
  3. Speech Therapy—instrumentation.   WM 475 S587c 1994]
    RC423.S517   1994
    616.85'5—dc20
    DNLM/DLC
    for Library of Congress   94-33135
                                               CIP

Printed in the United States of America
10 9 8 7 6 5 4 3 2   00 99 98 97 96

To my students, past and present,
American and Palestinian.

Contents

Preface

There are a number of children and adults with essentially normally hearing who are "locked-in" in the sense that their speech is inadequate for meeting their communication needs, at least temporarily. Their "speechlessness" could have resulted from one or a combination of several conditions including severe dysarthria, severe verbal apraxia, aphasia, glossectomy, tracheostomy, dysphonia, severe mental retardation, or childhood autism. During the past quarter century there has been considerable work on developing techniques and devices for augmenting the speech of such persons. Much of this work was reported after 1987 when the manuscript for the second edition of this book was completed. Based on reports in the literature, it would be difficult to conceive of a child or adult being so severely impaired that there would be no augmentative communication strategy or device that he or she could use.

This book is intended to acquaint the advanced undergraduate and masters-level graduate student in speech-language pathology as well as the professional speech-language pathologist and professionals in related fields (including special education, occupational therapy, physical therapy, physical medicine, biomedical engineering, electrical engineering, psychology, social work, vocational rehabilitation, and nursing) with the various strategies that have been developed for augmenting communication. It also is intended to serve as a key to the augmentative and alternative communication (AAC) literature. The reference/bibliography section contains a listing of more than 2,300 published and unpublished books and papers in English and other languages dealing with this topic through the beginning of 1993.

This revision continues to reflect my view that as wide a range of AAC options as possible should be considered when selecting the optimal one (or combination) for a client. Consequently, I have retained descriptions of "older" strategies that, while no longer "fashionable" (judging by the lack of attention paid to them in the recent AAC literature), have been demonstrated to be useful through research and/or clinical experience.

This revision also continues to reflect my view that, whenever possible, persons who initially report a phenomenon (finding) or whose research contributes to its being reported should be acknowledged for their contribution. Considerable information about AAC strategies and their impacts accepted as "factual" was first reported during the 1960s and 1970s. Consequently, many papers from this period are cited, particularly in chapters 2 and 4 and in the section on symbol sets in chapter 5.

Communication for the Speechless is divided into three parts. In the first, or introductory, part (chapters 1 and 2) I describe what is meant by an augmentative communication strategy; indicate how such strategies have been used with several clinical populations; describe the need for a "communication" rather than a "speech" orientation when dealing with persons from these populations; and summarize the outcome literature relevant to the impacts of intervention with these strategies on severely communicatively impaired children and adults. In the second part of the book (chapters 3 through 6) I describe and evaluate the various gestural (unaided), gestural-assisted (aided), and neuro-assisted (aided) communication strategies that have been developed. Finally, in part three (chapters 7 and 8) I describe an evaluation procedure for selecting the "optimal" communication strategy (or combination of strategies) for a client and indicate a number of considerations that were not dealt with in the second part of the book when developing an intervention program. All of the chapters have been updated and the material on intervention in chapter 8 has been expanded considerably.

It is impossible to give credit to all the sources from which the concepts presented in this book have been drawn. This book is the result of more than fifteen years of clinical experience with persons who are severely communicatively impaired. It is also the result of years of reading in the AAC literature (see the reference/bibliography section) and hundred of hours of conversations with students and colleagues about aspects of it. Thus, I cannot credit this or that concept to a particular person, but I can say "thank you" to all who have helped, particularly my students at Marquette University, the Medical College of Wisconsin, the University of Guam, and in the Gaza Strip, whose questions and criticisms through the years have helped me to clarify my own ideas.

FRANKLIN H. SILVERMAN

▶ 1

Need for Augmentative Communication Intervention

Imagine that you woke up tomorrow morning and found yourself unable to produce intelligible speech because your tongue was paralyzed (i.e., you had bilateral hypoglossal nerve damage). Your ability to understand speech and to think and reason would be unimpaired. What impacts would not being able to talk have on your life? Would you be able to continue working or preparing to work in the same field? If not, how would you support yourself? Would your relationships with family members change? If you had children, would they continue to regard you as an "authority figure"? Would your relationships with your friends change? Would they spend less time with you because it would make them uncomfortable being around someone who could not talk? Would you be depressed or possibly suicidal?

Being unable to speak is one of the most severe disabilities that a human being can experience. It is difficult to really understand what it is like to be speechless without actually experiencing the condition. To gain a little insight into what it is like to be speechless, Ricky Creech, a severely communicatively impaired person who is a speech-language pathologist (Creech, 1990c), suggests doing the following:

> *If you want to know what it is like to be unable to speak, there is a way. Go to a party and don't talk. Play mute. Use your hands if you wish but don't use paper or pencil. Paper and pencil are not always handy for mute persons. Here is what you will find: people talking; talking behind, beside, around, over, under, through and even for you. But never with you. You are ignored until finally you feel like a piece of furniture. (Musselwhite & St. Louis, 1988, p. 104)*

Many persons who are severely communicatively impaired with respect to speech are also similarly impaired with respect to writing. They are unable to write

1

well enough to meet their communication needs. Furthermore, some people who can speak well enough to meet their communication needs are unable to write well enough to do so (see Schultz-Muehling & Beukelman, 1990). They, like persons who are severely speech impaired, can be helped by augmentative communication.

To gain further insight into what it is like to be severely communicatively impaired, the following works are recommended: Brown (1954), Buck (1968), Creech (1984, 1988a), Creech and Viggiano (1981), Dahlberg and Jaffe (1977), Holmquist (1984), Huer and Lloyd (1988, 1990), Knox (1971), Moss (1972), Nolan (1981, 1987), Rush (1986), Sienkiewicz-Mercer and Costello (1992), Simpson (1988), Smith-Lewis and Ford (1987), Viggiano (1981, 1982), Weiss, Thatch, and Thatch (1987), Williams (1989), and Wint (1965).

Several conditions can cause natural speech to be inadequate for meeting communication needs other than deafness. Persons who suffer from these conditions are likely to benefit from intervention with what are known as *augmentative communication* (or *augmentative and alternative communication*, or *AAC*) strategies, symbols, aids, and techniques. Their development and utilization began during the 1960s (see McNaughton, 1990a; Zangari, Lloyd, & Vicker, 1994).

How large is the normal hearing, severely communicatively impaired population? Demographic information is limited. However, Blackstone and Painter (1985) estimated that approximately 900,000 people in the United States are nonspeaking as a result of congenital impairments. Shane and Anastasio (1989) estimated that the number of severely communicatively impaired persons in the United States who could benefit from augmentative communication is approximately 1.5 million. Bloomberg and Johnson (1990c) did a statewide survey in Victoria, Australia, and identified more than 5000 persons who were severely communicatively impaired for reasons other than deafness—0.12 percent of the state's population (4,164,700); for those below the age of 22, it was approximately 0.19 percent. Silverman and Meagher (1980) estimated this percentage for the United States as 0.09 percent. Their estimate included only those people who had been seen by ASHA-certified speech-language pathologists. Furthermore, an estimated 2.5 to 6.0 percent of children enrolled in special education programs are so severely speech impaired that they cannot be understood (Aiello, 1980; Blackstone, 1989b; Burd et al., 1988; Matas et al., 1985).

The objective of this chapter is to explain how augmentative communication intervention can be used in the habilitation and rehabilitation of such persons. To accomplish this end, I describe what is meant by augmentative communication, indicate conditions that might call for its use, and demonstrate why it would be both appropriate and advantageous for speech-language pathologists to assume responsibility for selecting and teaching such communication strategies—that is, demonstrate why it would be advantageous for them to function as *communication* therapists rather than as *speech* therapists.

WHAT ARE AUGMENTATIVE COMMUNICATION STRATEGIES?

Augmentative communication strategies can be defined operationally (Bridgman, 1927) as procedures for encoding and transmitting messages without their being written or directly encoded into phonemes by the vocal tract that can augment a person's ability to communicate. Such procedures are not intended to substitute for the residual abilities to speak and write a severely communicatively impaired person possesses. Rather, they are intended to be used in conjunction with them. That is, they are intended to augment, or increase, the abilities of such persons to meet their communication needs.

Almost all (if not all) severely communicatively impaired persons have some residual ability to communicate. In the most severe cases, it is limited to noises, gestures, or facial expressions that communicate being uncomfortable or wanting something. Thus, I prefer the term *augmentative communication* to augmentative and alternative communication.

Any approach to encoding and transmitting spoken messages that does not require a person to produce speech sounds *directly* would be classifiable by this definition as an augmentative communication strategy. The word "directly" is italicized because with some such approaches it is possible to encode a message *indirectly* into phonemes and transmit it as speech. Most indirect methods involve the use of microprocessors and speech synthesizers (see chapter 5).

Hundreds of approaches for encoding and transmitting messages have been developed that could be classified by this definition as augmentative communication strategies (Silverman, 1993a). There is, however, considerable variation in the level of refinement of these strategies. Although some have been tested and refined to the point where they can be regarded as both practical and dependable, others would have to be considered at least somewhat experimental. An example of the first type is American Sign Language, the manual communication system used by the deaf (see chapter 4). The other type includes strategies that use muscle action potentials and other electrical signals generated by the body to control typewriters and computers (LaCourse & Hludik, 1990) (see chapter 6).

Perhaps because the field of augmentative communication is so new, there is no universal agreement on terminology. Different terms sometimes are used for the same concept, and a given concept may be defined in different ways. The need for standardization of terms and definitions is recognized (see Lloyd & Blischak, 1992; Mirenda, 1991), as is the need to develop models of augmentative communication for exploring relationships among these concepts (e.g., Lloyd, Quist, & Windsor, 1990).

WHEN TO USE AUGMENTATIVE COMMUNICATION

Children and adults who have inadequate speech for communicative purposes, for a variety of reasons have benefited from augmentative communication. Its use with various conditions, either temporarily or permanently, are described briefly in this section. We discuss here dysarthria; verbal apraxia; aphasia; glossectomy; dysphonia, including laryngectomy; mental retardation; childhood autism; tracheostomy; intubation; Alzheimer's disease; and deafness. Although the size of the population with each condition (with the exception of deafness) who could benefit from such intervention is uncertain, evidence suggests that it is substantial (e.g., Matas et al., 1985; Silverman & Meagher, 1980). Papers describing the use of augmentative communication with persons having each of these conditions are cited.

Dysarthria

The term *dysarthria* refers to an impairment in the functioning of the musculature of respiration, phonation, and articulation caused by a lesion (or lesions) in the peripheral nervous system, central nervous system, or both. The degree of impairment can be so minimal that dysarthria would be difficult to detect during normal conversational speech, or so severe that any speech produced is completely unintelligible. Persons for whom the degree of neuromuscular impairment is so severe that there is no speech and eye movement is the only volitional motor activity sometimes are referred to as suffering from *locked-in syndrome* (McGann & Paslawski, 1991).

The impact of dysarthria on speech is a function of several factors, including the specific muscle groups affected and the extent to which the functioning of each affected muscle group is impaired. Whereas there is a negative relationship between the number of muscle groups affected and speech intelligibility (i.e., the more muscle groups affected, the poorer the speech intelligibility), the relationship is not perfect. An impairment in the functioning of only a few muscle groups (e.g., the adductors of the vocal folds bilaterally) can result in an inability to speak. (If the adductors of the vocal folds were paralyzed bilaterally and the abductors were unimpaired, the vocal folds would be fixed in the open position and phonation probably would be impossible.)

The extent to which the functioning of individual muscle groups is impaired also influences the impact of dysarthria on speech. Extent of impairment can range from being able to produce a desired muscle gesture (or movement) but at a slower rate than normal to being completely unable to produce that gesture. There is a negative relationship between the degree of impairment of muscle groups and speech intelligibility (i.e., the greater the degree of impairment, the poorer the speech intelligibility), but the relationship is not perfect. Relatively mild involvement of certain parts of the speech musculature (e.g., that of the tongue) can more adversely affect speech intelligibility than can moderate involvement of other parts of this musculature (e.g., that of the lips).

Specific deficits in muscle functioning are determined by the location of the lesion (or lesions) in the nervous system and its magnitude rather than by what produced it. A lesion of a given magnitude at a given point in the nervous system resulting from trauma, a tumor, or a degenerative disease process will produce the same deficit. If the lesion is in the lower motor neurons, the result will be flaccidity. If it is in the upper motor neurons, the result will be spasticity. If it is in the basal ganglia, the result will be involuntary movement. And if it is in the cerebellar system, the result will be dysmetria and other symptoms of ataxia. Thus, persons who have cerebral palsy can experience the same neuromuscular deficits as those who have had a stroke.

Most dysarthrias result in some reduction in speech intelligibility. In some cases this reduction is so great that speech is inadequate for most, if not all, interpersonal communication. In such cases augmentative communication can be used as a substitute for or as an adjunct to speech.

Involvement of certain of the muscle groups that control the vocal tract is particularly likely to result in speech that is not sufficiently intelligible to transmit most messages successfully. These muscle groups include those that control the tongue, the velum, and the vocal folds (particularly the adductors) bilaterally.

A number of neurological conditions frequently have a severe enough dysarthria associated with them to warrant the use of augmentative communication. Cerebral palsy, amyotrophic lateral sclerosis (Blackstone, 1988a), bulbar palsy, pseudobulbar palsy, cerebellar ataxia, Parkinsonism, dystonia, chorea, stroke (CVA), brain tumors, and trauma (Blackstone, 1989h) are examples. (For a description of these conditions, see Darley, Aronson, & Brown, 1975; and Mirenda & Mathy-Laikko, 1989).

Several types of augmentative communication strategies have been used with children and adults who are dysarthric. The following papers describe some of these strategies:

Blissymbolics, a symbol system that can be used with either electronic or nonelectronic communication devices (Australian News and Information Bureau, 1973; Harris-Vanderheiden et al., 1978; Hartley, 1974; Kates & McNaughton, n.d.; MacDonald, 1990; McNaughton, 1976a, 1976b; McNaughton & Kates, 1980; Nelms, 1986; Ross, 1979; Shenhav & Gorfil, 1990; Vanderheiden, Brown, MacKenzie, Reinen, & Scheibel, 1975).

Communication (conversation) boards (Angelo & Goldstein, 1990; Beukelman & Yorkston, 1977; Cohen, 1976; Cook, 1988; DeRuyter & Donoghue, 1989; Goldberg & Fenton, 1960; Handicapped youth . . ., 1974; Honsinger, 1989; Kladde, 1974; McDonald & Schultz, 1973; McNaughton, 1976b; Reichle & Yoder, 1985; Sayre, 1963; Vanderheiden, 1976; Vicker, 1974a, 1974b, 1974c, 1974d; Wu & Voda, 1985; Yorkston, 1989).

Electronic communication systems (Albanese et al., 1990; Alm, Arnott, & Murray, 1992; Alm, Arnott, & Newell, 1992a, 1992b; Alm et al., 1993; Angelo, 1992; Arruabarrena et al., 1989; Beukelman et al., 1986; Bruno & Stoughton, 1984; Bullock, Dalrymple, & Danca, 1975; Burnside, 1974; Butler & Fouldes, 1974; Carlson, 1976; Charbonneau, Cote, & Roy, 1974; Clappe et al., 1973; Combs, 1969; Computerized device . . . ., 1976; Copeland, 1974; Creech, 1984, 1988a, 1988b, 1990a, 1990b, 1990c; Creech et al., 1988; Creech & Viggiano, 1981; Dymond et al., 1988; Enderby & Hamilton, 1981; Ferrier, 1991; Foulds, 1982; Fried-Oken, 1985; Glennen, Sharp-Bittner, & Tullos, 1991; Gorhoff, Mitsuda, & Kenyon, 1981; Hagen, Porter, & Brink, 1973; Harmon, 1974; Harris-Vanderheiden, 1976b; Harris-Vanderheiden et al., 1973; He puffs . . ., 1974; Hill et al., 1968; Honsinger, 1989; Jack H. Eichler . . ., 1973; Jackson, Stirling, & Dixon, 1983; Jardine et al., 1984; Jefcoate, 1970, 1974, 1981; Johnson, Manning, & Lappin; 1972; Kilgallon, Roberts, & Miller, 1987; Lavoy, 1957; Maling & Clarkson, 1963; McGregor, 1991/92; McGuire, Palaganas-Tosco, & Redford, 1988; Perron, 1965; Pollak, 1982; Pollak & Gallagher, 1989; Seamone, 1982; Shahar, Nowaczyk, & Tervo, 1987; Shane & Melrose, 1975; Smith et al., 1989; Stassen, Soede, & Bakker, 1982; Steadman, Ferris, & Rhodine, 1980; Tolstrup, 1975; Vanderheiden, 1975, 1976a, 1976b, 1978; Vanderheiden et al., 1975; Vanderheiden & Luster, 1976; Vanderheiden & Smith, 1989; Vasa & Lywood, 1976; Weintraub, 1982; Wendt, Sprague, & Marquis, 1975; White, 1974).

Gestural Morse code (Adams, 1966; Clement, 1961).

Manual sign languages (Abkarian, 1981; Chen, 1971; Egan, Anthony, & Honke, 1976; Fenn & Rowe, 1975; Meline, 1980; Peters, 1973).

Yes-no gestures (DeRuyter & Donoghue, 1989).

Augmentative communication strategies also have been developed for children and adults who are dysarthric and are also deaf and/or visually impaired (Batstone & Bailey, 1990; Beukelman et al., 1984; Bristow & Pickering, 1990; Bristow, Pickering, & Ballinger, 1992).

Verbal Apraxia

Verbal apraxia prevents a person from normally producing the muscle gestures required for speech on a voluntary level. A person who has this condition is able to produce them normally, however, on a vegetative, or involuntary, level. This differentiates apraxics from dysarthrics, as the latter have some degree of motor deficit on both voluntary and involuntary levels. The condition can affect children as well as adults (Blackstone, 1989d; Culp, 1989; Cumley & Swanson, 1992a, 1992b; Mirenda & Mathy-Laikko, 1989).

Augmentative communication strategies have been used for two purposes with verbal apraxics: facilitating communication and facilitating speech. They facilitate communication by providing the apraxic with an additional channel (or channels) for encoding and transmitting messages—thus supplementing the three channels usually used for this purpose: speech, writing, and normal nonverbal communication. In regard to facilitating speech, there is some evidence (Skelly et al., 1974) that teaching verbal apraxics an augmentative communication strategy is likely to result in an increase in their attempts at speech. (The effect of teaching an augmentative communication strategy on subsequent attempts at verbalization is dealt with further in chapter 2.) Thus, teaching verbal apraxics an augmentative communication strategy may improve both their ability to speak and their ability to communicate.

Several augmentative communication strategies have been used with verbal apraxics. These include the following:

- *Blissymbols* (Lane & Samples, 1981).
- *Gesture* (Hanrahan & Odykirk, 1992).
- *Electronic communication devices* (Copeland, 1974; Perron, 1965).
- *Manual sign languages* (Chen 1968, 1971; Culp, 1989; Eagleson, 1970; Goldojarb, 1976; Goldstein & Cameron, 1952; Hanson, 1976; Helfrich, 1976; Skelly et al., 1974).
- *Nonelectronic communication, or conversation, boards* (Cohen, 1976; Culp, 1989; Nuffer, n.d.; Sklar & Bennett, 1956).
- *Pantomime* (Schlanger, 1976).

Manual sign language seems to be used more often with these patients than other augmentative communication strategies, perhaps partly due to the fact that many verbal apraxics are only hemiplegic. Because hemiplegics have one upper extremity that is normal motorically, it would be relatively simple for them to learn a one-hand manual sign language.

Aphasia

Aphasia is a neurological condition in which there is a deficit in one or more aspects of symbolic formulation and expression (Head, 1926). It is thought to result from a lesion (or lesions) in the cerebral cortex or associated subcortical structures. The aspects of language behavior in which there may be a deficit include speech comprehension, speaking, reading, writing, and computation. Also, there may not be an ability to comprehend and use gestures for communicative purposes (Christopoulou & Bonvillian, 1985; Davis, 1993; Duffy, Duffy, & Pearson, 1975; Kimura, Davidson, & McCormick, 1982; Peterson & Kirshner, 1981). The degree of deficit for a given language ability may be so mild that it only can be detected by a sensitive testing instrument, or so severe that it appears to be completely, or almost completely, absent.

Also, the degree of impairment of a given language ability may not remain constant over time; it may intensify (if the cause, e.g., is a tumor) or become less severe (by spontaneous recovery, the effects of therapies, or both). Note that verbal apraxia is classified by some authors as an aphasic disturbance. (For further information about the symptomatology and etiology of aphasia, see Davis, 1993.)

Augmentative communication can be used with aphasics on a temporary or permanent basis to facilitate communication (Blackstone, 1991c; Garrett & Beukelman, 1992; Garrett, Beukelman, & Low, 1987; Garrett, Beukelman, & Low-Morrow, 1989). Those with moderate to severe deficits in speech comprehension, speaking, reading, and writing may be able to communicate basic needs to persons taking care of them by pointing to pictures on a communication board, by pantomiming, or by using a manual sign language. The need for such communication strategies may only be temporary—perhaps during the first few months post-trauma—because speech comprehension, speaking, reading, and writing may improve sufficiently through spontaneous recovery and speech therapy to be adequate again for the person's communicative purposes. There is some evidence, incidentally, suggesting that the use of augmentative communication during the post-trauma period may facilitate the language recovery process (see chapter 2).

Several augmentative communication strategies have been used with aphasics. These include the following:

Blissymbols (Bailey, 1983; Johannsen-Horbach, Cegla, Mager, Schempp, & Wallesch, 1985; Lane & Samples, 1981; Nenonen, 1990; Rivarola & Risatti, 1990; Sawyer-Woods, 1992; Saya, 1979).

Communication (conversation) boards (Cohen, 1976; Jinks & Pashek, 1992; Merchant & Skarakis-Doyle, 1988; Nuffer, n.d.; Pashek & Jinks, 1992; Sklar & Bennett, 1956).

Drawing (Lyon & Helm-Estabrooks, 1987).

Electronic communication devices (Barron-Jadd & Weitzner-Lin, 1992; Colby et al., 1981; Copeland, 1974; DiSimoni, 1986; Enderby & Hamilton, 1983; Fagerberg & Raade, 1992; Friedrich, 1988; Goodenough-Trepagnier, Askey, & Koeppel, 1992; Hammons, Yager, & Swindell, 1989; Helm-Estabrooks & Walsh, 1982; Nielson, 1983; Perron, 1965; Steele et al., 1989; van Blom, 1990; van Blom & van Balkom, 1990; Yngvesson & Johnsen, 1990).

Manipulable symbols (Glass, Gazzaniga, & Premack, 1973).

Manual sign languages (Chen, 1968, 1971; Eagleson, Vaughn, & Knudson, 1970; Fawcus, 1986; Gardner et al., 1976; Goldojarb, 1976; Goldstein & Cameron, 1952; Guilford, Scheuerle, & Shirek, 1982; Hanson, 1976; Kiernan & Reid, 1984; Kirshner & Webb, 1981; Moody, 1982; Rao, 1986; Rao et al., 1979; Rao & Horner, 1980; Skelly et al., 1975; Wisocki & Mosher, 1980).

Pantomime and gesture (Foldi et al., 1976; Freiman & Schlanger, 1977; Hoit-Dalgaard, Newhoff, & Barnes, 1981; Koller, Schlanger, & Geffner, 1975; Schlanger, 1976; Schlanger & Schlanger, 1970; Tanenbaum & Schlanger, 1968).

Glossectomy

Glossectomy is the surgical excision, or removal, of all or part of the tongue, usually because of cancer. The amount of tissue removed may preclude the postsurgical learning of intelligible speech. Use of an augmentative communication strategy would obviously facilitate communication in such instances. (For further information on glossectomy and its impact on communication, see Skelly, Donaldson, & Fust, 1973.)

All the augmentative communication strategies described in this book are appropriate for glossectomy patients. The only one, however, that seems to have been used extensively with this population is American Indian Hand Talk, or Amer-Ind (Skelly et al., 1975).

Dysphonia (Including Laryngectomy)

Dysphonias are voice disorders. They often result from anatomic or physiological anomalies of the larynx that make normal phonation impossible. Such anomalies include absence of the vocal folds following laryngectomy; bilateral flaccid paralysis of the adductors of the vocal folds (which prevents them from approximating); or lesions on the vocal folds, such as vocal modules. (For additional information on the symptomatology and etiology of dysphonias, see Boone & McFarlane, 1988.)

Augmentative communication strategies have been used for several purposes with children and adults who have voice problems—for example, as a temporary communication mode for patients who are on vocal rest because of a lesion (or lesions) on their vocal folds (e.g., vocal nodules) resulting from vocal abuse. They also have been used as a permanent communication mode for patients who have permanently lost the ability to phonate, such as those with laryngectomies who are poor candidates for an electrolarynx or esophageal speech (included in this group would be persons who have had both laryngectomies and glossectomies). In addition, they have been used as a temporary communication mode for persons who have had laryngectomies, until they have acquired adequate esophageal speech for communicative purposes. They can provide such persons, for example, with a means of transmitting emergency and other messages over a telephone.

All the augmentative communication strategies described in this book are appropriate for dysphonic patients. The only type, however, that appears to have been used extensively with this population is manual sign language (Skelly et al., 1975).

Mental Retardation

Mental retardation is a condition that is presumed to result at least partly from organically based slowness in cognitive development—that is, slowness in the ability to solve problems and see relationships. Because this ability influences all aspects of functioning, the overall development of affected persons would be expected to be slow, including their use of speech for intrapersonal and interpersonal communication. The degree of slowness in cognitive development can be so little that it is unlikely to have a significant impact on the person's ability to cope with his or her environment, or so great that a person can cope only in a highly structured institutional environment that would make almost no demands on him or her. The cognitive development of persons with this condition rarely, if ever, catches up to that of normal persons. For additional information about this condition in the context of augmentative communication, see Mirenda and Mathy-Laikko (1989).

Many children who are mentally retarded (particularly those with IQs of less than 50) do not have enough speech to communicate all of their needs (Keogh et al., 1987). They attempt to communicate primarily by crying (or screaming or producing other noises), pointing, and/or using very concrete gestures. These behaviors often are not perceived as messages; or if they are perceived as such, are not appropriately interpreted. Considerable clinical evidence (see the papers cited in the next paragraph and Blackstone, 1990b, 1992b) indicates that augmentative communication strategies can not only improve the abilities of such persons to communicate but also can facilitate their acquisition of speech. (The impact of learning augmentative communication strategies on the verbal output of mentally retarded children and adults is discussed in chapter 2.)

Several types of augmentative communication strategies have been used with mentally retarded children and adults. The following are some of these strategies.

Blissymbolics (Australian News and Information Bureau, 1973; Fuller, 1992; Harris-Vanderheiden, 1976a; Hughes, 1979; Kalimikerakis, 1983; McNaughton, 1976a, 1976b; Song, 1979; Vanderheiden, Brown, MacKenzie, Reinen, & Scheibel, 1975).

Communication boards (Holst & Holmberg, 1990; House, Hanley, & Magid, 1980; Mirenda & Santogrossi, 1985; Reid & Hurlbut, 1977; Rotholz, Berkowitz, & Burberry, 1989; Taub, 1977).

Electronic communication devices (Armstrong, 1990; Cascella & Laurent, 1989; Cress & French, 1992; Kojima, 1990; Kostraba et al., 1992; Laurent & Cascella, 1989; Locke & Mirenda, 1988; Romski & Sevick, 1988c).

Eyegaze (Brown, Mineo, & Cavalier, 1986).

Manipulable symbols (Carrier, 1974a, 1974b, 1976; Carrier & Peak, 1975; Hodges & Schwethelm, 1984; Premack & Premack, 1974).

Manual sign languages (Anderson & Neuman, 1977; Bell et al, 1976; Bicker, 1972; Brenner, 1986; Bristow & Fristoe, 1987; Brookner & Murphy, 1975; Browder, Morris, & Snell, 1981; Bryen, Goldman, & Quinlist, 1988; Bryen & McGinley, 1991; Carr, 1981; Clark et al., 1984; Clarke, Remington, & Light, 1986, 1988; Dalrymple & Feldman, 1992; Duker, 1984; Duker & Michielsen, 1983; Duker & Moonen, 1985, 1986; Duker & Morsink, 1984; Fawcett & Clibbens, 1983; Fletcher & Havemeyer, 1977; Foxx et al., 1988; Fristoe, 1976; Fristoe & Lloyd, 1977, 1978, 1979a, 1979b, 1980; Gates, 1987; Gates & Edwards, 1989; Goodman & Remington, 1993; Goodman, Wilson, & Bornstein, 1978; Grecco, 1972; Green, 1975; Griffith & Robinson, 1980; Hall & Talkington, 1970; Hobson & Duncan, 1979; Hoffmeister & Farmer, 1972; Iacono & Parsons, 1986a, 1986b; Jones & Cregan, 1986; Kahn, 1977, 1981; Karlan, 1991b; Kent, 1974; Keogh et al., 1987; Kiernan, 1977; Kimble, 1975; Kohl, 1981; Kopchick & Lloyd, 1976; Kopchick, Romback, & Smilovitz, 1975; Kotkin, Simpson, & Desanto, 1978; Lake, 1976; Larson, 1971; Launonen & Kokkonen, 1990; Lebeis & Lebeis, 1975; Light, Watson, & Remington, 1990; Lloyd & Daniloff, 1983; Luftig, 1982, 1983; Malanga & Poling, 1992; Matson et al., 1988; McEntee, 1985; McIlvane et al., 1984; Miller et al., 1991; Nozaki et al., 1991; Oliver & Halle, 1982; Owens & Harper, 1971; Penner & Williams, 1982; Peters, 1973; Poulton & Algozzine, 1980; Prevost, 1983; Prinz & Shore, 1981; Reid & Kiernan, 1979; Remington & Clarke, 1993a, 1993b; Remington, Watson, & Light, 1990; Richardson, 1975; Romski & Ruder, 1984; Rotholz, Berkowitz, & Burberry, 1989; Roustan, Glazer, & Burbidge, 1986; Schaeffer, 1980; Schepis et al., 1982; Sedey, Rosin, & Miller, 1991; Sensenig, Mazeika, & Topf, 1989; Shaffer & Goehl, 1974; Shimizu, 1988; Sisson & Barrett, 1984; Sommer, Whitman, & Keogh, 1988; Spragale & Micucci, 1989, 1990; Stremel-Campbell, Cantrell, & Halle, 1977; Sutherland & Beckett, 1969; Topper, 1975; Topper-Zweibwan, 1977; Van Hook & Stohr, 1973; VanBiervliet, 1977; Watkins, Sprafkin, & Krolikowski, 1990; Wells, 1981; Wilson, 1974a, 1974b; Wilson, Goodman, & Wood, 1975; Zweiben, 1977).

Pantomime (Balick, Spiegel, & Greene, 1976; Levett, 1969, 1971a, 1971b).

Signaling behaviors (Carlson et al., 1987; Sternberg, McNerney, & Pegnatore, 1987).

Textured symbols for the visually impaired (Murray-Branch, Udavari-Solner, & Bailey, 1991).

Yerkish (LANA) lexigrams (Adamson et al., 1992; Abrahamsen, Brady & Saunders, 1991; Romski, 1984; Romski & Sevick, 1984, 1989; Romski et al., 1985; Romski, Sevcik, & Rumbaugh, 1985; Romski et al., 1984).

For augmentative communication strategies that have been used with cerebral palsied and other physically handicapped mentally retarded children and adults, see the papers cited in the section on *dysarthria* under the subheadings "Communication (conversation) boards" and "Electronic communication devices."

Childhood Autism

Autism appears to begin early in childhood. An autistic child is presumed to be in less than normal contact with his or her total external sensory environment, as children so diagnosed tend not to respond normally to most, if not all, forms of external sensory stimulation. There does not appear to be general agreement on the etiology of childhood autism—whether it is a learned response pattern, the result of abnormal functioning of some structure (or structures) within the central nervous system, both of these, or something else. (For additional information on childhood autism, see recent volumes of the *Journal of Autism and Childhood Schizophrenia* and Mirenda & Mathy-Laikko, 1989.)

Autistic children typically make little, if any, attempt to use speech for communicating with persons in their environments. Such children, in fact, are reported to make little, if any, use of vocalization or gesture for this purpose. Also, they typically do not respond normally to speech directed to them, and for this reason are sometimes misdiagnosed as having a hearing loss.

There is some evidence (see the papers cited in the next paragraph and Blackstone, 1991a) that the interpersonal communication of autistic children can be facilitated in two ways by augmentative communication strategies. First, at least some such children will attempt to communicate with persons in their environment more while using the strategies than they did previously. And, second, at least a few will begin to use speech for interpersonal communication. (The impact of augmentative communication strategies on the verbal output of autistic children is dealt with further in chapter 2.)

Several types of augmentative communication strategies have been used with autistic children, including the following:

Communication (conversation) boards (Howlin, 1989; Lapidus, Adler, & Modugno, 1984; Mirenda & Schuler, 1988; Ratusnik & Ratusnik, 1974, 1976; Reichle & Brown, 1986).

Computers and other electronic communication aids (Hendbring, 1985; Lakkanna & Kravitz, 1992).

Facilitated communication (Anderson & Harrison, 1992; Batt, Remington-Gurney, & Crossley, 1990; Beukelman, 1993; Biklen, 1988, 1990a, 1990b, 1992a, 1992b; Biklen & Crossley, 1990; Biklen et al., 1991; Bilkin & Schubert, 1991; Calculator, 1992a, 1992b; Crossley, 1991, 1992; Crossley & McDonald, 1984; Crossley, Remington-Gurney, & Batt, 1990; Cummins & Prior, 1992; Friedrich, 1992; Grandin, 1989; Hudson, Melita, & Arnold, 1993; McClennen & Gabel, 1992; McLean, 1992; Prior & Cummins, 1992; Prizant &

Schuler, 1987; Remington-Gurney, Crossley, & Batt, 1990; Rimland, 1992; Smith & Belcher, 1993). Facilitated communication usually involves an electronic device that has a keyboard such as a computer or a Cannon Communicator.

Manual sign languages (Barnes, S., 1973; Baron, Isensee, & Davis, 1977; Barrera, Labato-Barrera, & Sulzer-Azaroff, 1980; Barrera & Sulzer-Azaroff, 1983; Bebko, 1990; Benaroya et al., 1979; Benaroya et al., 1977; Bonvillian & Nelson, 1976, 1978; Bonvillian, Nelson, & Rhyme, 1981; Brady & Smouse, 1978; Carr, 1979, 1982; Carr et al., 1978; Carr & Kologinsky, 1983; Carr, Kologinsky, & Leff, 1987; Carr, Pridal, & Dores, 1984; Casey, 1978; Creedon, 1975; Fulwiler & Fouts, 1976; Haight, 1975; Hinerman et al., 1982; Hollander & Juhrs, 1974; Howlin, 1989; Karlan, 1991b; Kiernan, 1977, 1980, 1983; Kiernan & Reid, 1984; Kiesow, n.d.; Konstantareas, 1984, 1985, 1987; Konstantareas, Hunter, & Sloman, 1982; Konstantareas, Oxman, & Webster, 1977, 1978; Konstantareas et al., 1975; Konstantareas, Webster, & Oxman, 1979; Layton, 1988; Leibl, Pettet, & Webster, 1974; Lucas & Dean, 1976; Menyuk, 1974; Miller and Miller, 1973; Miller & Toca, 1979; Mirenda & Schuler, 1988; Offir, 1976; Ricks & Wing, 1975; Salvin et al., 1977; Schaeffer, 1980; Schaeffer et al., 1975; Schepis et al., 1982; Smith, 1975; Tatman & Webster, 1973; Watters, Wheeler, & Watters, 1981; Webster et al., 1973; Wetherby, 1989; Wherry & Edwards, 1983; Wills, 1981; Yoder & Layton, 1988).

Written language (Marshall & Hegrenes, 1972).

Tracheostomy

A person who has had a *tracheostomy*—an opening through the neck into the trachea with an indwelling tube inserted to prevent the opening from closing—is unable to speak. For some patients the tracheostomy is only temporary, as during the early stages of recovery from an accident while in intensive care. For others, it is long term or permanent, to allow them, for example, to be interfaced with a ventilator, a device that assists in breathing. Several augmentative communication strategies have been used by persons who have had a tracheostomy (Adamson & Dunbar, 1991; Blackstone, 1992a; Cumpata & Donahue, 1985; Dowden, 1986; Dowden, Beukelman, & Lossing, 1986; Dowden, Honsinger, & Beukelman, 1986; Easton, 1988; English & Prutting, 1975; Ferngren & Sundberg, 1990; Fried-Oken, Howard, & Stewart, 1991; Garrison, 1982; Gordan, Johnson, & Montague, 1979; Lee & Fina, 1985; Metz, Horst, & Kruger, 1984; Mitsuda et al., 1992; Simon, 1985; Sparker, 1989).

Intubation

Some patients, usually following trauma or during or after surgery, have a breathing tube inserted in the mouth or nose that passes through the larynx. The purpose of intubation is to ensure an airway for the delivery of an anesthetic gas or oxygen. Because the tube passes between the vocal folds, the patient is unable to speak. Intubated patients are often found in intensive care units. Augmentative strategies and devices have been used to facilitate communication for such persons (Fried-Oken, Howard, & Stewart, 1991; Honsinger, Yorkston, & Dowden, 1987; Mitsuda et al., 1992; Presley, 1980; Roodenburg, 1988; Sparker, 1989; Stovsky, Rudy, & Dragonette, 1988; Williams, 1992; Wyper, Evans, et al., 1986). Such patients' ability to communicate also has been augmented by encouraging them to mouth words (Fried-Oken, Howard, & Stewart, 1991).

Alzheimer's Disease and Other Types of Dementia

Many persons who have *Alzheimer's disease* and other types of dementia are severely communicatively impaired because of problems with memory and lexical retrieval (see Lubinski, 1991). They differ from the other populations discussed in that their communication impairment usually is not due to a lack of ability to speak. Portable communication boards (sometimes called memory books or memory bracelets) have been used by such persons as memory aids for facilitating communication (Bourgeois, 1990, 1991, 1992, 1993; Silverman & Schuyler, 1994). Other augmentative communication strategies may also facilitate their communication. Because dementia traditionally has not been considered a disorder that can be helped by augmentative communication intervention, its potential for helping persons with dementia is uncertain.

Deafness

Deafness is used to designate a profound hearing loss. Persons with this condition receive little or no information necessary to understand speech through the auditory channel. (They may, however, receive such information through the visual channel by speechreading.) Because they have both a profound interpersonal and intrapersonal hearing deficit for speech, the deaf usually do not learn to talk without special training. Even with such training, their speech may not become sufficiently intelligible for at least some communicative purposes. Many deaf persons, therefore, rely on augmentative communication as either a supplement to or substitute for speech.

The augmentative communication strategy used most often by the deaf is the manual gestural system known as American Sign Language, or Ameslan (Moores, 1974; this system is described in chapter 4). Ameslan has been used by the deaf in two ways. One is as a supplement to speech: Messages are encoded and transmitted simultaneously in manual sign and speech (this approach to communication for the deaf is referred to in the literature as "total communication"). The other is as a substitute for speech: Messages are encoded and transmitted in manual sign. Other augmentative communication strategies used with the deaf include ones involving Blissymbols (Goddard, 1977).

The only segment of the deaf population for which augmentative communication strategies other than manual gestural systems have been used extensively are those who are also intellectually impaired, physically impaired, and/or blind. Papers describing their use are Albanese, Sauer, and Jarrell (1990); Blackstone (1988d); Mathy-Laikko and Iacono (1988); Mathy-Laikko et al. (1989); Mathy-Laikko et al. (1987); Rowland (1988, 1990), Rowland and Schweigert (1989, 1990, 1992); Rowland, Schweigert, and Brummett (1988); Sauer, Albanese, and Jarrell (1992); and Thorley et al. (1991).

Although almost all the augmentative communication strategies that have been used with the deaf are described in this book, we do not treat their use with the deaf in depth here, for two reasons. First, there is already a very large literature describing their use, particularly Ameslan, with this population. (Representative bibliographies of this literature can be obtained from the Gallaudet College Bookstore, Washington, D.C.) And, second, a systematic review of this literature would not have been possible within the length restrictions of this book.

ROLE OF THE SPEECH-LANGUAGE PATHOLOGIST

An attempt has been made in this chapter to establish the need for augmentative communication by indicating that there are children and adults who are functionally speechless temporarily or permanently because of one or more of several conditions and by providing evidence that augmentative communication strategies can make functional communication possible for such persons. Assuming that the need for such communication strategies has been established, who should have the primary responsibility for selecting them and teaching their use?

This section presents the point of view advocated by the American Speech-Language-Hearing Association that the person who should assume this responsibility is the speech-language pathologist (American Speech-Language-Hearing Association, 1991a, 1991b, 1993; Competencies for speech-language pathologists providing services in augmentative communication, 1988; Position statement on nonspeech communication, 1981). At least half of all ASHA-certified speech-language pathologists do so (Shewan & Blake, 1991). This section also presents the point of view that speech-language pathologists, to discharge this responsibility successfully, have to function as *communication* therapists rather than *speech* therapists and consult when necessary with other professionals such as physical therapists, occupational therapists, physicians, psychologists, engineers (electrical or biomedical), social workers, vocational counselors, wheelchair seating specialists, nurses, special education teachers (see Locke & Mirenda, 1992), and clergy.

Professional Responsibilities of the Speech-Language Pathologist

The speech-language pathologist is responsible for diagnosing and treating (nonmedically) all communicative disorders except those arising from hearing loss. (The diagnosis and nonmedical treatment of communicative disorders resulting from hearing loss is the responsibility of the audiologist.) The speech-language pathologist assesses the communicative status of his or her clients and then develops intervention strategies that will, it is hoped, improve their ability to communicate. In most cases, such intervention strategies are intended to improve clients' ability to speak to the point where, if not within normal limits, is, nonetheless, adequate for their communicative purposes.

Following an assessment of their clients' communicative status, speech-language pathologists sometimes are forced to conclude that the prognosis for speech becoming adequate for communicative purposes is extremely poor. Or perhaps the prognosis is good for some future time but not for the immediate future. Under either circumstance, speech-language pathologists have a responsibility to help their clients develop augmentative communication strategies for meeting their communication needs. This responsibility has several aspects:

1. Selecting the augmentative communication strategy that will most likely meet the client's communication needs.
2. Securing necessary hardware and software.
3. Teaching the client how to use the strategy.
4. Periodically reassessing the client's cognitive, motor, and sensory abilities and communication needs to ensure that the strategy continues to meeting the client's communication needs.

The first part of the speech-language pathologist's responsibility to the severely communicatively impaired client is to select an optimum augmentative communication strategy (which may be a combination of augmentative communication strategies) for meeting his or her communication needs. The speech-language pathologist first determines which strategies the client has the motor, sensory, and cognitive abilities to use and then selects from this subset the one (or combination of several) that would be optimum for meeting the client's communication needs. An approach that can be used for these purposes is described in chapter 7.

Once an augmentative communication strategy has been selected, the speech-language pathologist is responsible for securing any necessary hardware or software. The concepts of hardware and software are adopted from computer terminology, where *hardware* refers to the instrumentation in a computer system, and *software* to the programs that are necessary for it to perform its functions. Thus, hardware refers to instrumentation, and software to the symbol system (or systems) required for it to perform its function.

Figure 1–1 illustrates the application of these concepts to augmentative communication. The device pictured is a simple conversation, or communication, board. The hardware component would be a piece of plywood, cardboard, Masonite, plastic, or other material of the desired size and shape, and the software component would be the symbols (in this case, words) attached to or printed on it. (Construction of communication boards is described in chapter 5.) Both the hardware and software components of augmentative communication aids often are considerably more complex than those illustrated in Figure 1–1. (The types of hardware and software components in augmentative communication aids are described in chapters 5 and 6.)

After a strategy has been selected and the necessary hardware and software have been secured, the speech-language pathologist is responsible for teaching the client how to use the strategy for encoding and transmitting messages. For some strategies, such instruction would take only a few minutes; for others, it could take a year or longer. An example of one that would probably take only a few minutes is teaching a glossectomy patient how to use a simple picture communication board. One that could take a year or longer is teaching a spastic quadriplegic how to use a sophisticated microcomputer-based Blissymbol communication aid.

One last aspect of the responsibility of the speech-language pathologist to severely communicatively impaired clients is periodically to reassess their cognitive, sensory, and motor abilities and communication needs to ensure that the strategies they use continue to help them meet their needs. Thus, the speech-language pathologist makes certain that the strategies used by clients continue to be optimum for them, helps clients maintain hardware and software, and counsels clients and those with whom they communicate as problems arise.

It is not safe to assume that what appears to be an optimal communication strategy when a client is first seen will continue to be so. There are several reasons. First, clients' communication needs may vary over time. An expressive aphasic, for ex-

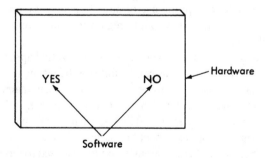

FIGURE 1–1   **Hardware and software components of an augmentative communication aid.**

ample, immediately following the stroke that caused her aphasia may be able to communicate necessary messages to hospital personnel by means of a relatively simple conversation board. After she is discharged from the hospital and returns home, however, the board may no longer be adequate for what she needs to communicate.

Another reason is that a client's sensory, cognitive, and motor abilities may not remain constant. They tend to become worse, for example, as some neurological conditions and diseases progress. Persons who have such a condition or disease may no longer be able at some point during its development to use effectively an augmentative communication strategy. In turn, clients also have to be reassessed periodically because of improvement in their motor, sensory, or cognitive abilities. With improvement in any of these areas, they may be able to use a more efficient and/or flexible strategy. A child who has cerebral palsy, for example, may show improvement in his cognitive, motor, and sensory abilities as he grows older. Consequently, a communication strategy (or combination of strategies) that would be optimal for such a child at age 3 may not be optimal for him or her at age 9.

It is necessary for speech-language pathologists periodically to contact severely communicatively impaired clients in order to help them maintain the hardware and software components of their communication aids. Such contact is particularly important if the aids have electronic components. Even the simplest electronic aid is likely to malfunction if it is used frequently or over a long period of time. Obviously, any malfunction will interfere to some extent with the client's ability to encode and transmit messages.

Also, speech-language pathologists should periodically contact their clients to provide necessary counseling. The attitudes of both the client and those with whom he or she communicates toward an augmentative communication strategy can influence the effectiveness of that strategy. If these attitudes are positive, the effectiveness of the strategy is likely to be enhanced. However, if they are negative, for either the client or those with whom he or she communicates, its effectiveness as a channel for encoding and transmitting messages is likely to be reduced. Although a client and his or her family may initially accept the use of an aid, their attitude may change with time, particularly if they rightly or wrongly regard the aid as only temporary until speech becomes adequate.

This is apt to happen with adults who have a severe verbal apraxia. Immediately following their stroke (or whatever was responsible for the lesion that precipitated the apraxia), they may have a positive attitude toward using an augmentative communication aid because it provides them with a way to communicate. If their speech does not return after a few months, however, and they sense that they may have to continue using the aid on a long-term or permanent basis, their attitude toward it may change from acceptance to rejection. There obviously would be a need for counseling in such a case. (Considerations in counseling users of augmentative communication aids and their families are dealt with in chapter 8.)

The Speech-Language Pathologist as Communication Pathologist

Speech-language pathologists would best serve their clients if their orientation were that of a communication pathologist rather than a speech pathologist. Having a communication orientation could influence their clinical functioning in several ways, including their goals for therapy and consequently their termination criteria and criteria for evaluating both therapy outcome and the adequacy of their own clinical performance.

From the *speech* orientation, the ultimate goal of therapy is either normal speech or speech that is adequate for the client's communicative purposes. (The latter would tend to be the ultimate goal for persons in the clinical populations that were mentioned earlier in this chapter.) The emphasis on therapy is on improving speech. Improving speech tends to be regarded as an end in itself rather than as a means to an end. Therapy usually is terminated when further improvement in speech seems unlikely. Therapy outcome is assessed primarily with regard to speech status, and clinicians tend to base judgments of the adequacy of their clinical performance on the amount of improvement in their clients' speech.

From the *communication* orientation, on the other hand, the ultimate goal of therapy would be developing the ability to communicate to a level adequate to meet communication needs. Because speech is almost universally regarded as the most flexible and efficient symbol system for encoding and transmitting messages, attempts would be made to improve speech as much as possible. Improving speech from this orientation, however, would tend to be regarded as a means to an end (i.e., achieving adequate ability to communicate) rather than an end in itself.

The emphasis in therapy from a communication orientation would be on developing an adequate ability to communicate. Several channels for encoding and transmitting messages usually are developed, including speech (Bodine & Beukelman, 1991). The client may be encouraged to combine speech with augmentative strategies while communicating. This approach to the habilitation and rehabilitation of severely communicatively impaired hearing clients is similar to the total communication approach used by teachers of the deaf.

Therapy would be terminated from a communication orientation when it appeared that further significant improvement in communication was unlikely. The point at which therapy would be terminated from this orientation sometimes would differ from the other. The discharge criteria used by a clinician having a communication orientation would include "no further significant improvement likely *at this time* in the client's ability to encode and transmit messages." Obviously, the possibility of there being further significant improvement at some future time cannot be eliminated. This aspect of the discharge criteria for clinicians having a speech orientation would tend to be more limited: "no further significant improvement likely at this time in the client's ability to encode and transmit messages *through speech*."

Therapy outcome from a communication orientation is assessed primarily in regard to communication status. The closer the clients' communication abilities come to meeting their communication needs, the better the therapy outcome is judged to be. Clients' speech status, of course, is considered when assessing therapy outcome from this perspective.

Clinicians who have a communication orientation tend to base judgments about the adequacy of their clinical performance on the amount their clients improve their ability to communicate. Whereas such clinicians would attempt to improve their clients' speech as much as possible, and would judge their clinical performance positively if they were able to improve their clients' speech significantly, they would not necessarily judge their clinical performance negatively if they were unsuccessful in helping them improve their speech. Because their goal for therapy is the improved ability to communicate, they would tend to judge the adequacy of their clinical performance positively if their clients significantly improved their abilities to encode and transmit messages, regardless of the contribution of speech to their clients' improved communication abilities. Because for most severely communicatively impaired persons the prognosis for developing adequate speech for communicative purposes tends to be poorer than that for developing adequate ability to communicate by augmentative means, clinicians are more likely to assess the adequacy of their clinical performance positively when working with such clients if they have a communication orientation than if they have a speech orientation.

Another way by which the orientation of clinicians can influence their clinical performance is the impact it can have on their attitude toward the role of augmentative communication in the habilitation and rehabilitation of clients who have inadequate speech for communicative purposes. From the speech orientation, augmentative communication would tend to be regarded as a last resort. It usually would not be introduced before attempts had been made to develop adequate speech for communicative purposes. Only after it became obvious that further speech therapy would be unlikely to facilitate adequate speech would augmentative communication tend to be considered. In some cases, augmentative communication would not be considered even then, as the speech-language pathologist may not consider developing and teaching the use of augmentative communication to be part of his or her professional responsibility. A speech-language pathologist is particularly likely to have this attitude if a client requires an aid more sophisticated than a simple nonelectronic communication board (e.g., one that uses a special switching mechanism to control a microcomputer).

In some cases, when a speech-language pathologist does not assume the responsibility for developing and teaching a client to use an augmentative communication system, someone else will (e.g., an occupational therapist or a special education teacher). In other situations, no one will assume this responsibility, and the client will remain unable to communicate adequately. Such a situation is unfortunate because there are currently augmentative strategies available through which the ability to communicate of almost any severely communicatively impaired person can be enhanced. (These are described in chapters 4, 5, and 6.)

From a communication orientation, augmentative communication strategies are not viewed as a last resort but as techniques that can assist a clinician in achieving his or her ultimate goal—the client's developing adequate ability to communicate. They may be introduced at the beginning of therapy before a reliable prognosis can be made about the likelihood of the client developing adequate speech for communicative purposes. When they are introduced at this stage of the habilitation or rehabilitation process, they may be regarded merely as temporary. Whether viewed as temporary or permanent, they do tend to improve the client's ability to communicate

If it appears at a later stage of therapy that speech alone is unlikely ever to be adequate for a client's communicative purposes, a speech-language pathologist with a communication orientation will attempt to select and teach the client to use the optimal strategy or strategies that alone or in combination with speech will allow adequate communication. This strategy or combination of strategies is likely to be more sophisticated than is that used by the client initially. One reason is that a client's communication needs may become more complex. Once stroke patients return home from the hospital, for example, they are apt to find that the messages they need to communicate are both greater in number and more complex than when they were in the hospital. The main point here is that communication-oriented clinicians will introduce augmentative communication strategies during the course of therapy whenever they feel such strategies are necessary.

These differences between the two orientations are summarized in Table 1–1.

The Speech-Language Pathologist as a Team Member

Although speech-language pathologists with a communication orientation usually would assume the primary responsibility for helping "speechless" patients communicate adequately, to discharge this responsibility they would frequently find it necessary to consult with and utilize the services of other professionals. Physical therapists, occupational therapists, engineers, psychologists, social workers, vocational counselors, wheelchair seating specialists, nurses, teachers, and clergy are examples of such professionals.

Physical and occupational therapists can contribute in several ways to the habilitation or rehabilitation of severely communicatively impaired patients. First, they can provide an assessment of muscle function of the extremities and other parts of the body—information needed when selecting a switching mechanism for a client and the muscle movement (gesture) to activate it. (Switching mechanisms are dealt with in chapters 3, 5, 6, and 7.) This information also would be needed when selecting a pointing technique (e.g., finger, eye, or head movement) that would enable a client to indicate message components on a communication board. (Pointing techniques are described in chapter 5.)

Another way physical and occupational therapists contribute to the habilitation or rehabilitation of severely communicatively impaired persons is by helping them to

TABLE 1–1 **Summary of Differences between Speech and Communication Orientations**

Speech Orientation	Communication Orientation
The ultimate goal in therapy is developing either normal speech or adequate speech for communicative purposes.	The ultimate goal of therapy is developing the ability to communicate at a level adequate to meet communication needs.
Improvement of speech is regarded as an end in itself.	Improvement of speech is regarded as a means to an end (i.e., achieving adequate ability to communicate).
The primary emphasis in therapy is on improving speech.	The primary emphasis in therapy is on developing adequate ability to communicate.
Therapy usually is terminated when it appears that further significant improvement in speech is unlikely.	Therapy usually is terminated when it appears that further significant improvement in communication is unlikely.
Therapy outcome is assessed primarily in regard to speech status.	Therapy outcome is assessed primarily in regard to communication status.
Clinicians tend to base judgments of the adequacy of their clinical performance on the amounts their clients improve their speech.	Clinicians tend to base judgments of the adequacy of their clinical performance on the amounts their clients improve their abilities to communicate.
Clinicians tend to regard augmentative communication strategies as "last resorts"; that is, they only tend to introduce them after attempts to improve speech have failed.	Clinicians tend to regard augmentative communication strategies as useful temporary or permanent techniques for achieving their goal, that is, adequate ability to communicate.

develop or refine muscle gestures that can be used for activating switching mechanisms or for indicating message components on a communication board. The more quickly and accurately the person is able to make these muscle gestures, the more flexible and efficient the communication aids he or she will be able to use.

A third way is by assisting in the design and construction of hardware components for communication systems, including

- Switching mechanisms
- Headsticks and other indicating devices for use with communication boards
- Braces for stabilizing an extremity or part of an extremity to permit the muscle gesture (or gestures) required to activate a switching mechanism or point to message components on a communication board
- Hardware components of communication boards and the frames for supporting them

(These components of communication aids are described in chapter 5.)

Another contribution of physical and occupational therapists (if no wheelchair seating specialist is available) is to construct inserts for clients' wheelchairs so that they will be aligned in space in a manner that is appropriate for facilitating communication. If a person is seated in a wheelchair, for example, and cannot easily see the symbols on his communication board, this obviously can interfere with his use of the device.

Engineers can recommend switching mechanisms that would be within the limits of the physical abilities of such patients to activate. Also, they can design, recommend components for, and construct (or arrange to have constructed) electronic communication aids that would meet particular patients' needs. And they can service (or arrange to have serviced) components of such aids when they malfunction. (Components of electronic communication aids are described in chapters 3, 5, and 6.)

Another professional group that can contribute in several ways to the communication habilitation or rehabilitation of speechless patients are nurses. They can suggest messages or message components that it would be important for a patient to be able to communicate to them; "doctor," "bedpan," "medication," "food," "water," and "nurse" are examples. Also nurses can make it possible for such patients to use their communication aids whenever they want to communicate. This involves, for example, making certain that a patient has his communication board available and positioned so that he can indicate message components on it. It also involves making certain, if the patient uses a headpointer to indicate message components, that the device is in place whenever he wishes to communicate. For patients who use a switching mechanism to control a display, this responsibility would involve making certain that the switching mechanism is positioned so that they can activate it whenever they wish. Finally, nurses can positively reinforce patients for communicating using their augmentative communication strategy or aid.

Another professional group that can be involved in the communication habilitation and rehabilitation of severely communicatively impaired persons, particularly children, are teachers. Their contributions are similar to those of nurses. Also, they can provide information about what messages a child would have to be able to communicate in a classroom in order to stand a chance of being successful academically.

In severely communicatively impaired persons, particularly adults who have aphasia or dysarthria, the clergy are important. For many such persons life no longer has much meaning. They can no longer do the things they did that made it meaningful. Unless they can find some reasons for renewing their interest in life, they are likely to remain depressed and not be motivated to communicate (Frankl, 1985). A priest, minister, or rabbi may be able to help them do this, thereby causing them to become less depressed and more interested in communicating.

Psychologists, social workers, and vocational counselors also can contribute: Psychologists can assess clients' level of cognitive functioning. Social workers can help clients and their families locate needed resources, particularly financial ones. And vocational counselors can provide information about occupations a client may be capable of pursuing and what communication abilities a particular occupation would require.

▶ 2

Impacts of Augmentative Communication Intervention on Behavior

Chapter 1 dealt with the need for augmentative communication. There it was argued that such intervention enables both children and adults who have insufficient speech for their communicative purposes to transmit messages. This chapter is concerned with the impacts of augmentative communication on the behavior of children and adults. When evaluating any therapy strategy, method, or technique, it is necessary to be concerned about its total impact on the person, not just its effect on the particular behavior (or behaviors) it is intended to modify or facilitate. Determining these impacts involves answering a series of questions (Silverman, 1993a, pp. 256-258):

1. What are the effects of the therapy upon specific behaviors that contribute to a client's communicative disorder at given points in space-time?
2. What are the effects of the therapy upon other attributes of a client's communicative behavior at given points in space-time?
3. What are the effects of a therapy upon a client other than those directly related to communicative behavior?
4. What are the client's attitudes toward the therapy and its effects on his or her communicative and other behaviors?
5. What are the attitudes of a client's clinician, family, friends, and others toward the therapy and toward its effects upon the client's communicative behavior and other attributes of behavior?
6. What investment is required of client and clinician?
7. What is the probability of relapse following termination of the therapy?

This chapter presents tentative answers to these questions for augmentative modes in general. The answers must be regarded as tentative because the data available for answering all except possibly the first question are insufficient or have levels of validity, reliability, and generality that are uncertain. (For a discussion of validity, reliability, and generality in this context, see Brodin, 1992; and Silverman, 1993a).

IMPACT ON COMMUNICATION

The first question deals with the impacts of a therapy strategy on a client's communicative disorder per se at various points in space-time. In the case of children and adults who lack adequate speech for their communicative purposes, this question would refer to the impact of the therapy strategy (i.e., intervention with augmentative communication) on their ability to communicate. (This, of course, assumes that the clinician has a communication rather than a speech orientation.) The space-time concept is used here to indicate that the impact of a therapy strategy on a client cannot be assumed to be the same at all points in time and in all situations. A simple picture communication board, for example, can allow an aphasic to communicate necessary messages to hospital personnel during the first few days following her stroke but may not adequately meet her communication needs after she returns home. There is a need, then, to include the space-time dimension when assessing the impacts of augmentative communication modes on clients.

How likely is augmentative communication to improve significantly a severely communicatively impaired client's ability to communicate, that is, to transmit messages? By "improve significantly" is meant sufficient progress that clients, their clinicians, and others (e.g., spouses and parents) judge that there has been real improvement in the clients' abilities to transmit messages in their environments. Note that the emphasis is on message transmission outside the therapy room. A client would not be regarded as having demonstrated significant improvement if he used augmentative communication only in the context of therapy.

Intervention with augmentative communication seems quite likely to improve significantly a severely communicatively impaired client's ability to communicate regardless of the reason for the client's inadequate speech. This conclusion is supported by a number of clinical case reports, representative examples of which are summarized in Table 2–1. Although the reliability and generality of the data in most of these reports are uncertain, the fact that they all conclude that a high percentage of the clients improved provides strong support. Of course, the probability of clients significantly improving their ability to communicate may not be quite as high as suggested by the data in Table 2–1 because successes rather than failures are more likely to be reported.

There is little question that augmentative communication can improve significantly the ability to communicate, but the amount of such improvement is not a constant. Some persons are reported to be able to transmit almost any message they wish through the use of such strategies, whereas others apparently are only able to learn to communicate a few basic needs with them. A number of factors seem to

TABLE 2–1 **Representative Reports of Impact of Augmentative Communication Strategies on Ability to Communicate**

Reference	Number of Clients	Children or Adults	Mode	Number Significantly Improving
Aphasia				
Chen (1971)	19	Adults	Manual alphabet and manual sign gestures	7
Eagleson, Vaughn, & Knudson (1970)	31	Adults	Hand signals	31
Glass et al. (1973)	7	Adults	Premack manipulable symbols	7
Goldstein & Cameron (1952)	?	Adults	Manual sign language	Most, if not all
Goodwin & Goodwin (1969)	2	Children	Edison Responsive Environment	2
Schlanger (1976)	5	Adults	Pantomime	5
Apraxia				
Elsworth & Kotkin (1975)	1	Child	Manual sign language	1
Helfrich (1976)	1	Child	Total communication	1
Skelly et al. (1974)	6	Adults	Amer-Ind gestural code	6
Autism				
Bonvillian & Nelson (1976)	1	Child	Ameslan	1
Creedon (1975)	30	Children	Total communication	30
Fulwiler & Fouts (1976)	2	Children	Ameslan	2
Gaines et al. (1988)	4	Children	Total communication	4
Konstantareas et al. (1975)	5	Children	Total communication	4
Lucas & Dean (1976)	1	Child	Ameslan	1
Miller & Miller (1973)	19	Children	Total communication	19
Offir (1976)	30	Children	Ameslan	30
Ratusnik & Ratusnik (1974)	1	Child	Communication board	1
Webster et al. (1973)	1	Child	Ameslan	1

Continued

TABLE 2-1 *Continued*

Dysarthria

Reference	Number of Clients	Children or Adults	Mode	Number Significantly Improving
Bullock, Dalrymple, & Danca (1975)	1	Child	Auto-Com communication board	1
Carlson (1976)	1	Child	Gestures, communication board, electronic system	1
Chen (1971)	5	Adults	Manual alphabet and manual sign gestures	4
Charbonneau, Cote, & Roy (1974)	5	Children	Comhandi electronic communication system	5
Clappe et al. (1973)	1	Adult	Electronic device	1
Computerized device . . . (1976)	5	Children	Electronic device	6*
Egan, Anthony, & Honke (1976)	1	Adult	Manual sign language	1
Feallock (1958)	12	Children	Communication boards	6
Fenn & Rowe (1975)	7	Children	Manual sign language	7
Gertenrich (1966)	1	Adult	Mouth-held writing device	1
Gitlis (1975)	1	Child	Total communication	1
Goldberg & Fenton (1960)	5	Children	Conversation boards	3
Hagen, Porter, & Brink (1973)	4	Children	Morse code oscillator	3
Handicapped youth . . . (1974)	1	Child	ETRAN chart	1
Harris-Vanderheiden (1976a)	5	Children	Blissymbolics	5
Harris-Vanderheiden (1976b)	7	Children	Auto-Com communication board	7
Hill et al. (1968)	1	Child	Two direct-selection aids	1
Jack H. Eichler . . . (1973)	1	Adult	ETRAN chart	1
Jenkins (1967)	1	Child	Possum typewriter	1
Kates & McNaughton (n.d.)	19	Children	Blissymbolics	"Nearly all"
Kladde (1974)	3	Children	Communication board	3
Levett (1971)	12	Children	Mime	7

Study	N	Population	Method	Improved
McDonald & Schultz (1973)	1	Child	Communication board	1
Nicol (1972)	1	Child	P.O.S.M.-controlled typewriter	1
Ontario Crippled Children's Centre Symbol Communication Programme (1974)	150	Children	Blissymbolics	122
Rice & Combs (1972)	4	Children	Myocom communication device	4 Children
	2	Adults		1 Adult
Vanderheiden & Harris-Vanderheiden (1976)	9	Children	Auto-Com communication board	9*
Vicker (1974)	23	Children	Communication boards	Most
Wendt, Sprague, & Marquis (1975)	1	Child	Auto-Com communication board	1
Glossectomy or Laryngectomy				
Chen (1971)	2	Adults	Manual alphabet and manual sign gestures	2
Skelly et al. (1975)	1	Adult	Amer-Ind gestural code	1
Mental Retardation				
Brookner & Murphy (1975)	1	Child	Total communication	1
Duncan & Silverman (1977)	32	Children	Amer-Ind gestural code	27
Gaines et al. (1988)	6	Children	Total communication	6
Hoffmeister & Farmer (1972)	8	Children	Ameslan	15
	8	Adults		
Kimble (1975)	4	Children	Signed English	3
Lebeis & Lebeis (1975)	27	Children	Ameslan	24
Richardson (1975)	9	Children	Ameslan	9
Topper (1975)	1	Adult	Ameslan	1
Vanderheiden et al. (1975)	5	Children	Blissymbolics	5
Wilson (1974b)	26	Children	Ameslan	26

*Report suggests, without directly saying so, that all subjects significantly improved their ability to communicate.

influence the amount of impact that use of augmentative communication strategies can have on a severely communicatively impaired child's or adult's ability to encode and transmit messages. Included are

- Cognitive status
- Motor status
- Sensory status
- Receptive language status
- Inner language status
- Desire or motivation to communicate
- The specific communication mode (or combination of modes) used
- Attitudes toward the communication mode used

Cognitive Status

The more normal the cognitive (intellectual) abilities of children and adults, the more impact augmentative communication is likely to have on their communication potential. Some support for this conclusion is found in the papers cited in Table 2–1 dealing with the impact of augmentative communication intervention on the mentally retarded. More manual signs, for example, tend to be acquired by the moderately mentally retarded than by the severely mentally retarded.

The cognitive status of adults who were not diagnosed mentally retarded as children also influences the probable impact. Persons who have neurological conditions that can adversely affect cognitive functioning, such as Alzheimer's disease, Huntington's chorea, and cerebral arteriosclerosis, may do less well with such communication strategies than those with comparable motor and sensory abilities (or disabilities) who do not have a condition of this type. Of course, as the cognitive status of persons with these conditions deteriorates, the impact of any augmentative strategy on their communication ability is likely to be reduced.

Motor Status

The more normal the motor abilities of severely communicatively impaired children and adults—particularly those of the upper extremities—the more impact augmentative communication is likely to have on their communication potential. Some levels of motor ability will support more flexible strategies than will others. A person whose upper extremities are normal motorically, for example, has the motor potential to use a highly flexible augmentative communication strategy such as American Sign Language (see chapter 4). On the other hand, a person whose upper extremities are not normal motorically may have to use a more limited strategy, such as a communication board (see chapter 5). The range of messages that can be transmitted by the latter tends to be more restricted than is that by the former.

Sensory Status

The more normal the sensory abilities of severely communicatively impaired children and adults, the more impact learning an augmentative communication strategy is likely to have on their communication potential. There are three sensory channels whose functioning can influence this potential: auditory, visual, and tactile-kinesthetic-proprioceptive.

The presence of a peripheral hearing loss (conductive, sensorineural, or mixed) or a central auditory disturbance (e.g., an auditory agnosia) can reduce the communication potential of any severely communicatively impaired person because it may interfere with his or her ability to decode and thereby understand speech. Such a reduction in communication potential could occur regardless of the augmentative strategy the person used unless a nonauditory communication strategy were also used for encoding and transmitting messages to him or her.

Any deficit in visual acuity, a visual field disturbance, or a visual agnosia can also reduce communication potential if the encoding or transmission process being used has to be monitored visually. The use of a communication board, for example, can be impeded by any of these disturbances. A person with a visual deficit may not be able to find and accurately indicate desired message components on the board.

Finally, a disturbance in tactile-kinesthetic-proprioceptive sensation, or feedback, could, for example, interfere with the accurate production of the manual gestures used in American Sign Language or in American Indian Hand Talk (both are discussed in chapter 4). It could also interfere with indicating message components on communication boards and activating the switching mechanisms of electronic communication aids (see chapter 5).

Receptive Language Status

The more normal the ability of a severely communicatively impaired child or adult to comprehend speech, the more impact learning and using augmentative communication are likely to have on the client's communication potential. Obviously, a person who does not understand a question is unlikely to respond appropriately. Some degree of receptive language deficit is likely to be manifested by aphasics and mentally retarded persons.

Inner Language Status

The term *inner language* is used here to refer to the accumulation of *units of experience*—things to which symbols refer (Myklebust, 1954). A person with a disturbance in inner language will also have a disturbance in receptive language, or speech comprehension. Hence, such clients may not respond appropriately to questions regardless of the symbol system, speech or nonspeech, used for transmitting messages to them.

Desire or Motivation to Communicate

The more highly motivated clients are, the more impact learning and using augmentative communication are likely to have. A person may become quite proficient at communicating using an augmentative strategy, but if he or she chooses not to communicate or to communicate only when absolutely necessary, the strategy is likely to have little impact. There are several reasons why a person may have little desire to communicate, including the three that follow:

1. *Depression.* People who are depressed usually are not highly motivated to communicate. A person who has inadequate speech because of aphasia, apraxia, dysarthria, laryngectomy, tracheostomy, or glossectomy is quite likely to be depressed, especially immediately following the onset of the condition. Such depression is apt to result from several factors, one being loss of ability to communicate and its implications. Teaching a person who is depressed for this reason to communicate using an augmentative strategy may help to reduce the depression.

2. *Little or no need to communicate.* Persons who have little or no need to communicate obviously will not realize their communication potentials. Two frequent reasons why persons tend to have little or no need to communicate are their needs are anticipated by those with whom they would ordinarily have to communicate and they have limited opportunity to communicate because they interact with very few people.

3. *Lack of positive reinforcement for communicating.* If a person does not regard communication as an enjoyable (or positively reinforcing) experience, his or her attempts to communicate will be limited.

Communication Strategy (or Strategies) Used

Some augmentative communication strategies are likely to have greater impact on a severely communicatively impaired person's ability to encode and transmit messages than are others. Some, for example, are more *portable* than others; they are relatively small and light in weight, and if they are electrical, they can operate on batteries. The more portable the components of an aid, the more likely users are to have it available when they wish to communicate and, hence, the greater its impact. Gestural strategies such as American Sign Language are, of course, the most portable of all because they require no hardware.

Also, some augmentative strategies have greater impact than others because they are more *flexible*, that is, they allow a greater number of messages to be encoded and transmitted. American Sign Language, for example, can be used to encode and transmit a greater variety of messages than can American Indian Hand Talk. (Both are described in chapter 4.) Also, a communication board containing letters of the alphabet and numbers has the potential for encoding a greater variety of messages than does one containing only Blissymbolics or pictures (see chapter 5).

Another variable that influences the relative impact of augmentative strategies is *efficiency*. Some strategies allow messages to be encoded and transmitted in less time and with less expenditure of energy than others. A strategy that requires each letter to be encoded and transmitted by Morse code is less efficient than one that uses fingerspelling. The reason is that the former requires more than one gesture (i.e., activation of a switch) to transmit a letter, whereas the latter requires only one. The more time-consuming and energy-consuming message transmission becomes, the fewer the messages that are likely to be transmitted; in turn, the fewer the messages that are likely to be transmitted, the less impact that augmentative strategy is likely to have.

A fourth variable is the *symbol system* used. Some symbol systems allow one to communicate with a greater variety of people than do others. A communication board on which words are spelled out would not permit communication with preschool children. And the use of American Sign Language would not permit communication with as many people as would the use of American Indian Hand Talk (see chapter 4).

Attitudes toward the Communication Strategy Used

The attitudes of the user and of those in his or her environment toward an augmentative strategy influence the impact it is likely to have on his or her ability to communicate (Creech & Viggiano, 1981). The more positive these attitudes, the greater the probable impact. If a person who could benefit from augmentative communication either refuses to use it or uses it only when absolutely necessary, its potential impact will be reduced. Also, if the members of the person's family and others do not respond positively, its frequency of use will probably be reduced. This is particularly likely to happen if members of the user's family feel that it is likely to reduce his or her attempts to speak. As research (summarized in the next section) indicates, learning an augmentative strategy is highly unlikely to impede the development of speech. In fact, there is at least one chance in three that such intervention will facilitate speech.

IMPACT ON SPEECH

Another question that needs to be answered when assessing any therapy method concerns its impact on aspects of communication behavior other than those it is intended to modify. An augmentative communication strategy, in addition to facilitating communication, may influence a person's communication behavior in other ways, either desirable or undesirable. Perhaps the most important aspect of communication behavior on which it would be necessary to determine the impact is verbal, or speech, output. Does learning and using an augmentative communication strategy appear to influence a person's attempts at speech communication? More specifically, does encouraging a client to use augmentative communication reduce his or her motivation for speech communication? If the answer were yes, a clinician might justifiably hesitate to teach a client to use augmentative communication if there were any chance that he or she could learn to communicate by speech.

I emphasize here: Teaching a severely communicatively impaired person to use augmentative communication does not appear to reduce his or her motivation for speech communication—a conclusion supported by more than 100 published and unpublished reports, some of which are summarized in Table 2–2. Thus, there seems to be little reason to be concerned about this aspect of augmentative communication strategies.

Can learning and using an augmentative communication strategy have any impact on verbal output? The answer to this question appears to be yes. The use of augmentative communication seems to facilitate speech (i.e., increase verbal output) in some children and adults (see Table 2–2). Judging by the data summarized in Table 2–2, the proportion of users who are likely to be so affected is at least 40 percent. Thus, intervention with augmentative communication strategies can be rationalized as being to facilitate speech as well as to improve message transmission. This form of intervention, in fact, appears as likely as any to be successful for facilitating speech in severely communicatively impaired children and adults.

The rationalization of augmentative communication strategies as speech facilitation techniques can be useful in gaining their acceptance by clients and their families. Speech-language pathologists' recommendations to their clients that they use augmentative communication may be interpreted by them and their families to mean that no further attempts will be made to develop or improve speech. This, obviously, could result in resistance. If augmentative communication were presented as a means for facilitating both communication and speech, such resistance would be minimized. (This topic is dealt with further in chapter 8.)

Although there appears to be general agreement among practitioners that intervention with augmentative communication can facilitate speech, there is no general agreement about why it does so. Almost all of our information about this phenomenon is from clinical case reports. Systematic research within the framework of coherent psychological theories would be needed to explain it (see Bowler, 1991).

OTHER IMPACTS ON USERS

Still another question necessary to answer when assessing a therapy method is concerned with its impacts other than those directly related to a client's communication behavior. An intervention strategy that influences communication behavior can influence other aspects of a person's functioning as well (see Warrick, 1988, for a discussion of augmentative communication from a sociocommunicative perspective). Such impacts can be classified as physical or behavioral (i.e., psychological) and as desirable or undesirable. An example of an undesirable physical impact would be a skin lesion at the location where a pointing or switching mechanism was attached to a

TABLE 2–2 **Representative Reports of Impact of Intervention with Augmentative Communication on Attempts at Speech Communication.**

Reference	Number of Clients	Children or Adults	Impact on Speech Attempts		
			Increased	Decreased	None
Aphasia					
Eagleson, Vaughn, & Knudson (1970)	31	Adults	"Success with this nonspeech mode of communication increased the apparent motivation of patients to persevere in learning verbal modes of communication."		
Goodwin & Goodwin (1969)	2	Children	2		
Schlanger (1976)	5	Adults	3		2
Apraxia					
Ellsworth & Kotkin (1975)	1	Child	1		
Skelly et al. (1974)	6	Adults	5		1
Autism					
Creedon (1975)	30	Children	"Some."		
Fulwiler & Fouts (1976)	1	Child	1		
Konstantareas et al. (1975)	5	Children	2		3
Miller & Miller (1973)	19	Children	2		17
Offir (1976)	30	Children	20		10
Schaeffer et al. (1976)	3	Children	3		
Dysarthria					
Gitlis (1975)	1	Child		1	
Kates & McNaughton (n.d.)	19	Children	"Symbol use appeared to encourage vocalization and speech."		

Continued

TABLE 2-2   *Continued*

Reference	Number of Clients	Children or Adults	Impact on Speech Attempts		
			Increased	Decreased	None
Kladde (1974)	3	Children	1		2
Levett (1971)	12	Children	1		11
Ontario Crippled Children's Centre Symbol Communication Programme (1974)	141	Children	45	2	94
Mental Retardation					
Balick, Spiegel, & Greene (1976)	5	Children	5		
Brookner & Murphy (1975)	22	Child			1
Duncan & Silverman (1977)	32	Children	15		17
Kimble (1975)	4	Children	2		2
Lebeis & Lebeis (1975)	27	Children	6		21
Linville (1977)	4	Children	2		2
Prinz & Shaw (1981)	17	Children	Most showed "increase in the use of speech."		
Schmidt, Carrier, & Parsons (1971)	10	Children	10		
Wills (1981)	—	Children	38%		
Wilson (1974)	26	Children	5		21

TABLE 2–3   **Representative Reports about Other Impacts of Augmentative Communication.**

Reference	Number of Clients	Children or Adults	Impacts
Apraxia			
Helfrich (1976)	1	Child	Reduced frustration behavior.
Autism			
Fulwiler & Fouts (1976)	2	Children	Increased social interaction; increased attentiveness.
Konstantareas et al. (1975)	5	Children	Increased "awareness, interaction with other persons, and improvements in self-care skills."
Konstantareas et al. (1979)	4	Children	Reported "measurable gains in social, self-care and related abilities."
Lucas & Dean (1976)	1	Child	"Disruptive behavior had dramatically decreased with increased appropriate attending and social behaviors."
Webster et al. (1973)	1	Child	Reduction in "bizarre behaviors."
Dysarthria			
Bullock, Dalrymple, & Danca (1975)	1	Child	Child "became more self-confident and independent." She also became a "more involved member of the class."
Hagen, Porter, & Brink (1973)	4	Children	3 became more relaxed physically.
Harris-Vanderheiden (1976b)	7	Children	Facilitated educational progress; enhanced self-confidence; increased independence.
Kates & McNaughton (n.d.)	19	Children	Children showed evidence of greater self-assurance and self-confidence.
Levett (1971)	12	Children	"All of the children were reported to be easier to handle both in and out of school."

Continued

TABLE 2–3   **Representative Reports about Other Impacts of Augmentative Communication.**

Reference	Number of Clients	Children or Adults	Impacts
Rowe & Rapp (1980)	2	Children	Observed "substantial emotional and behavioral improvements."
Vanderheiden & Harris-Vanderheiden (1976)	9	Children	Observed "a major beneficial effect on the students' educational progress, their productive educational time, . . . personal development, motivation and independence."
Mental Retardation			
Abrahamsen, Romski, & Sevcik (1989)	3	Adolescents	Attention span increased.
Balick, Spiegel, & Greene (1976)	5	Children	Attention span increased; hyperactivity decreased.
Brookner & Murphy (1975)	1	Child	Temper tantrums lessened.
Duncan & Silverman (1977)	32	Children	13 of the children were reported to have had noticeable changes in behavior—i.e., reduction in frustration behavior such as temper tantrums and being more willing to participate in language activities.
Kimble (1975)	4	Children	Increased willingness to interact with others; increased attention span.

client's body. (Interfacing people with pointing and switching mechanisms is dealt with in chapter 5.) An example of an undesirable behavioral impact would be depression arising from the need to rely on a device to communicate.

The noncommunication impacts of augmentative communication on users that have been reported are overwhelmingly desirable (see Table 2–3). Whether the paucity of reports of undesirable impacts is due to there not being any, or to a failure by clinician-investigators to evaluate for them and report them, is uncertain. Whatever the reason, the reports (Table 2–3; see also Carr & Durand, 1985, 1987; Carr & Kemp, 1989; Durand, 1990; Durand & Berotti, 1991; Durand & Carr, 1991) suggest that intervention with augmentative communication can have several desirable impacts on users, including decreased temper tantrums, increased willingness to participate in group activities, increased attention span, decreased hyperactivity, increased self-confidence, increased independence, and improved performance in the classroom.

ACCEPTANCE BY USERS AND OTHERS

Two more questions necessary to answer when assessing a therapy method concern its acceptability to the client and those with whom he or she interacts (e.g., parents or spouse). As already indicated, if a method is unacceptable to a client and those with whom he or she interacts, its potential impact will be reduced.

A few attempts have been made to determine systematically the level of acceptability of augmentative communication strategies to users and others (Gorenflo & Gorenflo, 1991; Gorenflo, Gorenflo, & Santer, 1994; Gorenflo, Eulenberg, & Casby, 1987; Raney & Silverman, 1992; Weatherill & Haak, 1992). Relevant data (e.g., Duncan & Silverman, 1977) suggest that such systems are likely to be acceptable to most users and those with whom they interact if they understand the following:

1. Intervention with augmentative communication does not necessarily mean that the speech-language pathologist has given up on improving the client's speech.
2. The augmentative communication strategy is intended to augment (supplement) the speech the person has; the goal is *total communication*. (The concept of total communication is dealt with in chapter 4.)
3. Learning and using an augmentative communication strategy is highly unlikely to result in reduced attempts at speech.
4. Learning and using an augmentative communication strategy appears to *facilitate* speech in some clients. The use of such a strategy may, in fact, be one of the most successful speech facilitation techniques for severely communicatively impaired children and adults.
5. It is important for the patient to have an alternative mode of message transmission to meet immediate communication needs if speech is not adequate.
6. People are unlikely to react more negatively to a severely communicatively impaired person if he or she uses augmentative communication than they are if the person attempts to communicate without it (Weatherill & Haas, 1992). In fact, the opposite is likely to be true.

INVESTMENT REQUIRED

Still another question concerns the investment required of the client and clinician. The investment can be of several kinds, including money, time, and willingness to use a communication mode that initially might make one feel uncomfortable.

Implementation of all augmentative communication strategies calls for some financial investment. If the strategy does not require a computer or other electronic devices, the cost is likely to be nominal. If it does contain such devices, the cost will be determined by their complexity or sophistication. The financial investment required can be thousands of dollars.

Time is invested when the clinician assembles the hardware and software components and teaches the client how to use them. The amount of time to do this ranges from a few hours (to construct and teach an apraxic adult to use a simple communication board) to hundreds of hours (to teach the use of American Sign Language to a mentally retarded child).

The client must be willing to tolerate being uncomfortable when first using the strategy. Some persons feel that using such a strategy will call unwanted attention to themselves. This is the same sort of concern that persons who are hard of hearing may have when first using a hearing aid. After a while, however, clients usually find that people are not reacting to them in the manner they had anticipated, and the problem solves itself.

LONG-TERM IMPACT

A final question is concerned with the impact of the therapy method on the client following termination of formal therapy. Does the impact tend to increase, decrease, or remain about the same? How likely are clients to continue using an augmentative communication strategy once they are no longer seeing a clinician on a regular basis? Answers to these questions obviously are important for assessing the impact of any augmentative communication strategy.

There have been only a few systematic follow-up studies (e.g., Beukelman et al., 1981; Culp et al., 1986; Enderby & Hamilton, 1981; Kiernan, 1983). However, there are a number of individual case studies that suggest that such communication strategies continue to be used and continue to have an impact following termination of therapy; their generality (or representativeness), however, is uncertain. Some clinicians may be reluctant to report and/or publish unsuccessful long-term outcomes (see Honsinger, 1989). There is a need, therefore, for clinicians to collect systematic follow-up data from clients using all types of augmentative communication strategies and to publish the information in the form of case studies. (See McEwen & Karlan, 1990, on how to write case studies. For a discussion of the role of the clinician in therapy outcome research, see chapter 2 in Silverman, 1993a.)

▶ 3

Classification of Augmentative Communication Strategies

All augmentative communication strategies can be assigned to one of three categories: gestural, gestural-assisted, or neuro-assisted. A strategy falls into a particular category on the basis of (1) whether any instrumentation were needed to encode or transmit messages and, (2) if instrumentation were needed, whether it is controlled by muscle gestures (patterned movements of muscle groups) or bioelectrical signals (electrical signals generated by the nervous system, such as muscle action potentials). The defining characteristics of these categories are summarized in Table 3–1.

GESTURAL STRATEGIES

The defining characteristic of a *gestural communication strategy* is that it requires no instrumentation, only patterned muscle gestures, or movements. Because they require no instrumentation, gestural strategies are sometimes referred to as *unaided* strategies. Messages are encoded into muscle gestures and transmitted visually. The muscle groups involved are primarily those of the upper extremities (one or both) and/or of the head and neck. Patterned movements of other muscle groups (such as those of the lower extremities) also could be used. The only requirement is that the gestural code be meaningful to the person using it and to those with whom the person is communicating.

Gestures are not an unusual strategy for encoding and transmitting messages. All persons use facial and body gesture to some extent for this purpose. We all, at times, indicate what we want by pointing. We answer questions by nodding or shaking our heads yes or no. We partially convey our messages through the facial and body gestures that accompany speech, including smiling. We all, therefore, use some form

TABLE 3–1   **Defining Characteristics of Gestural (Unaided), Gestural-Assisted (Aided), and Neuro-Assisted (Aided) Communication Strategies**

	Type of Strategy		
	Gestural (Unaided)	Gestural-Assisted (Aided)	Neuro-Assisted (Aided)
Instrumentation necessary	No	Yes	Yes
Muscle gesture control of instrumentation	No	Yes	No
Neuro-activity control of instrumentation	No	No	Yes

of total communication (see chapter 4). When we feel that we are not making ourselves understood (as when we attempt to communicate with someone who does not understand English well), we resort to pantomime. We shrug our shoulders to indicate we don't know. We may use hand signals while driving a car. We raise our right arm to signal someone to stop.

Persons who lack adequate speech for their communicative purposes are likely to use gestures to some extent to encode and transmit messages without being taught to use them. Some use smiling, for example, as an interaction maintenance strategy (Ruder & Sims, 1987). In fact, unless they are taught a formal augmentative communication strategy or are able to communicate by writing, this is probably the way they communicate.

Although almost all severely communicatively impaired persons exhibit some normal gestural communication, we cannot assume that their ability to communicate gesturally is normal. Their gestural communication may be limited for several reasons. For one, the musculature used to produce particular gestures may not function normally due to a neuromuscular disorder or apraxia. Such a condition is particularly apt to limit gestural communication if it affects the musculature of the upper extremities or head and neck.

Another reason is the presence of aphasia. Aphasics may have similar difficulties using gestures propositionally as they do using speech propositionally. They may not be able to signal yes or no reliably by shaking their heads or to communicate a message through pantomime. Such deficits have been observed in both aphasic children (e.g., Myklebust, 1954) and adults (Peterson & Kirshner, 1981; Davis, 1993).

One last reason for gestural communication being limited is the presence of developmentally inappropriate cognitive ability. Persons with this condition do not function intellectually (i.e., do not solve problems and see relationships) as well as would be expected for someone else their age. Included here are children and adults who are congenitally mentally retarded, as well as those who were developing normally but lost normal cognitive ability as a result of brain damage. Because the acquisition of the ability to communicate gesturally follows a predictable developmental sequence, such persons would be more limited in their use of some types of gestural communication than of others. The types that are most likely to be affected are those that develop last and are relatively abstract (e.g., pantomime).

Gestural communication strategies are taught to severely communicatively impaired persons to enhance their abilities to transmit messages gesturally. They can supplement normal gestural communication in two ways. First, they can provide additional information for messages than can be transmitted by normal gestural communication, thereby increasing the redundancy and hence the intelligibility of such messages. And, second, they can increase the number of messages that can be encoded and transmitted gesturally; that is, they can be used to encode and transmit messages that cannot be encoded and transmitted by normal gestural communication.

It should be noted that speech enhances normal gestural communication in the same manner as do gestural augmentative communication strategies. First, it increases the redundancy and hence the intelligibility of messages that can be communicated by facial and body gestures. And, second, it increases the number of messages that can be encoded and transmitted gesturally. Speech can be viewed as a gestural communication strategy because messages are encoded and transmitted by gestures of the articulators. The gestural nature of speech, incidentally, is particularly evident while speechreading.

How might the use of a formal gestural symbol system, such as fingerspelling, increase the redundancy of normal gestural communication? Suppose that a person were feeling depressed. He or she might communicate this by facial expression and overall bodily posture; he or she might "look depressed." If the person were to fingerspell the message "I feel depressed," this would increase its redundancy and thereby the probability that it would be understood. Fingerspelling, in this instance, would increase the probability that the message would be understood because the facial and bodily postural signs of depression may not be obvious to those to whom the message was being transmitted.

Gestural symbol systems also supplement normal gestural communication by providing a gestural means for encoding and transmitting messages that could not be encoded and transmitted by facial and other bodily gestures. The gestures used for this purpose (as well as for the previous one) are of two types. Those of the first type stand for, or signify, *linguistic units,* such as letters, phonemes, and morphemes. Messages (or message segments) that are encoded and transmitted by means of such gestures are directly translatable into a natural language such as English. Thus, gestures of the first type can be used to encode and transmit a message or message segment by

1. Spelling the words in it letter by letter (e.g., through the use of the manual alphabet)
2. Signaling the phonemes of the words in the message phoneme by phoneme (e.g., through the use of cued speech)

3. Signaling morphemic information contained, such as verb tense (e.g., through the use of Signed English)

Gestures of the second type stand for, or signify, *concepts.* Messages encoded by means of such gestures are not similar in structure to English or other Indo-European languages. They have a different linguistic structure; for example, they cannot be segmented into letters or phonemes. In addition, they may have a different syntactic structure (i.e., the ordering of signs for a message does not necessarily correspond to the ordering of the words used to express it). Finally, they may have a different semantic structure. There may not, for example, be a one-to-one correspondence between the number of words and number of gestures needed to encode and transmit a concept. For some concepts the number of gestures needed is less than the number of words, and for others the number needed is greater.

The gestures that signal morphemic information, such as verb tense, can be used with this second type of gestural system.

These two basic types of gestures are often used together for encoding and transmitting messages. When concept gestures exist, they are used; when they do not exist, the words necessary to communicate the concept are fingerspelled. Both types of gestures are combined in American Sign Language, the gestural symbol system used by the deaf in the United States.

Representative gestural augmentative communication strategies are described in chapter 4.

GESTURAL-ASSISTED STRATEGIES

The defining characteristic of *gestural-assisted communication strategies* is that they utilize a readout device (or display) that is activated directly or indirectly by muscle gestures or movements. Because they require instrumentation (a display), they sometimes are referred to as *aided* strategies. Users either point to or cause to be reproduced on the display the components of the message they wish to transmit. An example of a display that permits users to indicate message components by pointing is a communication, or conversation, board. (Several representative communication boards are reproduced in chapter 5.) An example of a device that permits users to reproduce message components is a computer.

Muscle gestures can be used to indicate message components directly or indirectly. Both approaches are diagrammed in Figure 3–1. With the first (number 1 in Figure 3–1), muscle gestures are used directly to indicate or reproduce message components on a display. The display is controlled directly by the person, not indirectly by an electronic switching mechanism. An example of a display that would use such an approach for indicating is a communication board. Muscle gestures that can be used to indicate directly message components include movements of one or both upper extremities, movements of the head (in conjunction with a headpointer), and movements of the eyes. The first two also can be used to reproduce message components directly. (This approach is described in depth in chapter 5.)

The second approach (number 2 in Figure 3–1) uses muscle gestures indirectly to indicate or reproduce message components on a display. The display is controlled by an electronic switching mechanism that is activated by one or more muscle gestures. Almost any movement resulting from the contraction of a muscle group can be used to activate a switching mechanism. Gestures used for this purpose include finger movements, head movements, foot movements, and eyebrow movements. (A number of gestures that can be used to activate electronic switching mechanisms are described in chapters 5 and 7.) The types of switches that can be activated by muscle gestures used to control electronic displays include mechanical microswitches, magnetic proximity switches, and photoelectric switches. (The use of these and others is dealt with in chapter 5.)

The control electronics (located in Figure 3–1 between the switching mechanism and display) make it possible for the switching mechanism to control the display. The functions performed by the control electronics are determined in part by the nature of the switching mechanism and display. In some instances a component of the control electronics is a microcomputer. (The functions of control electronics are discussed further in chapter 5.) Electronic switching mechanisms (with appropriate control electronics) can be used to indicate or reproduce message components on several types of displays or readout devices.

To be maximally effective in meeting each client's communication needs, gestural-assisted communication systems have to be individually designed. Although commercial communication boards can meet most clients' communication needs temporarily and those of a few permanently, they are not as functional for most clients as would be individually designed boards. (Factors that should be considered when developing a communication board for a client are indicated in chapter 5.) Also, standard combinations of switching mechanisms, control electronics, and displays are apt not be maximally effective in meeting most clients' communication needs.

Representative gestural-assisted communication strategies or aids that have been used with dysarthric, aphasic, tracheostomized, mentally retarded, and autistic children and adults are described in chapter 5.

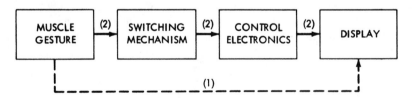

FIGURE 3–1   **Two approaches for indicating message components on a display with gestural-assisted communication aids. The first (1) is direct and the second (2) is indirect.**

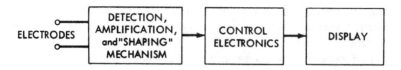

FIGURE 3–2   **Components of neuro-assisted communication aids.**

NEURO-ASSISTED STRATEGIES

The defining characteristic of *neuro-assisted* communication strategies is that they utilize a readout device or display that is activated by bioelectrical signals—electrical signals originating from within the body, such as muscle action potentials (electrical signals transmitted by lower motor neurons to muscle fibers, which causes them to contract). Because they require instrumentation, they, like gestural-assisted ones, are sometimes referred to as aided strategies.

The only way in which neuro-assisted communication strategies differ from electronic gestural-assisted ones (see Figure 3–1) is that they are activated by an electrical signal rather than by gestural manipulation of a switching mechanism. The components of neuro-assisted communication aids can be diagrammed as in Figure 3–2. Note that the only difference between this type of aid and that diagrammed in Figure 3–1 is that it interfaces with the user by means of an electro-activated signal detection, amplification, and modification mechanism rather than by a gesture-activated switching mechanism. The same displays are used by both types of aids. (Neuro-assisted communication strategies are discussed in chapter 6.)

Neuro-assisted communication strategies have not been refined to the same degree as have gestural and gestural-assisted ones. There appear to be several reasons for the relative lack of interest in them. One, the communication needs of almost all severely communicatively impaired children and adults can be met by gestural and gestural-assisted communication strategies. Also, neuro-assisted communication aids tend to be more sophisticated electronically and hence more expensive than comparable gestural-assisted ones. Finally, such aids (in part because they tend to be relatively complex electronically) are not as reliable as comparable gestural-assisted ones. We consider neuro-assisted communication strategies in this book because there are a few children and adults who are so involved motorically that they cannot communicate adequately with a gestural or gestural-assisted communication device.

▶ 4

Gestural Strategies

Chapter 3 outlined the characteristics of three classes of augmentative communication strategies: gestural (unaided), gestural-assisted (aided), and neuro-assisted (aided). This chapter discusses in more detail representative gestural communication strategies. (Representative gestural-assisted strategies are described in chapter 5, and neuro-assisted in chapter 6.) The descriptions include information about the following:

- Neuromuscular functions that must be intact for the strategy to be used
- Its intelligibility to untrained observers
- Its ability to convey messages concerned with the here and now
- Its ability to convey messages not concerned with the here and now
- Its syntactic and semantic structure
- The similarity of its linguistic structure to English
- Its ability to convey messages containing abstract concepts
- The time and energy investment required to learn to use it
- The time and energy investment required to learn to comprehend it
- The level of acceptability of the mode to users and interpreters
- The populations with which it has been used
- Examples of gestures—photographs or drawings
- Sources of dictionaries of gestures
- Sources of materials for teaching children and adults how to use the strategy

Specific applications of the strategies described are indicated at the end of the chapter.

AMERICAN SIGN LANGUAGE (AMESLAN)

American Sign Language, or Ameslan, is the manual gestural communication system used by the deaf in the United States. Each gestural sign in this system performs one of the following linguistic functions:

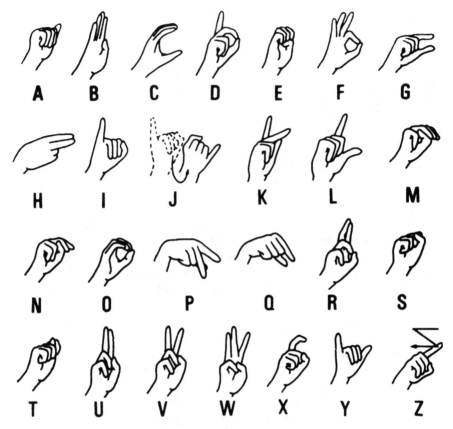

FIGURE 4–1   **American Manual Alphabet.**
Source: Bornstein, 1974.

1. It signals a *letter* of the alphabet. The set of 26 such signs is known as the American Manual Alphabet (see Figure 4–1).
2. It signals a *word* or *phrase*. There are more than 5000 such signs (Bornstein, 1974).
3. It signals *morphological* or *syntactic* information (e.g., verb tense). The 12 sign markers in Signed English (Bornstein, 1974) have this function (see Figure 4–2).
4. It signals a *phoneme*. The system known as Cued Speech (Lykos, 1971) contains such signs.

Signs having the first two functions are the most frequently occurring in messages transmitted by American Sign Language.

Communication with Ameslan usually involves the transmission of an ordered series of signs. When fingerspelling, signs are ordered to spell words. The ordering of the signs for a word corresponds to the ordering of the letters in it. Both words that are

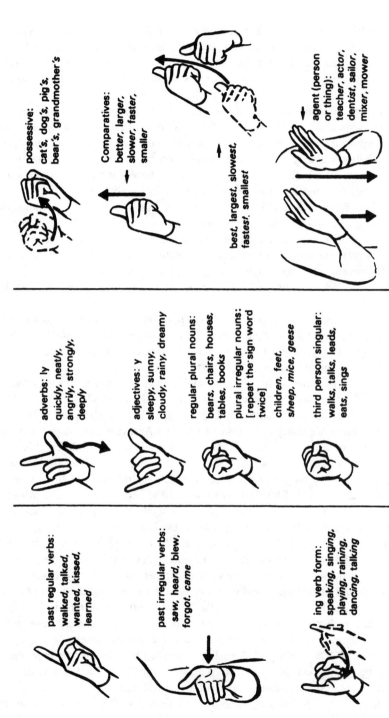

possessive:
cat's, dog's, pig's,
bear's, grandmother's

Comparatives:
better, larger,
slower, faster,
smaller

best, largest, slowest,
fastest, smallest

agent (person
or thing):
teacher, actor,
dentist, sailor,
mixer, mower

adverbs: ly
quickly, neatly,
angrily, strongly,
deeply

adjectives: y
sleepy, sunny,
cloudy, rainy, dreamy

regular plural nouns:
bears, chairs, houses,
tables, books

plural irregular nouns:
[repeat the sign word
twice]
children, feet,
sheep, mice, geese

third person singular:
walks, talks, leads,
eats, sings

past regular verbs:
walked, talked,
wanted, kissed,
learned

past irregular verbs:
saw, heard, blew,
forgot, came

ing verb form:
speaking, singing,
playing, raining,
dancing, talking

FIGURE 4-2 **Sign markers used in Signed English.**
Source: Bornstein, 1974.

signed as units and those that are fingerspelled are ordered on the basis of syntactic rules. However, these rules are not necessarily those of spoken English. The Signed English system (Bornstein, 1974; Bornstein, Saulnier, & Hamilton, 1983; Linville, 1977) is an attempt to develop a manual sign system with a syntax similar to spoken English.

Some users of Ameslan say their message at the same time that they sign it. Simultaneous speaking and signing is referred to as *total communication*. Presumably, communication is more successful than by speech or sign alone; even poor speech probably would provide some information that would help to interpret a signed message. Information transmitted by speech, however limited, would add to the redundancy of a message and, thereby, increase its intelligibility.

Ameslan, alone or in combination with speech, has been used as a communication medium by persons whose speech was inadequate because of deafness, mental retardation, childhood autism, and dysarthria. Its use as a communication medium for the mentally retarded, autistic, or dysarthric is relatively recent. Its use by persons in these three groups, incidentally, tends to be more limited than that by the deaf in that they tend to use fewer signs, and their signed utterances tend to be less complex syntactically.

The functioning of the musculature of both upper extremities must be reasonably good for Ameslan to be appropriate. It does not have to be normal, however. So long as a person is able to produce the signs at a reasonable rate of speed accurately enough for them to be recognizable, he or she can use the system.

The majority of Ameslan signs are not intelligible to untrained observers; that is, they have low transparency (Doherty, Karlan, & Lloyd, 1982; Dunham, 1989; Griffith & Robinson, 1980; Luftig & Lloyd, 1981; Snyder-McLean, 1978). The amount of training necessary to interpret a person's Ameslan signs depends on the number the person uses. For many mentally retarded and autistic children, this number will be relatively small (less than 200). When the number of signs used is small, people usually can be taught to interpret them in a short period of time. Clinical instruction, videotaped (or filmed) demonstration, microcomputer-based demonstration (with or without videodisk technology), and worksheets on which signs are illustrated by drawings, photographs, or both can be used for this purpose.

Ameslan is a very flexible sign system. It can be used to communicate any message concerning past, present, or future that could be communicated by English.

The time and energy investment necessary for a person to learn to use Ameslan is a function of several factors, including his or her mental age and the level of proficiency desired. The lower the mental age, the longer it will take to attain a given level of proficiency with Ameslan. And the higher the level of proficiency desired, the greater the time and energy investment necessary to attain that level.

The level of acceptability of Ameslan to persons who use it to communicate appears to be fairly good. Many persons who are mentally retarded or autistic have used Ameslan as a communication mode for a year or longer.

The level of acceptability of Ameslan to interpreters may not be particularly good. The problem is that many Ameslan signs cannot be understood by persons who have not been taught to interpret them. If a person used only a few such signs and interacted with only a few people (which would be the case, for instance, for some institutionalized mentally retarded persons), the training of interpreters probably would not be a serious problem. On the other hand, if a user had a relatively large Ameslan vocabulary, or had a need to communicate with persons who had not been trained to interpret the signs he or she used, or both, this could counterindicate the use of Ameslan. Of course, a person could be taught to use Ameslan only when communicating with those who understood it; when communicating with others, another augmentative strategy, such as a communication board, could be used. This situation, incidentally, is somewhat similar to that in which a person who spoke only English would find himself when visiting a country where English is not the national language. He would use English to communicate with those who understood it and something else (e.g., pantomime) to communicate with others.

A source for Ameslan dictionaries and other materials for teaching Ameslan (including Signed English) is the bookstore at Gallaudet College, in Washington, D.C., which publishes a list of such materials that can be ordered by mail. The materials are appropriate for all age groups, preschool through adult.

AMERICAN INDIAN HAND TALK (AMER-IND)

American Indian Hand Talk, or Amer-Ind, is a manual gestural communication system that was used by North American Indians for intertribal communication (Tomkins, 1969). It was also used to communicate with the early Spanish- and English-speaking European settlers. It functioned as what linguists refer to as an auxiliary international language, or interlanguage (Pei, 1965). Amer-Ind is probably one of the most successful such languages ever developed in that it was actually used for intercultural communication by large numbers of persons. It is interesting to note in this regard that

> the International Boy Scout movement . . . resolutely adopted the Indian sign language and proceeded to develop a science of pasimology, or gestures, which serves the Jamborees in perfect fashion. Representatives of as many as thirty-seven nations have met at various times and carried on both general business and private conversations in pasimology. The use of Indian sign language for international purposes has repeatedly been advocated. Sir Richard Paget and the American Tourist Association, in recent times, have both advocated the possibility of "handage" to replace language. (Pei, 1965, p. 17)

The gestural signs in Amer-Ind are (kinetic) pictographic and ideographic rather than phonetic. They represent ideas and in many cases are kinetic pictorial represen-

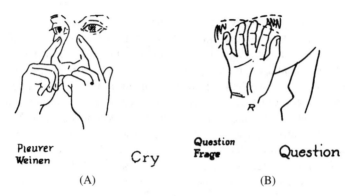

Pleurer
Weinen

Cry

Question
Frage

Question

(A)   (B)

FIGURE 4–3   **Amer-Ind signs. (A) Amer-Ind sign for cry. With both hands at eyes tears are indicated as flowing by tracing their course down the face. (B) Amer-Ind sign for question. Right hand is held palm outward at height of shoulders with fingers and thumb extended, separated, and pointed upward. The hand is turned slightly by wrist action two or three times.**
Source: Tomkins, 1969.

tations of the ideas conveyed. The Amer-Ind sign for "cry" (see Figure 4–3A) illustrates the pictographic and ideographic nature of the signs in this system.

The Amer-Ind signs for some words or concepts consist of an ordered series of gestures rather than a single gesture. The meanings of the individual gestures indicate the meaning of the composite. This process, called *agglutination*, greatly increases the number of words or concepts that can be communicated. The entries in Table 4–1 illustrate the agglutination process.

The syntactic structure of Amer-Ind is less complex than that of English and other spoken languages. Its grammatical rules, according to Tomkins (1969), include the following:

1. "Every question begins with, or is preceded by, a question sign (see Figure 4–3B). Thus, "Where are you going?" in Amer-Ind sign would be QUESTION YOU GOING? "The sign for 'question' covers the words WHAT, WHY, WHERE and WHEN. It is made to attract attention, to ask, to inquire, to examine" (pp. 7–8).
2. "Present time is expressed by adding the sign for NOW or for TODAY. Past tense is expressed by adding LONG TIME" (p. 8).
3. "What we understand to be the first person singular is indicated by pointing to one's-self. The plural WE is made by the signs ME and ALL. YOU, ALL, means WE; while HE, ALL means THEY" (p. 8).
4. "Gender is shown by adding the signs MAN or WOMAN" (p. 8).
5. "Such words or articles, as A, THE, AN, IT, etc., are not used" (p. 8).

TABLE 4–1 **Agglutinated Amer-Ind Sign Sequences for 10 Words or Concepts**

Word or Concept	Amer-Ind Sign Sequence
Aid	WORK, WITH
Bachelor	MAN, MARRY, NO
Boil	WATER, KETTLE, FIRE
City	HOUSE, MANY
Cook	MAKE, EAT
Generous	HEART, BIG
Hospital	HOUSE, SICK, MANY
Midnight	NIGHT, MIDDLE
Read	BOOK, LOOK
Store	HOUSE, TRADE

Source: Tomkins, 1969.

The items in Table 4–2 illustrate several aspects of the syntactic structure of Amer-Ind gestural code. (For other examples of Amer-Ind sign equivalents of English utterances, see Tomkins, 1969, pp. 97–100.)

Many Amer-Ind signs stand for more than one English word. The question sign (see Figure 4–3B), for example, can be interpreted as WHAT, WHERE, WHY, or WHEN. The intended meaning of this type of Amer-Ind sign is inferred from context.

Amer-Ind, at first, was adapted for use with severely communicatively handicapped adults (Rao et al., 1979; Skelly, 1979; Skelly et al., 1975; Skelly et al., 1974) and then, later, it was adapted for severely communicatively handicapped children, particularly those who are mentally retarded (Duncan & Silverman, 1977; Lloyd &

TABLE 4–2 **Amer-Ind Sign Equivalents of 10 English Utterances**

English	Amer-Ind Sign Equivalent
I want a drink of water.	I WANT WATER.
Do you understand Indian Sign Language?	QUESTION YOU KNOW INDIAN SIGN LANGUAGE.
Look, it is raining.	SEE RAIN.
When do we eat, at noon?	QUESTION FUTURE-TIME ME ALL EAT, SUN HIGH?
What is your name?	QUESTION YOU CALLED?
Don't wait for me, I'll come pretty soon.	WAIT ME NOT. I COME SHORT-TIME FUTURE.
Be quiet, listen to the speaker.	QUIET: LISTEN: MAN TALK.
We like to walk.	ME ALL FOND WALK.
The girl is running.	GIRL RUN.
I do not eat much for breakfast.	I EAT NOT MUCH SUNRISE.

Source: Tomkins, 1969.

Daniloff, 1983; Skelly, 1979). Signs not applicable to present-day use were eliminated, and signs were developed for contemporary activities (e.g., driving a car, going to McDonald's). Many of the signs that were developed, incidentally, were judged by native American users of Amer-Ind for compatibility with the system. In addition, a one-hand version was developed for use by hemiplegics. Both the one-hand and two-hand versions, as adapted by Madge Skelly and her associates, are demonstrated in a series of eight videotapes that were produced by the Learning Resources Center of the St. Louis Veterans Administration Hospital and are illustrated in Skelly's *Amer-Ind Gestural Code* (1979).

To use Amer-Ind, a person must have essentially normal neuromuscular functioning of at least one upper extremity. Although Amer-Ind signs are usually formed using two hands, many can be encoded with one hand. (The one-hand version of Amer-Ind is demonstrated in the fourth tape of the *Amer-Ind Video Dictionary*.) It also is desirable, but not essential, that the functioning of the musculature of the face and neck be essentially normal because facial expression appears to be a component of some Amer-Ind signs (e.g., BAD ODOR).

Amer-Ind can be used to convey messages about the here and now as well as the past and future. Although it can be used to convey both abstract and concrete concepts, one probably would tend to be more successful using it to convey the latter than the former.

The time and energy investments required to learn to use Amer-Ind are not excessive. Based on reports in the literature, most children and adults can acquire enough Amer-Ind to have a significant impact on their ability to communicate in two months or less. Obviously, the speed at which a given person would achieve a particular level of proficiency with Amer-Ind would be influenced by several factors, including intellectual level. The *Amer-Ind Video Dictionary* (1975), which presents demonstrations of 193 two-hand and 42 one-hand Amer-Ind signs, can be used both to reduce the time necessary for a client to learn Amer-Ind (assuming that the dictionary is used for self-instruction) and to minimize the clinician's time investment (see Skelly, 1979, for illustrations).

Although some Amer-Ind signs are more transparent (likely to be understood without special training) than others (Doherty, Daniloff, & Lloyd, 1985), the time and energy investments necessary for learning to comprehend Amer-Ind are usually minimal (and less than necessary for learning to comprehend Ameslan) for several reasons. For one, it is more than 40 percent intelligible to most untrained observers (Bady & Silverman, 1978; Daniloff, Lloyd, & Fristoe, 1983; Imhoff & McMillen, 1984; Skelly et al., 1975). Also, its syntactic structure is relatively simple; there are only a few rules governing the ordering of signs in utterances. Finally, Amer-Ind signs tend to be relatively easy to learn because almost all are concrete or representational. The representational nature of some Amer-Ind signs may not be obvious at first glance. However, once you are told, you usually are able to perceive how they are suggestive or representational of their meanings. The same is true for agglutinated signs. After you learn what one means, you usually can understand how the meanings of the individual signs that make it up concretely indicate its meaning. The *Amer-Ind*

Video Dictionary can also be used to improve comprehension of Amer-Ind signs. Some persons can learn the meanings of relatively large numbers of Amer-Ind signs merely by viewing these videotapes several times (Bady & Silverman, 1978).

Amer-Ind is relatively acceptable to most users and interpreters (Duncan & Silverman, 1977; Skelly, 1979; Skelly et al., 1975; Skelly et al., 1974). The majority of persons who are taught it appear to use it for communicating outside the therapy room. Duncan and Silverman (1977) have reported that it was sufficiently acceptable to the parents of a group of 32 mentally retarded children who were being taught it for them to request that their children continue receiving instruction after a 10-week experimental program in which they had been enrolled terminated. There may be some initial resistance, however, because using it may at first make the person feel uncomfortable, or as one aphasic put it, feel "crazy" (Melvin Cohen, personal communication). Such resistance probably can be reduced or overcome by positive experiences with Amer-Ind and by counseling. (Counseling users of augmentative communication and their families is dealt with in chapter 8.) Resistance from this source, incidentally, can occur with the introduction of any augmentative communication strategy.

There are several dictionarylike compilations of Amer-Ind signs. One is the *Amer-Ind Video Dictionary,* produced by Skelly and her associates. In it are demonstrated 193 two-hand and 42 one-hand Amer-Ind signs. Another such compilation is also by Skelly (1979) that illustrates, by drawings and verbal descriptions, the Amer-Ind signs in the *Amer-Ind Video Dictionary.* There is also a videotape of Amer-Ind signs, *Amer-Ind Code Repertoire,* published by Auditec, 330 Selma Avenue, St. Louis, MO 63119.

OTHER GESTURAL COMMUNICATION STRATEGIES

Head and Eye Movements, Facial Expressions, and Hand Gestures

Head movements, eye movements, facial expressions, and hand gestures are the ways that many severely communicatively impaired persons who do not have an augmentative technique or aid communicate. Many who do have one also, at times, communicate in these ways. Using them, some persons are able to construct relatively complex messages. Adamson and Dunbar (1991, p. 279), for example, have reported the following message from a young child who has a tracheostomy.

> *At 20 months Amy conveyed the message "You [one of several adults present in the room] give me that [a glass of water]," by orienting toward her potential partner, staring intently at her and then, once the communicative channel was open, pointing with one hand to the agent, the other to the object.*

It sometimes is possible to train clients to use such gestures more effectively.

Pantomime (Mime)

Pantomime, or mime, can be defined as "the art or technique of portraying a character, mood, idea, or narration by gestures and bodily movements" (Stein, 1966, p. 911). It differs from manual gestural systems, such as Ameslan and Amer-Ind, in several ways. First, it uses the musculature of the entire body, not just that (or primarily that) of the upper extremities. Second, the gestures tend to be dynamic rather than static. Meaning is conveyed primarily by the sequential relationships between gestures, rather than by the configurations of individual gestures. Third, more gestures are usually needed to convey a message than with the manual systems. And, fourth, the gestures are an analog of the message; that is, they are a dramatization of the message. Their structure is similar (or isomorphic) to that of the message. Because a pantomime tends to be similar in structure to what is being pantomimed, its meaning will be conveyed to most observers without training.

All persons use pantomime. It is a medium for message transmission (an aspect of nonverbal communication) as well as a theatrical art form. It occurs in interpersonal communication both alone and simultaneously with speech.

Pantomime has been used with both children and adults who lack adequate speech for their needs to facilitate communication (Balick, Spiegel, & Greene, 1976; Beukelman, Yorkston, & Waugh, 1980; Brown, 1988; Christopoulou & Bonvillian, 1985; Hoit-Dalgaard, Newhoff, & Barnes, 1981; Levett, 1969, 1971; Schlanger, 1976; Schlanger, Geffner, & DiCarrado, 1974). The clinical populations with which it has been used include children who have cerebral palsy, mentally retarded children, and aphasic adults. The purposes for which it has been used with persons in these populations are

1. To provide a means for encoding and transmitting messages.
2. To facilitate speech. Users are encouraged to speak their message as they pantomime it. Some aphasics have reported that this activity helps them to formulate more complete sentences and minimize word-finding problems. Communicating by pantomime also seems to increase the verbal output of some persons.
3. To facilitate receptive and expressive manual communication. Pantomime is more concrete than is either Ameslan or Amer-Ind. It usually can provide a more complete (or representational) impression of an idea or concept than can either of them. For this reason, mime is easier to understand and do than Ameslan or Amer-Ind. It is not surprising, therefore, that it has been used as an initial gestural communication strategy: A person is first taught to mime a relatively small set of concepts (usually fewer than 100). Manual signs are then slowly introduced, the first ones being primarily for abstract concepts that are difficult to mime. With the passage of time, a smaller and smaller percentage of the person's gestural communication would consist of mime.
4. To increase spontaneity and attention span and improve auditory and visual memory (Balick, Spiegel, & Greene, 1976).

The concepts it is possible to mime range from the relatively concrete to the relatively abstract. The concrete end of the continuum includes the following: above, big, can, broken, down, good, hungry, knife, light, mother, nurse, plate, shut, small, tired, train, where, bad, boat, cup, father, heavy, house, letter, long, money, on, open, sleep, spoon, toilet, up, who, both, bus, book, doctor, fork, I, I don't know, in, love, no, pain, quick, quiet, stop, tomorrow, and wash (from Levett, 1969). The following pantomime, which a person used to communicate that someone he knew had adopted a baby, is representative of the other end of the continuum:

> *Mr. M. outlines a large store window. He looks into the window and watches what appears to be moving objects on display. He waves at them, smiles and emits a vocalization that sounds like "kitchy, kitchy koo." He then outlines a door which he opens. He goes into the room and summons someone out to show her something in the window. He gives the woman money from his wallet as he continues pointing at one thing in the window. He goes into the store, picks up the object from the window, cuddles it, uses his forefinger to stimulate a smile from the baby in his arm. (Schlanger, 1976, pp. 3–4)*

The musculature of the entire body is used in mime. However, muscle function does not have to be completely normal. Some cerebral-palsied children have used mime successfully (Levett, 1969, 1971). Mime does not require as high a level of functioning of the musculature of the upper extremities as do Ameslan or Amer-Ind.

Mime, if done reasonably well, should be highly intelligible to untrained observers. Photographs, drawings, and/or videotaped demonstrations (that can be viewed on a home videotape recorder) of the mime used by a person can be made available to those with whom he interacts to improve their understanding of it.

Mime can convey messages concerning the past and future as well as the present. Although it can convey messages containing either abstract or concrete concepts, it is more suited to the concrete, particularly when the user is relatively inexperienced. Mime does not have a standard, nationally accepted semantic or syntactic structure. No dictionarylike compilations illustrating standardized mime-gesture sequences for specific concepts are available. Also, there are no formal, generally accepted sets of rules for ordering mime-gesture sequences.

The time and energy investments usually required for learning to use and comprehend mime are not excessive (see Table 1 in Levett, 1971). The level of acceptability of mime by at least some users and interpreters appears to be quite high (Balick, Spiegel, & Greene, 1976; Levett, 1971; Schlanger, 1976).

There are a number of books about mime as an art form that may provide information useful for teaching it. Also, the services of a professional mime can be useful both for training clients to use the technique and for training clinicians to teach it (Balick, Spiegel, & Greene, 1976). The theater department in a local college or a theater group may be able to help you locate such a person.

Left-Hand Manual Alphabet

Aphasia resulting from a stroke, or CVA, usually is accompanied by right hemiplegia. This is because the left half of the cerebral cortex is dominant for speech for almost everyone. Persons who have this condition who were right-handed prior to their stroke probably would not have adequate control of the musculature of their right hand to use the American Manual Alphabet (see Figure 4–1). Chen (1968, 1971) has devised a left-hand manual alphabet for such persons (see Figure 4–4). His manual alphabet is more concrete than the American Manual Alphabet because the finger gestures used in it more closely approximate printed letters. This should make it easier for many aphasics to learn. The linguistic and other characteristics of Chen's system are about the same as for the American Manual Alphabet (see the section on Ameslan).

Limited Manual Sign Systems

Several limited manual sign systems have been developed for use with aphasic, dysarthric, and dysphonic adults. These systems are limited in the sense that they are intended primarily for communicating basic needs in a hospital or nursing home setting. The systems of Chen (1968, 1971), Eagleson, Vaughn, and Knudson (1970), and Goldstein and Cameron (1952) are representative.

Manual Shorthand

Chen (1968, 1971) has devised a gestural system for basic needs, which he refers to as manual shorthand, by combining letters from his left-hand manual alphabet (Figure 4–4) and other gestures. All gestures in this system can be made with the left hand. Needs that cannot be communicated by manual shorthand can be spelled out using the left-hand manual alphabet. Chen refers to the combination of the manual shorthand and left-hand manual alphabet as the "talking hand" system.

The following gestures are included in Chen's manual shorthand system (1971, pp. 381, 383):

O.K.—Make a sign of "O" and "K."

Water—Make a sign of "W" and then point the finger to mouth.

Milk—Make a sign of "M" and then point the finger to mouth.

Tea—Make a sign of "T" and then point the finger to mouth.

Coffee—Make a sign of "C" and point the finger to mouth.

Juice—Make a sign of "J" and point the finger to mouth.

Open—Palm up and extend all fingers and then point to the object to be opened.

Close—Flex all fingers to make a fist and then point to the object to be closed.

Light on—Make a sign of "L" and then palm up with extend fingers.

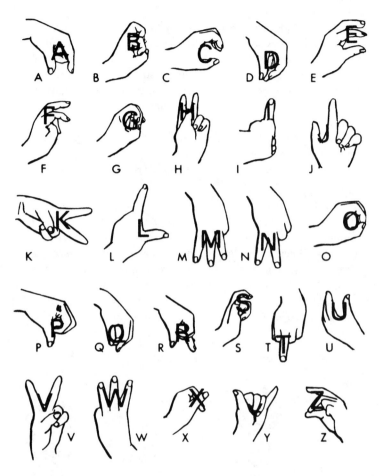

FIGURE 4–4 **Left-hand manual alphabet.**
Source: Chen, 1968.

Light off—Make a sign of "L" and then flex fingers to make a fist.

Too cold—Make a sign of "C" and put left hand at right shoulder and shrug the shoulders.

Too hot—Make a sign of "H" and then wipe the forehead with left hand.

Thirsty—Make a sign of "T" and "H" and then point the finger to mouth.

Pain—Make a sign of "P" and then point to the site of pain.

Urinal—Make a sign of "U."

Bedpan—Make a sign of "B" and "P."

Bathroom—Make a sign of "B" and "R."

Chen used his talking hand system with aphasic, dysarthric, and dysphonic patients. Approximately 50 percent were "able to learn all the manual alphabet and to communicate using manual shorthand or to spell out any words that . . . [they] wanted" (1971, p. 383). Results were poorest for aphasics, particularly sensory aphasics. Chen does not report outcome data for the manual shorthand separately, but it seems reasonable to assume that the success rate would be higher for it than for the entire system.

Chen's system probably would be usable in at least some hospital and nursing home settings. Training patients to use it and staff to interpret it should not require much time or energy investment. (See Chen, 1968, 1971, for relevant data.)

Manual Self-Care Signals

Eagleson, Vaughn, and Knudson (1970) devised 12 self-care signals for use as an interim communication system for expressive aphasics who have right hemiplegia (see Figure 4–5). All can be made with the left hand. They attempted to teach the signals to 31 expressive aphasics, and felt they were successful in all cases.

This system, like Chen's talking hand system, probably would be usable in at least some hospital and nursing home settings. The training required to teach patients to use it and staff to interpret it should be minimal. An enlarged copy of Figure 4–5

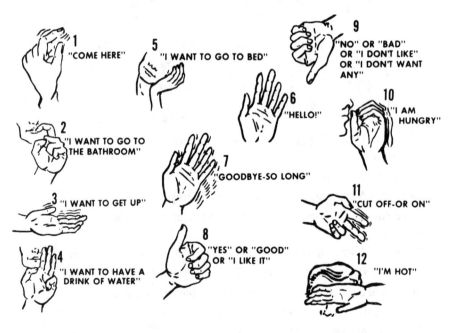

FIGURE 4–5   **Manual self-care signals.**
Source: Eagleson, Vaughn, & Knudson, 1970.

could be attached to the patient's bed or wheelchair to facilitate his and the staff's use of the system.

Hand Talking Chart

Goldstein and Cameron (1952) have devised a set of 20 self-care hand signals. They are reproduced on a chart (see Figure 4–6) that also functions as a communication board. A copy of the chart is given to the patient. He uses it to learn the hand signals and to communicate by pointing to the letters of the words in his message with his left hand (assuming that he has right hemiplegia). The chart also is used by physicians, nurses, family members, and others to interpret the patient's hand signals. All can be made with the left hand. The system is reported to have been used successfully with more than 200 aphasics (Goldstein & Cameron, 1952).

This system, like the previous two, should be usable in at least some hospital and nursing home settings. The training required to teach patients to use it and staff to interpret it should be minimal, in part because of the presence of the chart. Making the chart large (e.g., 1 foot by 2 feet) may facilitate its use by patients who have visual acuity problems.

Gestures for Yes and No

It is extremely important for any severely communicatively impaired person, child or adult, to develop reliable gestural signs for yes and no as quickly as possible. Once these signals are developed, the person can communicate by answering questions, if his or her ability to understand speech is relatively intact (Sappington et al., 1989). A frequently used strategy to facilitate such communication is similar to the game "Twenty Questions." After a person indicates he or she wants something, the "listener" asks a series of questions, beginning with the carrier phrase "Do you want _____?" The questioning continues until he or she signals yes. Obviously not a highly efficient communication strategy, it may be the only one that can be used with some patients who are severely involved motorically.

A second reason why it is important for a person to develop reliable yes and no signals is to make it possible for him or her to use a communication board with a scanning response mode (see chapter 5).

The term "reliable" has two meanings when applied to gestural signals for yes or no. First, it refers to the patient's use of them. He must signal yes when he means yes and no when he means no. Some severely communicatively impaired persons, particularly those who are aphasic, may not signal yes and no reliably. And, second, it refers to the observer's interpretation of them. They must be distinctive enough for an observer to perceive their presence reliably and different enough for him or her to differentiate reliably between them. Obviously, if an observer cannot detect when a patient is attempting to answer a question or determine whether his or her answer is yes or no, reliable communication is impossible.

How might yes and no be signaled gesturally? Any two gestures are usable for

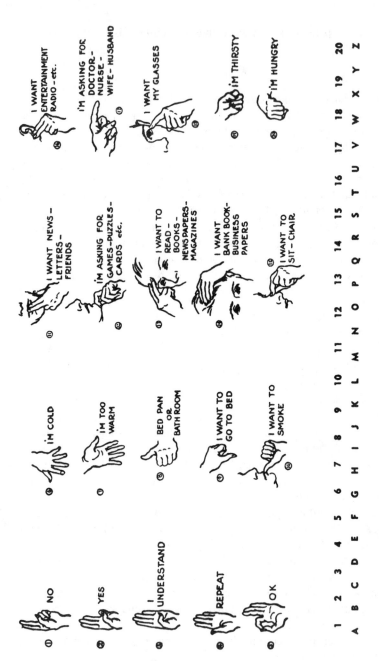

FIGURE 4–6 **Hand talking chart. The sign language in the designs speaks for itself. By pointing with pencil or finger to the letters or figures needed to further a conversation, communication between patient and friend can be amplified even to the "dictation" of a letter by the patient who otherwise would remain completely inarticulate.**

Source: Goldstein & Cameron, 1952.

this purpose so long as they can be produced and interpreted reliably. Those that have been used include

1. Moving head from side to side for a no and up and down for a yes (this set of signals, if usable, is the most satisfactory because its meaning is universally understood)
2. Turning head or directing gaze to right for a yes and to the left for a no (Carlson, 1976)
3. Looking up for a yes and down for a no (Easton, 1988)
4. Blinking right eye for yes and left eye for no
5. Blinking once for a no and twice for a yes
6. Forming a fist with the thumb pointing up for a yes and pointed down for a no (see Figure 4–5)
7. Moving the right foot for a yes and the left foot for a no (Schreiber, 1979)

An attention-getting sign describing the patient's yes and no signals should be attached to his bed, wheelchair, or both.

A patient who can signal yes and no gesturally and can comprehend speech and spell fairly well can communicate messages without instrumentation if the listener can be taught to scan letters of the alphabet vocally. The listener says letters and the patient indicates by signaling yes after the listener says the one needed for the message. The main limitation of this strategy is that it is slow. It can be made more efficient by asking two questions before beginning the scanning process for each letter: Is it a vowel sound? Is the letter between "B" and "N"? (Easton, 1988). Because vowels occur more often than consonants, a yes to the first question makes it unnecessary to ask the second. A no to both questions indicates that it is a letter between "P" and "Z." This strategy can be particularly useful with patients who are visually impaired.

Eye-Blink Encoding

A person may be able to communicate a few basic needs by means of an eye-blink encoding system (Adams, 1966). A specific number of eye-blinks would signal a particular need. Here is one such set of signals (adapted from that illustrated in Figure 4–5):

Number of Eye Blinks	Meaning
1	No.
2	Yes.
3	I want to go to the bathroom.
4	I want a drink of water.
5	I am hungry.
6	I am uncomfortable.

Cards describing the signals would be placed where they could be seen by the patient and the person with whom he or she is attempting to communicate. A phonatory grunting could be used instead of an eye blink (Adams, 1966).

Gestural Morse Code

The Morse code, which encodes letters and digits in dots and dashes (see Table 4–3), can be used as a gestural communication strategy. Dots and dashes can be signaled gesturally in two basic ways:

1. Producing a single gesture at two durations (e.g., a brief eye blink for a dot and one approximately twice as long for a dash)
2. Producing two gestures—one signaling a dot and the other a dash (e.g., a blink of the left eye signaling a dot, and one of the right eye a dash)

Also, Morse code can be used in conjunction with switching mechanisms to control the functioning of microcomputers (see discussion in chapter 5).

To use gestural Morse code, it is only necessary that a person be sufficiently intact neuromuscularly to produce a single muscle gesture at two rates or two muscle

TABLE 4–3   **The International Morse Code**

Symbol	Code	Symbol	Code
A	. -	V	. . . -
B	- . . .	W	. - -
C	- . - .	X	- . . -
D	- . .	Y	- . - -
E	.	Z	- - . .
F	. . - .	1	. - - - -
G	- - .	2	. . - - -
H	. . . .	3	. . . - -
I	. .	4	. . . . -
J	. - - -	5	. . . . .
K	- . -	6	- . . . .
L	. - . .	7	- - . . .
M	- -	8	- - - . .
N	- .	9	- - - - .
O	- - -	0	- - - - -
P	. - - .	Period	. - . - . -
Q	- - . -	Comma	- - . . - -
R	. - .	?	. . - - . .
S	. . .	Error	. . . .
T	-	Wait	. - . . .
U	. . -	End	. - . - .

gestures at a single rate. Any gestures can be used so long as they can be made and interpreted reliably.

Whereas Morse code can be used to convey any message to an observer who can interpret it, it is unintelligible to an untrained observer. The time and energy investment necessary for learning to use and interpret it should not be excessive, particularly if cards on which the code is reproduced are available to both users and interpreters while messages are being transmitted. The linguistic structure of a Morse code message, of course, is that of English.

The level of acceptability of Morse code communication to at least some potential users and interpreters probably would be fairly high because it only would be used with persons who are severely involved motorically and it would permit such persons to communicate. Morse code would be a particularly viable communication medium for persons who had learned it prior to the onset of their condition. Patients who are FCC-licensed amateur radio operators, for example, are likely to know the code.

Pointing

A severely communicatively impaired person may be able to signal a need or desire by pointing to something related to it. This communication strategy tends to be used frequently by such persons who do not have a formal communication system. Most point with either a hand or an eye (by directing gaze). Although pointing by itself is a very limited communication strategy (it only can be used to signal needs and desires that are related to something in the immediate environment), when it is combined with a communication board it can become a relatively flexible communication strategy. (The use of pointing responses to indicate message components on communication boards is dealt with in chapter 5.)

WHICH STRATEGY TO USE?

Salient features of more than 10 gestural strategies have been summarized in this chapter. These strategies (as well as those discussed in chapters 5 and 6) make different demands on users and interpreters and vary in flexibility and efficiency (Bristow & Fristoe, 1984; Daniloff, 1984; Daniloff et al., in press; Hodges & Schwethelm, 1984; Imhoff & McMillen, 1984). With whom would each be used and when? The comments in this section are designed to answer this question. All circumstances under which each would be used of course are not indicated, and the uses indicated are not necessarily applicable to all persons in the populations mentioned. The names of the strategies are italicized to facilitate locating comments about particular ones.

1. All severely communicatively impaired persons should be taught *gestures for yes and no* if they do not have them. This should be done regardless of the other communication strategies they are going to be taught. One of the first goals of therapy for clients who do not have these gestures should be to teach them. Once a client can reliably signal yes and no, he or she can communicate by answering questions.

2. *Ameslan* would be the most appropriate for the client (child or adult) who needs a communication strategy that approaches speech in flexibility and efficiency—provided that the client can learn to produce the gestures and at least some of the persons with whom he or she needs to communicate can interpret them or learn to do so.

3. For the client (child or adult) who needs a communication strategy that will allow him or her to communicate reasonably effectively with persons who have had little or no training in interpreting the gestures being used, *Amer-Ind* probably would be the most appropriate, provided the client could learn it. Although it is not as flexible a system as *Ameslan, Amer-Ind* signs tend to be easier to learn because of their concreteness, and they are more intelligible than *Ameslan* signs to untrained observers.

4. For the client, particularly the expressive aphasic with right hemiplegia, who needs an interim strategy for communicating basic needs while in a hospital or nursing home, the *Manual Shorthand, Manual Self-Care Signals*, or *Hand Talking Chart* should be appropriate.

5. The communication ability of almost any client who can spell, and who has at least one hand that is normal motorically, can be enhanced by teaching the *American Manual Alphabet* or the *Left-Hand Manual Alphabet*. These manual alphabets can be used in combination with *Ameslan* signs, *Amer-Ind* signs, or *mime*.

6. *Mime* may be useful for introducing gestural communication to clients (particularly mentally retarded ones). It is more concrete than either *Ameslan* or *Amer-Ind* and, thus, is easier to learn. Once a client has developed a basic *mime* vocabulary, *Ameslan* or *Amer-Ind* signs can be introduced.

7. The *mild* quadriplegic whose use of his or her hands is not adequate for *Ameslan* or *Amer-Ind* may find *mime* to be a usable communication strategy.

8. The *moderate or severe* quadriplegic may find *eye-blink encoding* or *gestural Morse code* to be a usable communication strategy. The latter, of course, is more flexible than the former.

9. It is desirable that a person who will use a communication board develop a *pointing* gesture. This is also desirable for use of an electronic communication aid. A pointing gesture can be used to activate the switching mechanism that controls such aids.

▶ 5

Gestural-Assisted Strategies

A number of representative gestural-assisted augmentative communication strategies are discussed in this chapter. Those included here were selected because they illustrate salient features of such strategies.

All gestural-assisted strategies have three types of components:

1. A symbol system for encoding messages
2. A display on which elements of the symbol system are reproduced (e.g., a computer monitor screen)
3. A means of indicating (or reproducing) on the display in an appropriate sequence the elements of the symbol system that encode a message

The displays used and the means of indicating symbols on a display tend to be different for electronic and nonelectronic systems, and thus those for each type are discussed separately. The symbols used for encoding messages with both types are essentially the same.

The description of each type of gestural-assisted strategy includes the following information:

- Its components
- The manner in which its components are assembled
- Its portability, cost, and commercial availability
- Sources of plans and components
- Neuromuscular functions that must be intact for it to be usable
- The time and energy investment required to learn to use it
- Its level of acceptability to users and interpreters
- The speed at which messages can be communicated with it
- The populations with which it has been used

Specific guidelines for selecting components are also presented.

SYMBOL SETS

A *symbol set* is a group of sensory (visual, auditory, or tactile) images, or signs, that suggest, or stand for, something else by reason of relationship (association) or convention. Visual signs that singly or in combination can function as symbols for encoding messages with augmentative communication aids are photographs, drawings, Blissymbols, rebuses, Yerkish lexigrams, the alphabet, printed words, and tokens (e.g., plastic symbols used in the Non-SLIP Program). Auditory signs that can serve this function include both phoneme sequences (e.g., synthesized speech) and noise sequences (e.g., patterned bursts of noise used for communication by Morse code). Tactile signs include the raised-dot configurations of the Braille alphabet. Some of these message-encoding techniques are more effective than are others (Beukelman & Yorkston, 1984; Bray & Goossens', 1991; Goossens', Elder, & Bray, 1990; Light & Lindsay, 1991b; Light et al., 1990; Schwartz, 1988).

A sign can function as a symbol because of a structural relationship (isomorphism) between it and what it symbolizes or by reason of convention (it being assigned a particular meaning or meanings). A sign bears a structural relationship to its referent (or is isomorphic to its referent) if it is somehow similar to it in appearance, or is somehow associated with (or suggestive of) it, or both. A drawing of a house can serve as a symbol for the concept "house" because it is similar in appearance to this referent. A photograph of a person who looks unhappy can serve as a symbol for the concept "pain" because it is suggestive of its meaning. And a drawing of a person drinking something can serve as a symbol for the concept "thirsty" because it is both similar in appearance to and suggestive of this referent.

Many signs function as symbols because of convention. Any sign can have any meaning that all who use it wish it to have. Conventional signs usually are not related to their referents by appearance or association. Examples are words and some types of pictographs (e.g., Yerkes symbols).

The description of each symbol set includes information concerning the following:

- Its intelligibility to untrained observers
- Its ability to convey messages concerning the here and now
- Its ability to convey messages not concerned with the here and now
- Its ability to convey abstract concepts
- Its syntactic and semantic structure
- The similarity of its linguistic structure to English
- The time and energy investment required to learn to use and interpret it
- The populations with which it has been used

Objects

The most concrete symbol set that can be used for augmentative communication consists of objects. A user transmits a message by pointing to (e.g., looking at) an object that would somehow suggest it to the person with whom he or she is trying to communicate. A person could look at a glass, for example, to signal that he or she was thirsty. This is one of the main ways that severely communicatively impaired persons, particularly those who have not been interfaced with an augmentative system, communicate. In a sense, they are using a "natural" communication board on which the symbol set consists of all the objects in their environment to which they can point. A clinician can facilitate the use of this strategy by encouraging caregivers to place objects in the person's environment that suggest various messages that he or she may need to communicate.

Miniature versions of objects (such as dollhouse furniture) can also be used as symbols. They can be placed loose in the person's environment, or they can be attached to something (as to a sheet of plywood or a piece of fabric). This type of symbol should be considered for clients with vision problems but who have sufficiently good control of an upper extremity to identify objects by touch. It also should be considered for clients with abstract-concrete imbalance for whom photographs or drawings are too abstract to use as symbols.

For further information about the use of objects as symbols, see Rowland and Schweigert (1989, 1990).

Photographs and Drawings

Photographs and drawings are frequently used with persons who cannot speak, write, or read English. Users include severely communicatively impaired children and adults who (1) have not learned to read, (2) are dyslexic because of cortical damage, and (3) are able to read one or more languages but not English. A patient in a hospital or nursing home who is unable to speak or write English could use such symbols for communicating basic needs to the staff.

Sets of pictures used as symbols in gestural-assisted communication schemes vary on several dimensions, including size, level of abstraction, degree of complexity, degree of ambiguity, and number of messages that can be encoded.

Size

Pictures used as symbols should be large enough to be seen by both users and interpreters, but no larger than necessary, so that the display on which they appear can be kept as small as possible. Picture size is a particularly important variable when users or interpreters have visual acuity or visual field disturbances or when the display is located at a distance from them.

Level of Abstraction

The level of abstraction is a function of the amount of detail (or information) present in the object or event depicted that is included in the picture. The more detail (or information) omitted, the higher the level of abstraction. Suppose you wanted a picture for a communication board to which a patient could point to indicate that she is thirsty. The following pictures, which are ordered from a relatively high level of abstraction to relatively low level, might be used for this purpose:

A line drawing of a woman drinking from a glass

A line drawing of a woman drinking from a glass that resembles the one the patient uses

A black and white photograph of a woman drinking from a glass that resembles the one the patient uses

A color photograph of a woman drinking from a glass that resembles the one the patient uses

A color photograph of the patient drinking from the glass she uses

There are, of course, many more gradations possible; these were selected only to illustrate what is meant by the abstraction continuum.

Is the level of abstraction an important consideration when selecting picture symbols for gestural-assisted communication aids? It appears to be, particularly for patients who have cortical damage. Some patients who have such lesions tend to exhibit what has been referred to as abstract-concrete imbalance. They are more concrete than normal in their conceptual functioning, and, consequently, have more difficulty than usual in recognizing relatively abstract representations of objects and events. They might not, for example, recognize a line drawing of a glass.

Persons with abstract-concrete imbalance also tend to have difficulty with categorization. They may fail to perceive the abstract quality that results in objects and events that do not look alike being assigned to the same category. They do not abstract similarities and ignore differences as much as most people do. Consequently, they may not realize that, by pointing to a photograph of a glass that does not look like the one they use, they can communicate that they wish to drink from their glass.

The first pictures presented to patients with cortical damage should be as concrete as possible. For a picture symbol to which a patient with this condition can point to indicate he is thirsty, you might use a Polaroid photograph of him drinking from his glass. Its use should place only a minimal demand on his ability to recognize and categorize objects and events. Such ability is called into play because he would have to recognize that a two-dimensional, static representation of a three-dimensional, dynamic event can portray, or symbolize, that event.

Following a period of therapy, spontaneous recovery, or both, it may be possible for a patient to utilize more abstract picture stimuli as symbols than those he or she was able to use initially. Increasing the abstraction level of picture stimuli usually should be done in relatively small steps.

Degree of Complexity

The degree of complexity of a picture is partly a function of the extent to which its foreground stands out from its background. The foreground of a picture is the part that has symbol value—that is, the part necessary for encoding the concept the picture is intended to communicate. All other details or lines in a picture would constitute its background. The greater the separation between foreground and background, the lower the level of complexity. A photograph of a patient drinking from a glass (intended for encoding "thirsty") that was taken against a white background probably would be less complex than would one of the same person drinking from the same glass with kitchen cupboards in the background.

It is desirable to keep the level of complexity of picture symbols as low as is practical. Backgrounds of photographs can be deemphasized by spraying them with a light coating of white watercolor paint using an airbrush. A masking material can be used to cover foreground objects as the paint is being sprayed. This can also be done by scanning the photographs into a computer and using retouching software to simulate airbrushing.

Degree of Ambiguity

The degree of ambiguity of a picture is a function of the number of concepts it could be used to encode. The more meanings that could reasonably be assigned to it, the greater its ambiguity. A picture of a person sitting at a kitchen table that has a glass of milk on it could be used to encode a number of concepts—drink, milk, person, kitchen, sit, table. It is, of course, desirable to select picture symbols that would have only the desired meaning to most persons. Reducing complexity, incidentally, is one way of reducing ambiguity.

Number of Messages

The dimensions that have been discussed thus far are relevant to individual pictures. A dimension that applies to sets of pictures is the number of messages that can be encoded. Some sets can encode more messages than others. Several factors influence the number of messages a set of pictures can encode, for example:

The number of pictures in the set

The possibility of message expansion by agglutination (e.g., pointing to a picture of a glass and a picture of a carton of milk to encode a glass of milk)

The possibility of combining concepts encoded by several pictures into an utterance (e.g., pointing to a picture of a person carrying something, a picture of a milk carton, and a picture of a glass to encode the message "Bring me a glass of milk")

The smallest set of pictures should be selected by which necessary messages can be encoded.

Picture symbols should be intelligible to untrained observers, particularly if an effort is made to minimize their complexity and ambiguity. Any question regarding their intelligibility can be eliminated by printing above each picture the concept it is intended to encode (assuming that the observers can read).

Pictures usually are better suited for encoding messages about the here and now than the past or future. The ability of a set of picture symbols to encode messages about the past and future can be enhanced by including in it a picture that would signal past time (e.g., a caveman) and one that would signal future time (e.g., a space colony on another planet).

Pictures are better suited for encoding concrete than abstract concepts, but they can be used for encoding both. The more abstract a concept, the more ambiguous a picture depicting it tends to be. Pictures suitable for encoding many relatively abstract concepts can be found in the Peabody Picture Vocabulary Test (Dunn and Dunn, 1981) and other picture tests of receptive-language functioning.

The linguistic structure of a message encoded in picture symbols usually differs from one encoded in English on morphological, syntactic, and semantic levels. Pictures depicting specific morphemic forms in English (e.g., singular vs. plural) usually are not used; appropriate English morphemic forms are inferred from context. Also, the ordering of picture symbols in a message does not necessarily correspond to that for English words. (A message encoded in picture symbols, though, may have a subject-predicate form; pictures that encode a noun and a verb may be used together.) In addition, picture symbols do not necessarily correspond to individual English words. A message encoded by a picture symbol may require two or more English words to encode. It may, in fact, be equivalent to an entire English utterance (e.g., pointing to a picture of someone drinking from a glass could be equivalent to "I'm thirsty. I want a drink").

The time and energy investments required for learning to use and interpret picture symbols should be minimal, particularly if their levels of complexity and ambiguity are relatively low and the messages they are intended to encode are printed above them.

What picture symbols should be included in the set intended for a particular child or adult? Although this decision would be partly determined by the client's environment (home, hospital, etc.) and specific communication needs, some of the following picture symbols may be used:

Picture	*Message Encoded*
Person eating	I am hungry.
Person drinking	I am thirsty.
Person sleeping	I am tired.
Person near fire	I am too warm.
Person sitting on ice	I am too cold.
Smiling face	I am happy.
Sad face	I am unhappy.
Bedpan, urinal, toilet	I want (bedpan, urinal, toilet).
Television set	I want the TV turned on/off.
Nurse	I want a nurse.
Doctor	I want a doctor.
Photographs of family members	I want (family member).
Wheelchair	I want my wheelchair.
Eyeglasses, dental plate, or hearing aid	I want my eyeglasses (dental plate, hearing aid)

Picture	*Message Encoded*
Pills, hypodermic needle	I want my medication.
Book, magazine	I want to read.
Pencil, pen	I want to write.
Pictures of foods the person might want to eat	I want ____ to eat.
Pictures of things the person might want to drink	I want ____ to drink.
Caveman	Past (time)
Space colony	Future (time)
Line drawing of front, back, and side of body on which the person can indicate where he hurts by pointing (see Figure 5–1) or scanning (see Figure 5–2)	My ____ hurts.

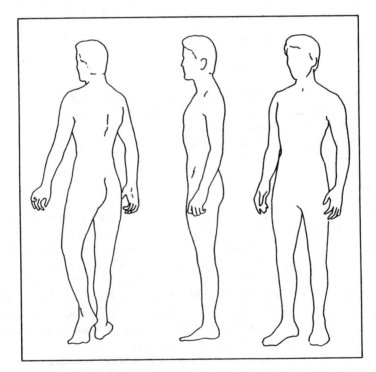

FIGURE 5–1 **Line drawings of back, side, and front of body on which sites of pain can be indicated by pointing.**
Source: Courtesy of Cleo Living Aids, Cleveland, Ohio.

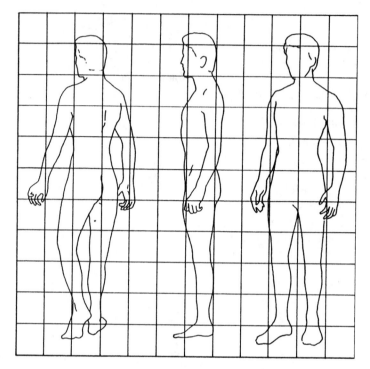

FIGURE 5–2   **Line drawings of back, side, and front of body superimposed on a matrix on which sites of pain can be indicated by linear scanning (see section on strategies for indicating message components in this chapter).**
Source: Courtesy of Cleo Living Aids, Cleveland, Ohio.

Picsyms

A clinician who wishes to use drawings as symbols on communication boards has to decide, first, how to represent the various concepts she wants her client to be able to communicate and then she has to be able to draw them on the board in the appropriate size. Picsyms is a graphic symbol set intended for use on communication boards that can be used for simplifying both of these tasks (Carlson, 1981, 1984; Carlson & James, 1980; Carlson & Kovarik, 1985; Mizuko, 1987b; Mizuko & Reichle, 1988a). The symbols, which are line drawings (see Figure 5–3), are both ideographic and pictographic. A dictionary containing more than 1800 of the symbols, arranged alphabetically, is available (Carlson & James, 1980; Carlson, 1984).

The symbols can be drawn in almost any size by someone who has even minimal artistic ability by copying them on a six-row by eight-column grid containing appropriate size cells. Picsyms is open-ended, and new symbols may be created using the logic of the system. Included are symbols that represent verbs, nouns, and prepositions. The English word equivalent of each Picsym usually is printed above or below

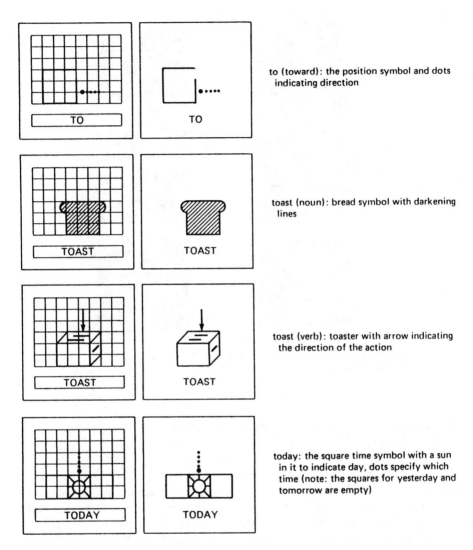

FIGURE 5–3 **Representative Picsyms.**
Source: Carlson, 1984.

it. These symbols have been used with children as young as 20 months (Carlson & Kovarik, 1985).

PIC Symbols

The PIC (Pictogram Ideogram Communication) symbol set consists of approximately 400 drawings intended for use on communication boards (Maharaj, 1980). These

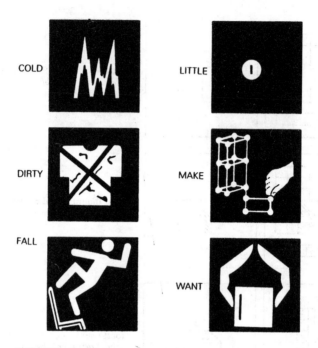

FIGURE 5–4   **Representative PIC symbols.**
Source: Blackstone, 1986.

drawings differ from the others described in this chapter in that they are white on a black background (see Figure 5–4). They were drawn in this manner to make them more conspicuous, but whether white on black drawings have a visual saliency advantage over black on white ones is uncertain (Campbell & Lloyd, 1986; Meador et al., 1984). All these symbols are ideographic, and some are also pictographic. Although the symbols in this set can be supplemented by the clinician, they are difficult to draw because of the white on black feature. Whether PIC symbols would be more easily guessed than the others described in this chapter has not been established.

Sigsymbols

Sigsymbols (Cregan, 1980, 1982, 1984; Cregan & Lloyd, 1984a, 1984b, 1988; Cregan & Lonnquist, 1990; Kangas & Lloyd, 1988a; Lloyd & Cregan, 1984; Vanderheiden & Lloyd, 1986), like Picsyms and PIC symbols, are pictographic and/or ideographic line drawings intended for use on communication boards. They differ from those in these two symbol sets in that some are linked to Ameslan or another manual sign symbol set. In fact, Sigsymbol is a contraction of sig from manual sign and symbol from graphic symbol (Cregan, 1980). Examples of Ameslan-linked Sig-

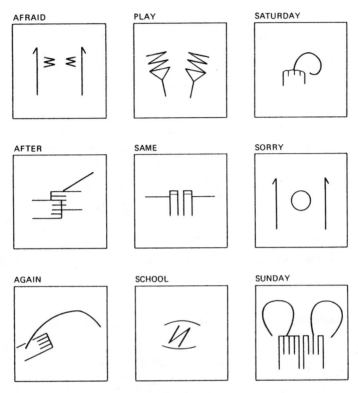

FIGURE 5–5   **Representative Ameslan-based Sigsymbols.**
Source: Blackstone, 1986.

symbols are presented in Figure 5–5. The use of Sigsymbols may be particularly attractive in classrooms and other settings in which both manual signs and communication boards with graphic symbols are used. That is, their use may facilitate teaching persons who use one type of symbol to comprehend the other. Because these symbols do not contain a lot of detail, they are relatively easy to draw.

Traditional Orthography

If the user of a gestural-assisted communication aid and those with whom he or she intends to communicate can read English (or another language), *traditional orthography* probably would the most advantageous symbol set to use. It can encode as many messages as any of the other symbol sets. In fact, it can be used to transmit any message if the sender can spell the words used accurately and the receiver can read them. In addition, if the sender can spell fairly well, it requires a smaller number of symbols for encoding a given number of messages (as long as this number exceeds

36) than any of the other symbol sets. An English-language symbol set usually would contain a minimum of 36 elements: 26 letters and 10 digits. Although the digits are not essential, they increase the efficiency of communication. One consequence of needing only a small number of symbols is that they can be displayed in a relatively small area. This increases both the portability of a display and its usefulness to persons who have a restricted range of movement.

Although an English-language message can be encoded with a symbol set containing as few as 26 elements, the use of such a set would be relatively inefficient because every word would have to be spelled out. For this reason, English symbol sets intended for gestural-assisted communication systems usually contain some frequently used words and phrases in addition to letters and digits. The words and phrases on the communication board reproduced in Figure 5–6 are representative.

An English symbol set can be used by itself or in combination with other symbol sets. If it is combined with another set, the English symbols may be printed above those of the other set (e.g., pictures or Blissymbols) to assist observers in interpreting them, or they may be used to encode messages that cannot be encoded with the other

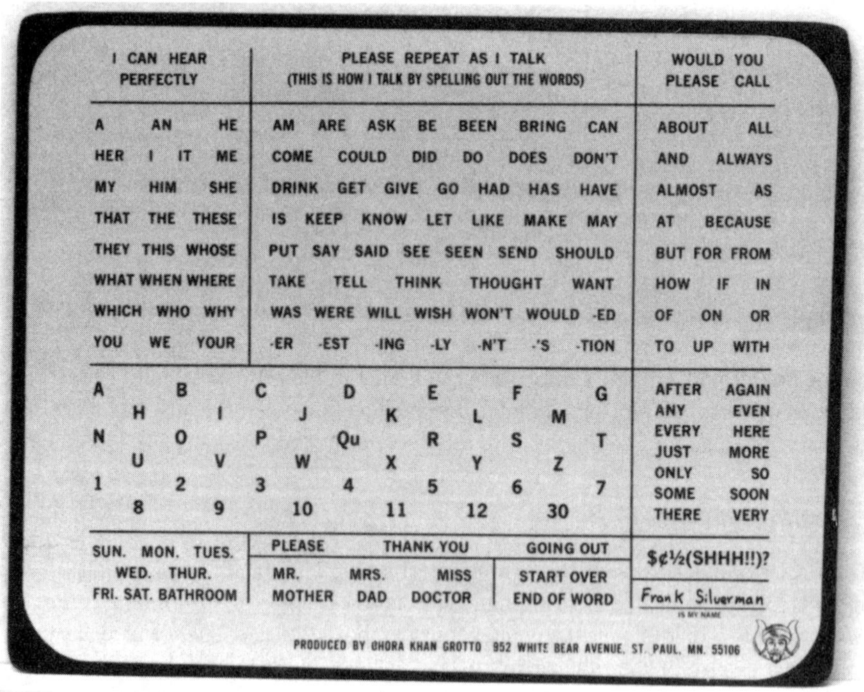

FIGURE 5–6 Representative English-language communication board.
Source: Courtesy of Ghora Kahn Grotto, St. Paul, Minnesota.

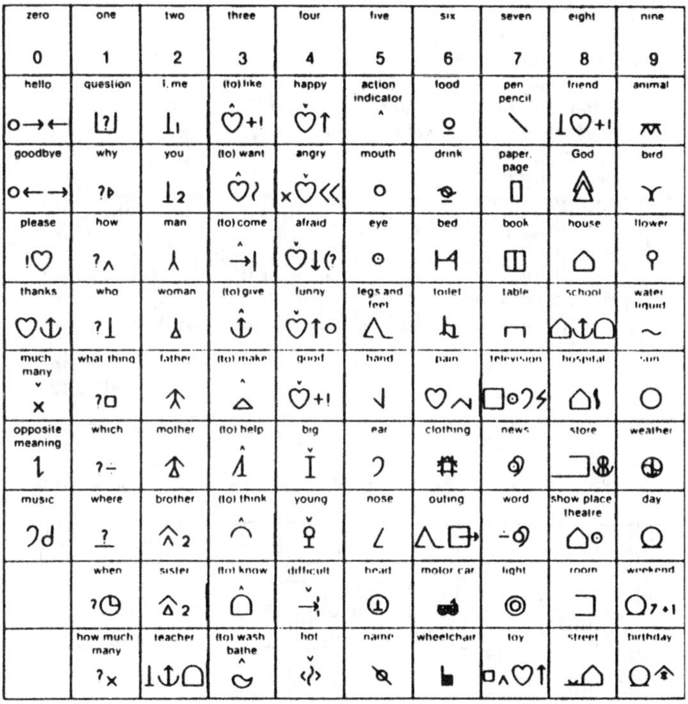

zero	one	two	three	four	five	six	seven	eight	nine
0	1	2	3	4	5	6	7	8	9
hello	question	i, me	(to) like	happy	action indicator	food	pen pencil	friend	animal
goodbye	why	you	(to) want	angry	mouth	drink	paper, page	God	bird
please	how	man	(to) come	afraid	eye	bed	book	house	flower
thanks	who	woman	(to) give	funny	legs and feet	toilet	table	school	water liquid
much many	what thing	father	(to) make	good	hand	pain	television	hospital	sun
opposite meaning	which	mother	(to) help	big	ear	clothing	news	store	weather
music	where	brother	(to) think	young	nose	outing	word	show place theatre	day
	when	sister	(to) know	difficult	head	motor car	light	room	weekend
	how much many	teacher	(to) wash bathe	hot	name	wheelchair	toy	street	birthday

FIGURE 5-7 **Representative Blissymbolics communication board.**
Source: Courtesy of Blissymbolics Communication International, Toronto, Ontario.

set. The first mode of combining English with those of another set (Blissymbolics) is illustrated by the communication board reproduced in Figure 5–7 and the second by that reproduced in Figure 5–8.

Capital and/or lowercase letters can be used in displays. The letters should be large enough to be readable by both users and interpreters and printed in a relatively plain (unembellished) type style. The letters can be drawn with black ink or generated with a microcomputer, or black rub-on letters or vinyl letters can be used (both of which can be purchased at an art supply or stationery store).

SPEEC

The SPEEC (Sequences of Phonemes for Efficient English Communication) symbol set consists of "phoneme sequences which have a high frequency of occurrence in the spoken language, along with a full set of single phonemes, represented in a simplified, consistent orthography" (Goodenough-Trepagnier & Prather, 1981, p. 322). A por-

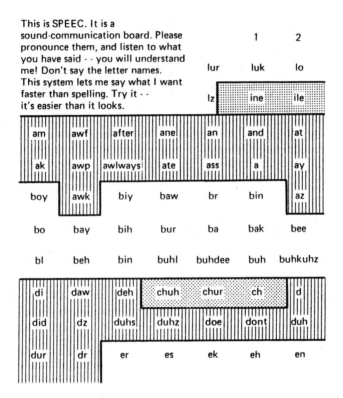

FIGURE 5–8   **Portion of a communication board with SPEEC symbols.**
Source: Goodenough-Trepagnier & Prather, 1981.

tion of a communication board with these symbols is reproduced in Figure 5–8. (A French-language version of this board is also available.) Messages are transmitted by pointing in the appropriate sequence to the phonemes and phoneme sequences for the words contained in it. A severely communicatively impaired person who can understand speech but cannot spell very well may be more successful communicating with this symbol set than one consisting of the alphabet. A SPEEC symbol set, like an alphabet-based one, could be used for encoding any message.

Blissymbolics

Blissymbolics (or Semantography) is a pictographic, ideographic writing system developed by Charles K. Bliss (1965) that can be read (decoded) in all languages. It is intended to function as an auxiliary language for written international communication. As such, it is one of a relatively large number of auxiliary languages intended for international communication constructed during the past 500 years. None, with the possible exception of Esperanto, have been widely accepted, even though few people seem to view learning such a language as undesirable. This may be partly because few people know that they exist (see Silverman & Silverman, 1979). Blissymbolics has been adapted for use as a communication medium for prereading, severely communicatively handicapped children (e.g., Archer, 1977; Guttman, 1990; Haynes & Quist, 1992; McNaughton, 1975, 1976a, 1976b, 1978, 1981, 1982, 1985, 1986a, 1986b, 1990b, 1990c, 1990d; McNaughton & Kates, 1974, 1980; McNaughton, Kates, & Silverman, 1976, 1978; McNaughton et al., 1988; McNaughton, Reid et al., 1988; McNaughton & Seybold, 1990; McNaughton & Warrick, 1984, 1986; McNaughton & Wood, 1986; Silverman, McNaughton, & Kates, 1978).

The Blissymbolic symbol set consists of approximately 100 pictorial ideographic and arbitrary symbols that when used singly (see Figure 5–9 for the 70 most frequently used symbols) or when combined in various ways (see Figure 5–10) can encode almost any message.* The structure of Blissymbolics (see Figure 5–7) is comparable to that of printed ideographic Chinese characters. Bliss views his system as a simplified Chinese writing system: This ideographic system has been understood and used for thousands of years by persons living in China, who do not speak a common language.

Most Blissymbols encode information on a semantic, or meaning, level (a few encode grammatical information). Each symbol element represents a general idea or concept. This general idea or concept usually includes a set of related ideas or concepts that would be encoded in English (or another language) by more than one word. The symbol for "water" with the addition of other elements (see Figure 5–10) can mean rain, steam, snow, cloud, lake, ocean, freezing, thawing, hail, current, river, or cloudburst.

The specific concept or idea encoded by a Blissymbol is indicated by the manner in which it has been manipulated or modified. Following are 14 of the ways that a symbol may be manipulated or modified to change its meaning:

1. *Agglutination* (see Figure 5–10a). Symbols are combined by superimposing or sequencing elemmments to form compound symbols. The meaning of such a symbol can be inferred from the meanings of its elements plus context. If a cross-out symbol, for example, is combined with the symbol for ear, the result would be a compound symbol that could encode the concept deaf. Likewise, if the symbols for person, mouth, and musical note are combined, the result would be a compound symbol that could encode the concept singer.

Many symbols may have more than one interpretation. Their meaning in a par-

---

*The Blissymbols illustrated here are in accordance with B.C.I.-approved symbols as of January 1979. Copyright by C.K. Bliss and exclusive worldwide licensee, Blissymbolics Communication International, Toronto, Ontario, Canada.

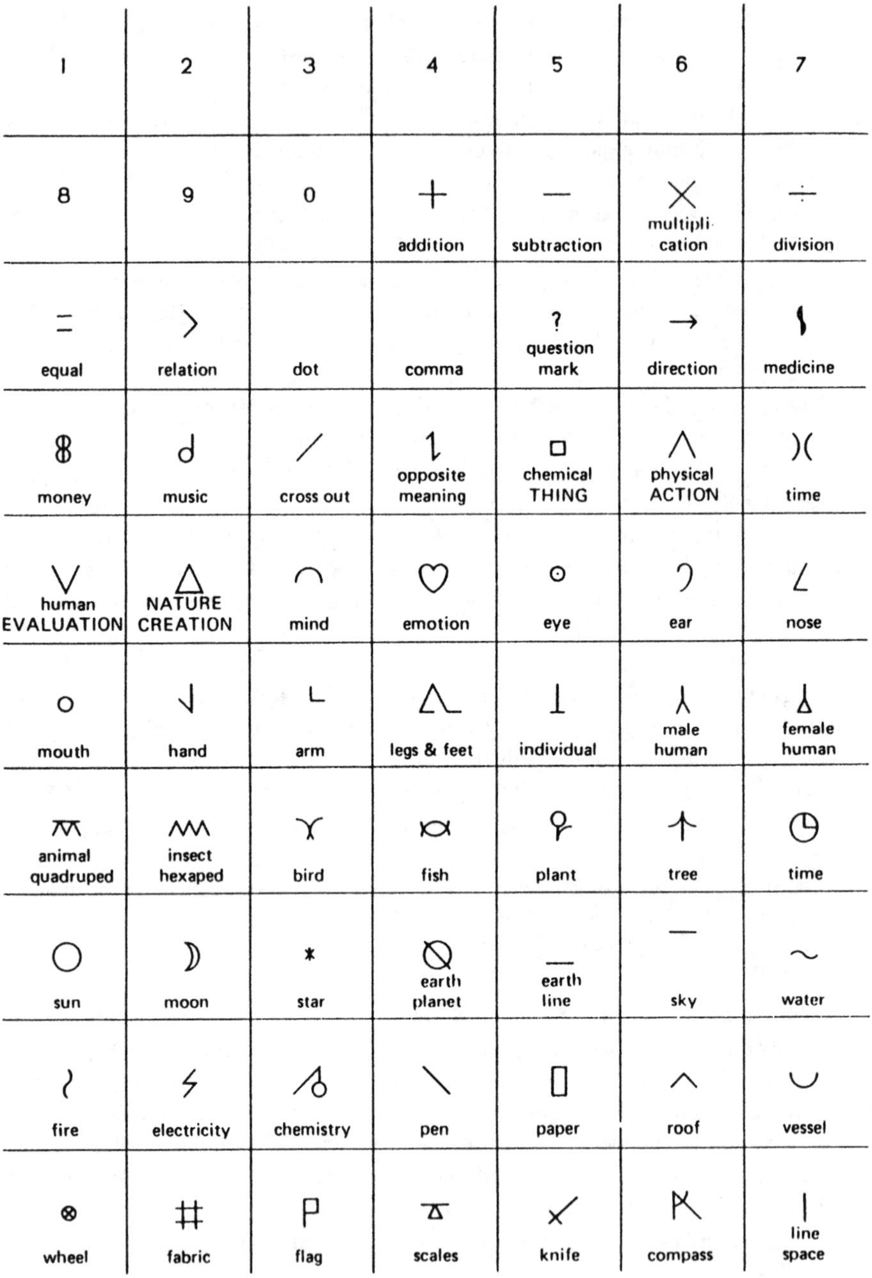

1	2	3	4	5	6	7
8	9	0	+ addition	— subtraction	× multipli-cation	÷ division
= equal	﹥ relation	dot	comma	? question mark	→ direction	∫ medicine
₿ money	♩ music	/ cross out	↿ opposite meaning	□ chemical THING	∧ physical ACTION	)(time
∨ human EVALUATION	△ NATURE CREATION	⌢ mind	♡ emotion	⊙ eye	⌐ ear	∠ nose
○ mouth	√ hand	L arm	∧ legs & feet	⊥ individual	λ male human	▲ female human
⼈ animal quadruped	⋀⋀ insect hexaped	Υ bird	⋈ fish	♀ plant	⊥ tree	◷ time
○ sun	☽ moon	✳ star	⊘ earth planet	— earth line	— sky	~ water
⟨ fire	⚡ electricity	⟋ chemistry	＼ pen	▯ paper	⌃ roof	∪ vessel
⊗ wheel	♯ fabric	ꟼ flag	⊼ scales	✗ knife	Ҡ compass	∣ line space

FIGURE 5–9 **The main basic Blissymbol elements.**
Source: Bliss, 1965.

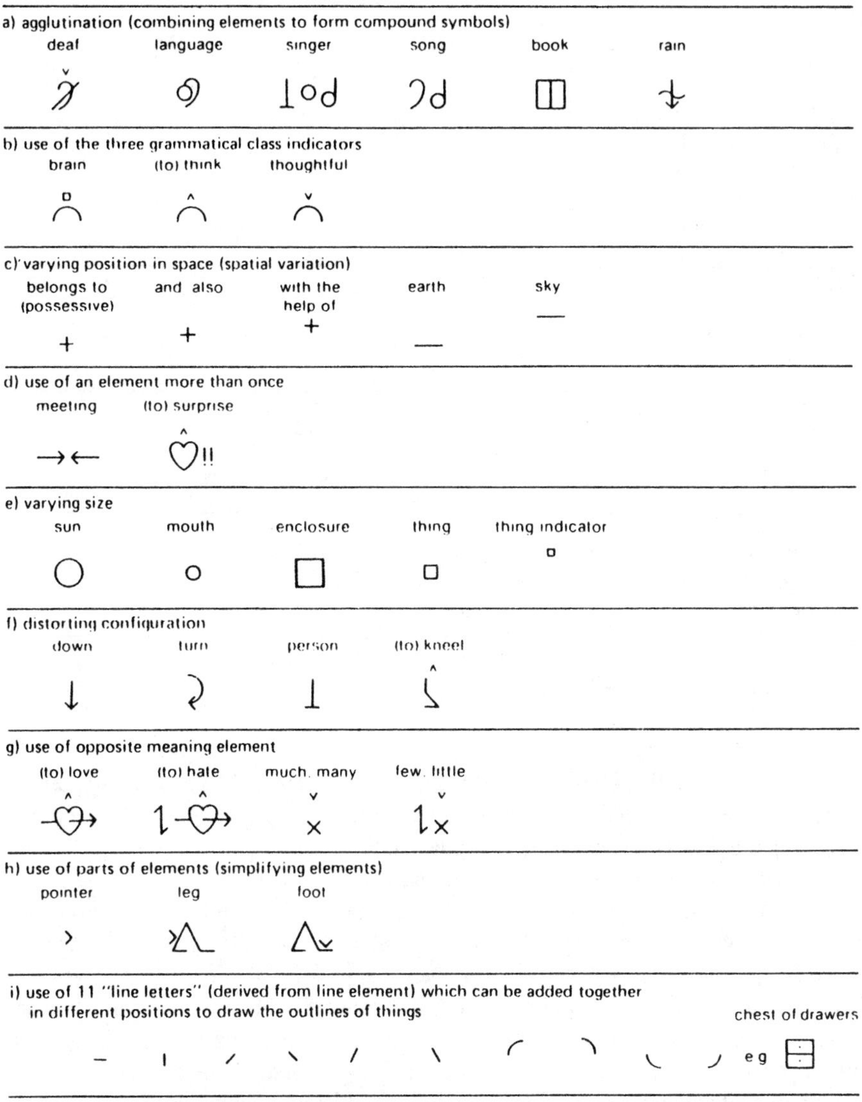

a) agglutination (combining elements to form compound symbols)

deaf	language	singer	song	book	rain

b) use of the three grammatical class indicators

brain	(to) think	thoughtful

c) varying position in space (spatial variation)

belongs to (possessive)	and also	with the help of	earth	sky

d) use of an element more than once

meeting	(to) surprise

e) varying size

sun	mouth	enclosure	thing	thing indicator

f) distorting configuration

down	turn	person	(to) kneel

g) use of opposite meaning element

(to) love	(to) hate	much, many	few, little

h) use of parts of elements (simplifying elements)

pointer	leg	foot

i) use of 11 "line letters" (derived from line element) which can be added together in different positions to draw the outlines of things   chest of drawers

FIGURE 5–10   **Strategies for vocabulary expansion by manipulation of Blissymbol elements.**

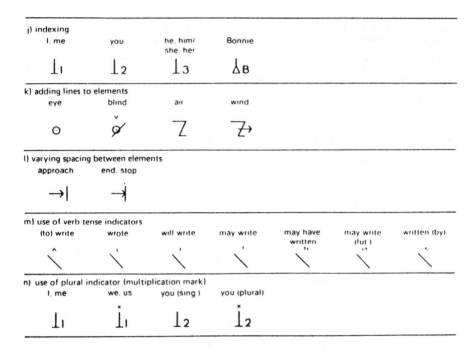

FIGURE 5–10 *Continued*

ticular message usually can be inferred from context. Also, the English equivalent is almost certain to be printed with it. (Bliss insists that all reproductions of his symbols be accompanied by English or other language equivalents.)

2. *Use of the three grammatical class indicators* (see Figure 5–10b). A given Blissymbol can function as the English equivalent of a noun, verb, adverb, or adjective. Its grammatical class is specified by the indicator that appears above it. A small square (which indicates a "chemical THING") appearing above a signal gives it a concrete noun meaning. A small cone pointing upward (which indicates a "physical ACTION") appearing above a symbol gives it a verb meaning. And a small cone pointing downward (which indicates a "human EVALUATION") appearing above a symbol gives it an adjective or adverb meaning. (The rationale underlying the use of these three indicators is outlined in Bliss, 1965.) If there is no indicator above a Blissymbol that could function as a noun, verb, adverb, or adjective, it is assumed to be a noun. Thus, the Blissymbol for mind with a square above it would mean brain; with the upward cone above it would mean (to) think (or some form of this verb); and with the downward cone above it would mean thoughtful (or some other adjective or adverb pertaining to thinking). The specific English equivalent (translation) of a Blissymbol is inferred from context.

3. *Varying position in space* (see Figure 5–10c). The position of a symbol in its allocated space can influence its meaning. If a small cross appears at the bottom of its allocated space, it means belongs to (possessive); if it appears at the top of its allocated space, it means with the help of; in midposition, it means and also. Similarly, a long line at the bottom means earth; on the top, it means sky. English equivalents of symbol elements in atypical positions can be inferred from their usual meanings, the nature of their atypical position, and context. Rarely will there ever be any question about their meanings because their English equivalents will be printed with them.

4. *Use of an element more than once* (see Figure 5–10d). The same element may appear in a compound symbol two or more times. It may appear each time in approximately the same position in its allocated space or in different positions in this space. The latter is illustrated in Figure 5–7d (the two arrows of *meeting* are pointing in opposite directions). The meaning of symbol elements that are used more than once in a compound symbol, such as (to) surprise, can be inferred from their meaning when used alone, the number used and their relationship to each other, and context.

5. *Varying size* (see Figure 5–10e). A given symbol may occur in more than one size, and the size in which it is drawn influences its meaning. A circle can be used to encode either sun or mouth, depending on its size. The square can encode enclosure in full size, thing in half size, and in a quarter size, is used to designate a concrete noun. The meanings of symbol elements that are smaller or larger than normal can be inferred from their meaning when a normal size, how their size differs from normal, and context.

6. *Altering configuration* (see Figure 5–10f). The configuration of a symbol may be distorted in some manner (e.g., a straight line may be curved). Thus, curving the straight-line portion of the arrow (as in Figure 5–10f) changes it meaning from down to turn. The shape of a person is visible in (to) kneel. The meanings of distorted symbol elements can be inferred from their meanings when unaltered, the nature and pictographic significance of the alteration, and context.

7. *Use of the opposite meaning symbol* (see Figure 5–10g). Placing the opposite meaning symbol before another symbol changes its meaning to the opposite of what it would be without it. Thus, placing an opposite meaning symbol before the symbol for (to) love changes its meaning to (to) hate; and the opposite meaning symbol plus much, many becomes few, little.

8. *Use of parts of symbols* (see Figure 5–10h). A part of a symbol may appear in a compound symbol. The part will have either the same meaning as the entire symbol or a related meaning. The tip of the arrow can be used as a pointer to indicate locations on other symbols. The location of the pointer determines the meaning of the symbol.

9. *Use of 11 "line letters"* (see Figure 5–10i). There are 11 types of line segments (derived from the line element) that can combined in different positions to draw the outlines of things. These segments, called *line letters*, can be used by themselves or combined with other symbol elements (e.g., the wheel element to outline a vehicle). Blissymbols formed from line letters are pictographic; their outlines indicate their meaning (see the chest of drawers in the figure).

10. *Indexing* (see Figure 5–10j). Digits can be used as subscripts with other symbols to indicate a specific subpopulation, or subset, of the objects or events referred to by them. (This strategy was adopted from general semantics; see Korzybski, 1933.) The symbol for an individual with the subscript 1 means I; with the subscript 2, you; and with the subscript 3, he or she.

Another type of indexing that is sometimes used is placing the first letter of the name of a person referred to after the symbol for man or woman.

11. *Adding lines to elements* (see Figure 5–10k). Lines can be added to symbol elements to indicate pictographically a specific subpopulation, or subset, of the objects or events referred to by them (lines used in this manner perform the same function as indexing). Thus, eye plus the symbol for cross out means blind; the symbol for air plus the forward symbol (arrow) means wind.

12. *Varying spacing between elements* (see Figure 5–10l). The amount of spacing between the elements in a compound symbol can influence its meaning. The combination of an arrow and a vertical line means approach, if there is a space between the tip of the arrow and the line, and end, if there is no space between them.

13. *Use of verb tense, mood and voice indicators* (see Figure 5–10m). The tense of a Blissymbol (functioning as a verb) can be designated by placing the appropriate tense, mood, or voice indicator above it. Verb indicators are small time action and question mark symbols (see Figure 5–6), used singly or in combination.

14. *Use of the plural indicator* (see Figure 5–10n). The placement of a small multiplication sign above a Blissymbol functioning as a noun changes it from singular to plural. Thus, placing a multiplication sign above the Blissymbol for I changes its meaning to we, and you (singular) changes its meaning to you plural.

Blissymbols vary with regard to their degree of *iconicity*—that is, the degree of visual relationship a symbol has to the unit of experience (concept) it represents (Fuller & Lloyd, 1992). Three degrees of iconicity have been identified: transparency, translucency, and opaqueness:

> *A transparent symbol is easily guessable even when its referent is not present. A translucent symbol may not be easily guessable, but a relationship between symbol and referent is generally perceived once the referent is known. An opaque symbol is not guessable, nor is the symbol-to-referent relationship understood once the referent has been revealed. (Fuller & Lloyd, 1992, p. 1376)*

Translucent and opaque graphic symbols and manual signs are not only less easily guessable than transparent ones but are also harder for users to learn (Bloomberg, Karlan, & Lloyd, 1990; Doherty, 1985b; Dunham, 1986, 1989; Fristoe & Bristow, 1982; Fried-Oken, 1987; Fuller, 1987, 1988, 1992; Fuller & Lloyd, 1987, 1988, 1991, 1992; Fuller, Lloyd, & Schlosser, 1992; Fuller & Stratton, 1991; Goossens', 1983; Granlund, Strom, & Olsson, 1989; Griffith & Robinson, 1980; Johnson, 1989; Konstantareas, Oxman, & Webster, 1978; Lloyd, 1985; Lloyd &

Blischak, 1992; Lloyd & Fuller, 1986, 1990; Lloyd & Kangas, 1988a, 1990; Luftig, 1982, 1983, 1984; Luftig & Bersani, 1985a, 1985b; Luftig & Lloyd, 1981; Luftig, Lloyd, & Page, 1982; Luftig, Page, & Lloyd, 1983; Mirenda & Locke, 1989; Mizuko, 1986, 1987a, 1987b; Mizuko & Reichle, 1988b; 1989; Musselwhite, 1987b; Musselwhite & Ruscello, 1984; Page, 1981; Sevcik, Romski, & Wilkinson, 1991; Yovetich, 1985; Yovetich & Paivio, 1980; Yovetich & Young, 1988).

For further information about Blissymbols, see Bliss (1965, 1975) and the film *Mr. Symbol Man* (Film Board of Canada); for its application, publications of the Blissymbolics Communication International, Toronto, Ontario, Canada.

Blissymbolics has been used since the early 1970s, originally as a symbol set for prereading children who were nonspeaking due to physical handicaps. It is now being used for all ages, with its use being explored for the mentally retarded, dysarthric (or both), and stroke victims (Bristow & Fristoe, 1984; Burroughs et al., 1990; Carlson, 1976; Clark, 1981; Elder, 1980; Harris-Vanderheiden, 1976; Hooper, Connell, & Flett, 1987; Hughes, 1979; Hurlbut, Iwata, & Green, 1982; Johannsen-Horbach et al., 1985; Kates & McNaughton, 1975; Kiernan & Jones, 1985; Lane & Samples, 1981; Luftig & Bersani, 1985; McDonald, 1980, 1984; McNaughton, 1976a, 1976b, 1981, 1982, 1985; McNaughton & Kates, 1974, 1980; McNaughton, Kates, & Silverman, 1975, 1976; McNaughton & Warrick, 1984; Mizuko, 1987; Morningstar, 1981; Musselwhite & Ruscello, 1984; Olson, 1976; *Ontario Crippled Children's Centre Symbol Communication Programme*, 1974; Ross, 1979; Vanderheiden, Brown, MacKenzie, Reinen, & Scheibel, 1975; Vanderheiden & Kelso, 1982; Warrick, 1982; Zangari & Lloyd, 1987). Their use with handicapped children originated at the Ontario Crippled Children's Centre. They have been used on communication boards (see Figure 5–7) and on the displays of electronic communication aids (Fairhurst & Stephanidis, 1985, 1989). They have also been used for writing children's stories and other narrative materials (e.g., Theriault, 1993).

Blissymbols by themselves may not be highly intelligible (transparent) to untrained observers. However, when used on communication boards and electronic aids, they are highly intelligible to almost all observers, because the English or other language equivalent of each Blissymbol is printed by it (usually above it). Thus, to understand Blissymbols, it is only necessary that the observer be able to read English (or other language used).

Blissymbols can be used to convey messages about the here and now as well as the past and the future. It can encode both abstract and concrete concepts. In fact, it can be used to encode such sophisticated material as poetry and the Bible.

The linguistic structure of Blissymbolics can be made comparable to that of English. The order of the Blissymbols in a sentence or utterance can correspond to that for English words. Though the morphological structure of Blissymbolics differs from that of English, morphological variations in Blissymbolics have English equivalents. There are Blissymbols for most, if not all, English words that should be in the vocabulary of a prereading child.

A substantial time and energy investment appears necessary for a child to learn to use Blissymbolics as a communication medium. However, this investment appears to be less than would be required to achieve any given level of proficiency with written English. Children seem to be able to learn to comprehend pictographic, ideographic symbol systems such as Blissymbolics more easily than phonetically based ones such as written English.

The use of Blissymbolics appears to facilitate learning to read English. Children often acquire a sight vocabulary just through frequent exposure to the English words that are printed with the Blissymbols they use.

There are several dictionarylike compilations of Blissymbols. One of the most comprehensive is in Bliss's book Semantography (1965). The Blissymbolics Communication Institute has published a compilation of Blissymbols, *Blissymbols for Use*, that have been used with handicapped children. Materials for teaching the Blissymbol system are distributed by the Blissymbolics Communication International.

Rebuses

Rebuses are predominantly pictographic symbols (e.g., line drawings) that represent whole words or parts of words (see Figure 5–11). The object or event depicted in a rebus may indicate its meaning or how all or a part of the equivalent English word "sounds"—that is, the phoneme sequence of the entire word or one or more of its syllables. The rebuses in Figure 5–11 for boot and breakfast are representative of the first type, and those for bottleneck and boxer of the second type. The part of a word represented by a drawing can be a morpheme. Thus, rebuses can have phonological, morphological, or semantic significance.

A rebus may consist of a single drawing, several drawings, or a combination of letters of the alphabet and drawings. The rebuses in Figure 5–11 for boot, bowl, and breakfast are representative of the first type; those for bookshelf, boyfriend, and breadboard of the second type; and those for boxer, brain, and breaker of the third type.

Variants of root words (morphemic variations) are indicated by adding an appropriate English suffix to a rebus (see Figure 5–12), such as those the following (from Clark, Davies, & Woodcock, 1974, pp. 8–9):

1. Adding an *s* to a rebus to indicate more than one (see Figure 5–12a)
2. Adding an *'s* to a rebus to indicate the possessive case (see Figure 5–12b)
3. Adding *s, ed,* or *ing* to a rebus for a verb to indicate its tense (see Figure 5–12c)
4. Adding *er* or *est* to a rebus to indicate a comparative form (see Figure 5–12d)
5. Adding *y* or *ly* to a rebus to denote an adjective or adverb (see Figure 5–12e)

Special rebuses are used for irregular verbs and nouns that do not form the plural by adding *s*.

Rebuses are easier to learn and remember than are spelled words (Clark, Davies, & Woodcock, 1974). Consequently, they have been used as a first symbol set for

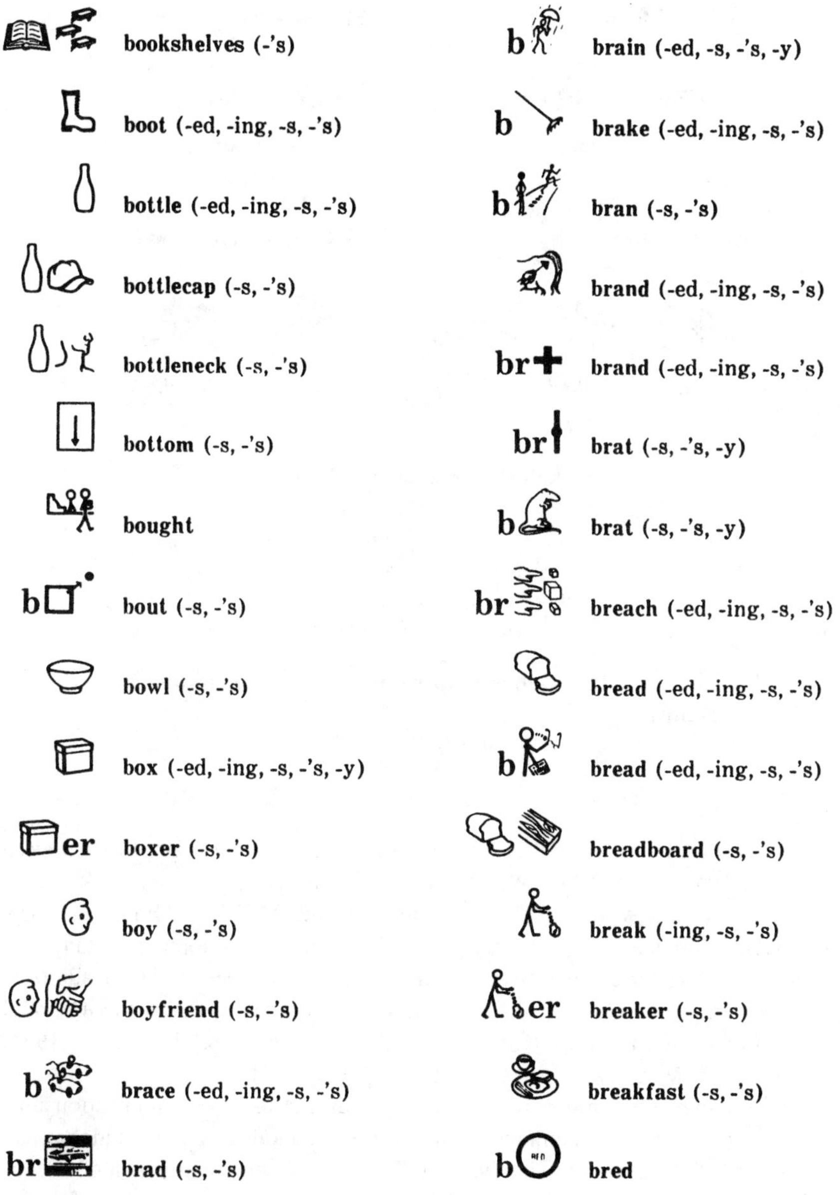

bookshelves (-'s)

boot (-ed, -ing, -s, -'s)

bottle (-ed, -ing, -s, -'s)

bottlecap (-s, -'s)

bottleneck (-s, -'s)

bottom (-s, -'s)

bought

b☐• bout (-s, -'s)

bowl (-s, -'s)

box (-ed, -ing, -s, -'s, -y)

☐er boxer (-s, -'s)

boy (-s, -'s)

boyfriend (-s, -'s)

b brace (-ed, -ing, -s, -'s)

br brad (-s, -'s)

b brain (-ed, -s, -'s, -y)

b brake (-ed, -ing, -s, -'s)

b bran (-s, -'s)

brand (-ed, -ing, -s, -'s)

br+ brand (-ed, -ing, -s, -'s)

br brat (-s, -'s, -y)

b brat (-s, -'s, -y)

br breach (-ed, -ing, -s, -'s)

bread (-ed, -ing, -s, -'s)

b bread (-ed, -ing, -s, -'s)

breadboard (-s, -'s)

break (-ing, -s, -'s)

er breaker (-s, -'s)

breakfast (-s, -'s)

b bred

FIGURE 5–11 **Representative rebuses.**
Source: Clark, Davies, & Woodcock, 1974.

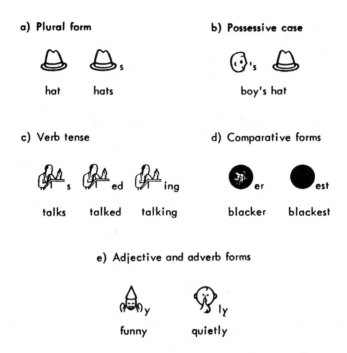

FIGURE 5–12   **Representative morphemic variations of rebuses.**
Source: Clark, Davies, & Woodcock, 1974.

teaching reading to both normal preschool children and mentally retarded children (Woodcock, 1958, 1965, 1968; Woodcock, Clark, and Davies, 1968, 1969). Also, they have been used with Ameslan vocabulary in the MELDS (Minnesota Early Language Development Sequence) program to facilitate the development of language skills in children who use Ameslan (Clark, Moores, & Woodcock, 1973). In addition, because they are easier to decode than spelled words, they have been used as a symbol set on communication boards (Clark, 1981; Clark, Davies, & Woodcock, 1974; Goossens', 1983; Musselwhite & Ruscello, 1984; Pecyna, 1988).

Rebuses can be used in several ways with gestural-assisted communication aids. They can be used alone (not combined with symbols of another system), and they can be combined with English word equivalents. The English word equivalent of a rebus could be printed above it, as is done with Blissymbols. Also, rebuses can be combined with English words that are not equivalents of the rebuses used. Rebuses would be substituted for English words that the person using the aid could not read. Presumably, the rebuses would be replaced by English word equivalents once he or she could read them.

Most rebuses should be intelligible to untrained observers even without English word equivalents printed above them. Of course, when printed above them, messages encoded in rebuses would be intelligible to any observer who could read English. Rebuses can be used to encode messages concerning the here and now as well as the past and future. Also, they can be used to encode both abstract and concrete concepts. The morphological, syntactic, and semantic structures of messages encoded in rebuses can be made to correspond to those encoded in English. Messages can, in fact, be encoded with a combination of rebuses and English words.

The time and energy investments ordinarily required to learn to decode rebuses appears to be minimal. In one study (Woodcock, 1958) the subjects (children) took only 30 to 45 minutes to learn the meanings of 72 rebuses.

A dictionarylike compilation of rebuses has been published (Clark, Davies, & Woodcock, 1974). In it are rebuses for more than 2000 alphabetically listed words, including those for almost all the objects and events one may wish to symbolize on a communication board. There are no restrictions on the right to reproduce and use the rebuses in this publication other than making appropriate acknowledgment of their source, as they are not copyrighted.

A few studies have suggested that rebuses are easier for children and adults to learn than are less pictographic symbol sets, such as Blissymbolics (Burroughs et al., 1990; Clark, 1981; Ecklund & Reichle, 1987; Hurlbut, Iwata, & Green, 1982; Musselwhite & Ruscello, 1984). However, a rebus symbol set is not as flexible—it cannot be used to encode as many messages—as can Blissymbolics (Burroughs et al., 1990). Therefore, in spite of the fact that rebuses are easier to learn than Blissymbols, Blissymbols probably would be a better choice for someone whose communication needs are relatively complex.

Yerkish Language (LANA Lexigrams)

The Yerkish lexigram language was developed by Ernst von Glaserfeld (1977) for the LANA Project (LANA is an acronym for Language Analog Project as well as being the name of a chimpanzee) of the Yerkes Regional Research Center (see Rumbaugh, 1977, for a detailed description of the project). The purpose of the project was to develop a computer-based language-training system for investigating the ability of chimpanzees to acquire language. The LANA technology, including Yerkish lexigrams (with different meanings than those for chimpanzees), has been used as a communication medium for persons who are severely or profoundly retarded and have little or no functional speech (Adamson et al., 1992; Adamson, Romski, & Sevcik, 1989; Brady & Saunders, 1991; Parkel, White, & Warner, 1977; Romski, 1989; Romski & Sevcik, 1981, 1989; Romski, Sevcik, & Joyner, 1984; Romski et al., 1985; Romski, Sevcik, & Rumbaugh, 1985; Romski et al., 1984; Romski et al., 1994; Sevcik & Romski, 1984). A portable electronic conversation board has been developed that utilizes LANA lexigrams for encoding messages (Warner, Bell, & Brown, 1977).

The Yerkish language consists of nine design elements (see Figure 5–13) that

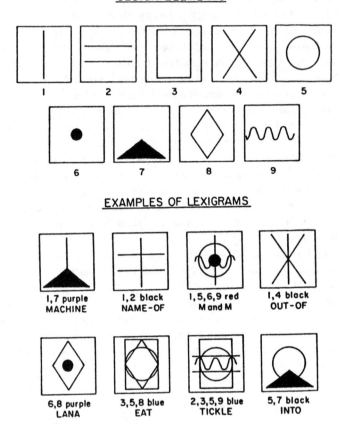

DESIGN ELEMENTS

EXAMPLES OF LEXIGRAMS

1,7 purple
MACHINE

1,2 black
NAME-OF

1,5,6,9 red
M and M

1,4 black
OUT-OF

6,8 purple
LANA

3,5,8 blue
EAT

2,3,5,9 blue
TICKLE

5,7 black
INTO

FIGURE 5–13 **Yerkish (LANA) design elements and representative lexigrams.**
Source: von Glaserfeld, 1977.

when used singly and in combinations of two, three, and four yield 255 different lexigrams (von Glaserfeld, 1977). See Figure 5–13 for representative lexigrams. The design elements used were selected because they were readily discernible from each other, could be superimposed on one another, and once superimposed, would yield combinations that were still discernible. Lexigrams are reproduced with one of seven background colors; the color-coding categorizes the lexigrams on the basis of meaning (e.g., a green background designates lexigrams that can encode a part of the body).

Each Yerkish lexigram has only one meaning, and this meaning almost always corresponds to that of an English word (the English equivalents of a few lexigrams are phrases). The meaning assigned to a Yerkish lexigram usually is not associated with its configuration in any way. Thus, Yerkish lexigrams differ from Blissymbols and rebuses in not being pictographic. They are similar to them, though, in being ideographic.

Yerkish lexigrams can be combined to form utterances. Most Yerkish utterances are between three and seven lexigrams in length. The ordering of the lexigrams in an utterance corresponds generally to that for English words. The following are English equivalents of four representative Yerkish utterances (von Glaserfeld, 1977):

Please Tim make window open.

?Tim make machine give Coke.

This piece of apple black.

Lana want apple.

For an in-depth description of Yerkish syntax, see von Glaserfeld (1977).

Because Yerkish lexigrams are conventional symbols (i.e., they have assigned meanings), they are not intelligible to untrained observers. They were designed to convey a small number of relatively concrete messages concerning the here and now. The time and energy investments required for adults to learn to decode messages in Yerkish should not be very great, but the investments required to teach it to severely and profoundly retarded children could be considerable.

When this chapter was written, insufficient data were available to assess the potential of Yerkish as a symbol set for gestural-assisted communication aids. Even though it is reasonable to inquire whether the fact that it can be mastered by a chimpanzee indicates it is within the ability range of a mentally retarded child, it is not necessarily safe to assume that the language potential of a brain-damaged child is similar to that of a neurologically intact chimpanzee (Mayberry, 1976).

Premack-Type Plastic Word Symbols

To investigate the ability of the chimpanzee to learn several aspects of human language ("reading and writing"), David Premack designed a symbol set consisting of pieces of plastic, each representing a specific word (Premack, 1971a, 1971b; Premack & Premack, 1972, 1974). The plastic symbols varied in color, shape, and size. Each was backed with metal so that it would adhere to a magnetic board. Sentences were "written" by arranging symbols vertically on the magnetic board in the proper sequence from top to bottom.

Premack's symbols are ideographic but not pictographic. Each stands for a specific word or concept, but its configuration is not related to or suggestive of the word or concept it represents. (These symbols, therefore, are conventional symbols because their meanings are assigned.) The syntactic rules for sequencing these symbols were adopted from English. (For illustrations of some of these symbols and the manner in which they are sequenced, see Premack & Premack, 1972.)

Premack taught a young chimpanzee named Sarah to "read" and "write" using the plastic symbols. Sarah developed a receptive-expressive vocabulary of more than 130 "words." She was able both to encode (write) messages using the symbols and decode (read) messages that have been encoded with them. Premack described the program used to teach her to read and write in considerable detail (Premack, 1970, 1971a, 1971b; Premack & Premack, 1972, 1974). This program can be adapted for the teaching of humans.

Adaptations of Premack's plastic language and the program developed for teaching it have been used with several populations of severely communicatively impaired persons including global aphasics (Glass, Gazzaniga, & Premack, 1973), autistic children (Premack & Premack, 1974), and mentally retarded children (Carrier, 1974a, 1974b, 1976; Carrier and Peak, 1975; Hodges & Schwethelm, 1984; Premack & Premack, 1974). In most instances they have not been taught to provide a symbol set for communication but as an introduction to the strategies involved in using symbol systems or languages. The assumption is made that learning this communication strategy will facilitate the acquisition of others, such as speech or manual sign. This assumption is reflected in the name that Carrier (1974a, 1974b, 1976) has given to his adaptation of Premack's symbol system—the Non-Speech Language Initiation Program (Non-SLIP)—and in the following statement: "Non-SLIP is not intended to be a comprehensive communication training program. Rather, it is a very carefully structured, finely graded, set of procedures for starting children through the process of learning communication skills" (Carrier & Peak, 1975, p. 10).

Because Premack-type plastic symbols have not been used much as a communication medium does not necessarily mean that they are unusable for this purpose. They have several features that tend to make them desirable for use with certain clients:

1. They can be identified either by sight or by touch; their configuration can be both seen and felt. This would tend to make them more usable with patients who have visual problems than the other symbol systems described in this section, with the exception of Braille.
2. They place minimal demands on a patient's memory. He or she does not have to remember the portion of a message that has already been encoded, because it is visible on a display.
3. It may be easier to learn and remember these symbols than strictly visual ones because they are recorded in both tactile and visual memory.

Premack-type plastic symbols can be fabricated quite easily from 1/8-inch sheet Plexiglas. The protective paper covering should not be removed from the Plexiglas until after the pieces have been cut out and their edges sanded. Some shapes that can be used for symbols are illustrated in Figure 5–14. The size of the symbols depends on several factors, including the potential user's ability to grasp and his or her visual functioning. A height of 3 inches would be sufficient for most persons. The symbols

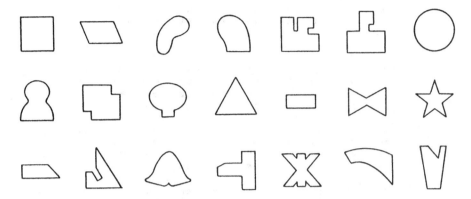

FIGURE 5–14   **Representative Premack-type word symbols.**

can be the same color or can be color-coded based on grammatical function (e.g., red for symbols functioning as nouns and blue for verbs). The English word equivalent of each should be printed on it. The symbols can be backed with small magnets so that they can be displayed on a magnetic board, or they can be displayed (without being backed) horizontally on a tabletop or vertically on a board with a ledge at the bottom (like a blackboard).

Premack-type plastic symbols would be intelligible to untrained observers only if English word equivalents were printed on them. They could be used to encode messages about the here and now as well as the past and the future if appropriate verb tense indicators were available. And they could be used to encode both abstract and concrete concepts. (Of course, the physical size of the symbols imposes a limit on the maximum number a person can use and, hence, the maximum number of messages that can be encoded with any set of such symbols.)

The time and energy investments required for learning to use Premack-type symbols are a function of several variables, including the user's level of conceptual functioning and the complexity of the program being taught. If the English equivalents of the symbols are printed on them, no training should be necessary to learn to interpret them (unless the person to whom messages are being sent cannot read English).

Braille

Occasionally a patient is encountered who lacks adequate speech for communicative purposes and whose vision is inadequate for use of the symbol sets described in this section (with the possible exception of Premack-type plastic symbols). The patient may be completely blind or have a visual field problem, a visual acuity problem, or a visual agnosia. The visual problem may have antedated the condition responsible for the communicative disorder, or it may have resulted from this condition or one that

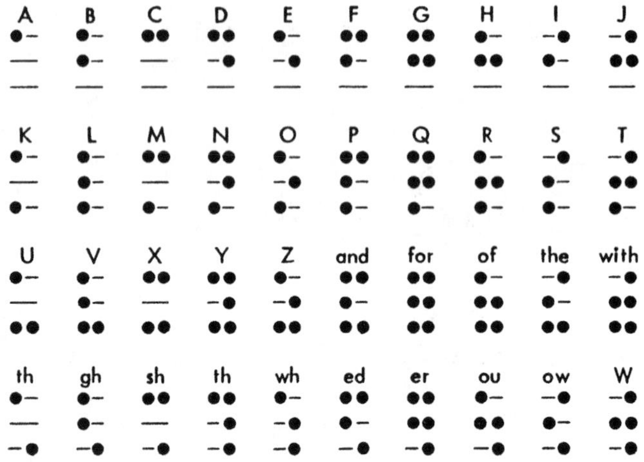

A	B	C	D	E	F	G	H	I	J

K	L	M	N	O	P	Q	R	S	T

U	V	X	Y	Z	and	for	of	the	with

th	gh	sh	th	wh	ed	er	ou	ow	W

FIGURE 5–15 **The Braille character set.**
Source: Courtesy of the *Encyclopaedia Britannica*.

followed it. Such a patient would probably find a tactile symbol set more advantageous than a visual one. Braille is the most widely used and flexible tactile symbol set.

The Braille Symbol Set, which was invented by Louis Braille in 1824, consists of 63 characters, each made up of a one to six raised-dot pattern in a six-position (i.e., cell) matrix (see Figure 5–15). These characters encode letters of the alphabet, digits, punctuation marks, and frequently used words (e.g., "and") and letter combinations (e.g., "ed"). They are embossed in lines on paper and are read by passing the fingers lightly over them. Their structure is as follows:

> To aid in identifying the 63 dot patterns, or characters, that are possible within the six-dot cell, Braille numbered the dot positions 1-2-3 downward on the left and 4-5-6 downward on the right. The illustration [see Figure 5–15] shows the formation of each cell and its simplest designated meaning. The first ten letters of the alphabet are formed with dots 1, 2, 4, and 5. When preceded by the numeric indicator, these signs have number values. The letters k through t are formed by adding dot 3 to the signs in line 1. Five of the remaining letters of the alphabet and five very common words are formed by adding dots 3 and 6 to the signs in line 1. When dot 6 is added to the first ten letters, the letter w and nine common letter combinations are formed (see line 4). Punctuation marks and two additional common letter combinations are made by placing the signs in line 1 in dot positions 2, 3, 5, and 6. Three final letter combinations, the numeric indicator, and two more punctuation marks are formed with dots 3, 4, 5, and 6. (Encyclopaedia Britannica, *15th ed., Volume 3, 1974, p. 110*)

Braille can be embossed ("written") on a sheet of paper by hand with a device called a slate or with a typewriterlike machine. A microcomputer with an embossing printer also can be used.

Because Braille is a system for writing English, the linguistic structure of messages encoded in Braille is that of English. Any message that can be encoded in English can be encoded in Braille.

Braille is not intelligible to untrained observers. However, if the English equivalents of Braille characters are printed above them, messages encoded in Braille can be decoded by anyone able to read English. A communication board could be constructed on which each message component appears in both Braille and printed English. The user would locate message components by scanning the board with his fingers. When he located a component he wanted to transmit, he would point to it. The person to whom he was transmitting the message would note the English letter, letter combination, digit, word, or punctuation mark printed above it. The user would then locate the next message component, and the process would continue until the entire message had been transmitted.

The time and energy investments necessary to learn to decode Braille well enough to identify a finite number of message components encoded in it on a communication board should not be too great. Learning it well enough to be able to read and write it fluently would, of course, take a great deal of training.

Machine-Generated Speech

Machine-generated (recorded or synthesized) spoken English has been used with electronic gestural-assisted communication aids for encoding messages (e.g., Bedrosian & Hoag, 1992; Bruno, 1989; Carlson et al., 1981; Dabbagh & Damper, 1985; Ehrlich, 1974; Evans et al., 1985; Graff & Wotus, 1985; Jackson, Stirling, & Dixon, 1983; Karjalainen, Laine, & Rahko, 1980; Keating et al., 1989; Microprocessor-based voice synthesizer . . . , 1977; Murray, Bedrosian, & Higginbotham, 1992a, 1992b; Nielson, 1983; Quist & Blischak, 1992; Rahimi & Eylenberg, 1973; Record-player . . . , 1977; Rentschler, 1985; Reuter, 1974; Sevcik & Romski, 1985; Trefler & Crislip, 1985). Communication aids that generate speech are known as VOCAs (Voice Output Communication Aids). Some of these aids contain speech synthesizers that generate messages by stringing together phonemes. Others generate messages from recorded, prestored words and phrases (and possibly letters, prefixes, and suffixes). The speech elements are sequenced to create utterances that structurally are equivalent to those of spoken English. Some aids can generate only a male voice and others can generate either a male or female voice (Crabtree, Mirenda, & Beukelman, 1989, 1990). While the intelligibility of speech generated by VOCAs is poorer than of natural speech (Mitchell & Atkins, 1988), the intelligibility of that generated by some VOCAs is significantly better than that generated by others (Kannenberg, Marquardt, & Larson, 1988; Mirenda & Beukelman, 1990).

When messages are generated from prestored information, the user must be taught a strategy for retrieving them. The one used most frequently is *Minspeak*, an acronym for minimum effort speech (Baker, 1982, 1983, 1985, 1986; Bruno, 1988, 1989; Bruno & Baker, 1986; Dobres, White, & Haight, 1991; Ferrier, 1991; Frumkin & Foley, 1987; Musson, 1987; Rothchild & Collier, 1986; Stump, 1986; White & Dobres, 1992; White et al., 1990). It is a semantic compaction technique. The user accesses prestored information by generating icon (symbol) sequences. Almost any type of symbol—words, Blissymbols, line drawings—can be used as an icon. The symbol sequences have a semantic and/or syntactic relationship to the prestored information. They are a code that enables the user to generate grammatically correct speech with minimum effort. The following symbol sequences and sentences (from Bruno, 1989) illustrate the process:

Symbol Sequence	*Sentence Spoken*
you + joke	You're funny.
I + eat	I'm hungry. What can I eat?
question + you	How are you?
I + sick	I don't feel good.

The symbols or icons are ideographic; they represent concepts rather than words. The process of defining icons and icon sequences is under the control of the user. This system can be used with children as young as 4 years (Bruno, 1989; Bruno & Goehl, 1991). This form of semantic compaction has also been used with gestural systems (Frumkin, 1986).

Machine-generated speech can enable severely communicatively impaired persons to communicate by telephone without a telecommunication relay service (Silverman, 1993c). They can even do it with an inexpensive audiocassette tape recorder so long as the device has a counter and the user does not have a neuromuscular disorder affecting his or her upper extremities. Messages are recorded by the clinician at specific locations on the tape. The user utilizes the counter to locate the one that he or she wants to "say." It is, of course, impractical to generate a large number of messages in this way. One vocabulary set designed specifically for use with such a device (Record-player "voice". . . , 1977) contains the following words: yes, no, OK, hello, goodbye, maybe, correct, wrong, right, true, untrue, definitely, fine, too bad, why, when, what, how, where, who, good, and bad. It also contains the following phrases: please repeat; how are you; I'm fine, thanks; my name is _____; my address is _____; I feel ill; please come as soon as possible; and I am using a device to speak because I have a voice problem.

Morse Code

The international Morse code (see Table 4–3) has been used as a symbol system for generating messages with microprocessor-based gestural-assisted communication aids. Messages are encoded in Morse code but are translated into and displayed in another symbol system, usually printed English. There are microcomputer-based gestural-assisted communication aids, for example, that will translate messages encoded in Morse code (by activation of a switching mechanism) and display them on a monitor screen, cause them to be "spoken" by a speech synthesizer, and/or printed by a computer printer. Hardware and software components of such systems are described later in this chapter.

When to Use Each Symbol Set

Eleven symbol sets are described in this section. When might it be advantageous to use each of them? The recommendations made here are intended to provide a tentative, partial answer to this question. The answer is tentative because data from clinical research may require some of the recommendations to be modified; it is partial because all possible applications of these symbol systems obviously are not mentioned and the uses indicated are not necessarily applicable to all persons in the populations specified. The names of symbol sets are italicized to facilitate locating comments about particular ones.

1. The most flexible and efficient symbol system for gestural-assisted communication aids is printed *English* or another natural language. It can transmit any message that the user can spell and those with whom he or she is communicating can read.

2. The most concrete symbol set other than one consisting of *objects* and probably the easiest to learn to use would consist of *photographs, drawings,* or a combination of the two. These can be used and understood by almost anyone who is sufficiently intact visually to identify the objects and events depicted. This type of symbol set is particularly useful for communicating basic needs in hospitals and nursing home settings and as an initial symbol set for children's communication boards. One source of line drawings for such applications is *Picsyms.*

3. *Blissymbolics* is the most flexible symbol set for persons who are unable to read or spell *English* words well enough to encode the messages they wish to transmit. It can encode almost any message that can be encoded in English, and it is easier for most persons to learn to "read" than English. Also, it tends to facilitate learning to read English because the English equivalent of each *Blissymbol* is printed with it.

4. *Photographs* and *drawings* (or *Picsyms* or *Pic symbols*), *Blissymbols,* and printed *English* can be used sequentially. A person could begin with photographs, drawings, or a combination of these. Blissymbols could be gradually introduced and used along with photographs and drawings. Blissymbols, in turn, could be replaced by English words as the person's ability to read improved.

5. *Rebuses* can supplement symbol sets consisting of *photographs* and *drawings* (or *Picsyms*) or *English* words. They can be particularly useful with adults who have normal or nearly normal ability to understand spoken *English* and are dyslexic. Rebuses can be useful by helping persons to remember the auditory symbol (spoken word) for the concepts or ideas that they are used to encode.

6. *Premack-type plastic symbols* or *Braille* can be used with persons who lack adequate vision to identify and discriminate between symbols visually. The latter, of course, can encode more messages than can the former.

7. *Machine-generated speech* can be used with almost any severely communicatively impaired person to facilitate telephone communication. It also can be used to enhance face-to-face communication, particularly with young children and others who cannot read.

8. The *Non-SLIP* adaptation of the *Premack symbol system* can be used to introduce children (particularly severely or profoundly mentally retarded children) to the nature of symbols and the strategies involved in using them. A program combining *Lana lexigrams* with a computer system also can be used for this purpose.

9. *Morse code* can be used by quadriplegics to generate message components with microcomputer-based communication aids.

10. *SPEEC* can be used with severely communicatively impaired persons who cannot spell well enough to use an *English*-language symbol set but are able to identify the phonemes in words. This would permit such persons to encode any message that could be encoded in English.

11. *Sigsymbols* may be useful in facilities where there are persons who sign using *Ameslan,* as well as persons who use a communication board with pictographic symbols because many Sigsymbols graphically depict Ameslan signs.

NONELECTRONIC GESTURAL-ASSISTED COMMUNICATION STRATEGIES

There are three types of nonelectronic gestural-assisted communication strategies:

1. Strategies in which the symbols are reproduced on a display known as a communication board (or conversation board) and in which messages are transmitted by the user, who indicates in the appropriate sequence the symbols on the board that encode them
2. Strategies in which the symbols are manipulable, and messages are transmitted by the user, who arranges the symbols that encode them in the appropriate sequence on a magnetic board, tabletop, or other surface
3. Strategies in which the symbols are drawn or written, and messages are transmitted by the user, who writes or draws the symbols that encode them in the appropriate sequence on a piece of paper or other material

Representative strategies of these three types are described in the following sections.

Communication (Conversation) Boards

Communication, or *conversation*, *boards* consist of one or more sheets of some type of material—paper, cardboard, cloth, plastic, Masonite, plywood—on which the elements of a symbol set are reproduced. The symbol elements may be reproduced on a single sheet of material or on several sheets (e.g., in booklet form). Each sheet may contain a single symbol element (see Figure 5–16) or a number of symbol elements (see Figures 5–6, 5–7, and 5–8). The symbol elements may be reproduced directly on the board or on pieces of material (usually paper or cardboard) that are attached to it. The symbol sets described in the first section of this chapter, except for Premack-type plastic symbols and Morse code, can be used on communication boards.

Aside from the symbol set to be used, a number of factors must be considered when designing a communication board for a client:

Construction Material
Communication boards can be fabricated from various materials. That chosen for a particular client would be determined by several factors:

1. The size of the board: The larger the board, the sturdier the material needed.
2. The length of time the board is to be used: The longer a board is to be used, the more durable the material needed.
3. How portable the board has to be: The more portability needed, the lighter the weight of the construction material.
4. How the board is to be mounted: A board that is to be used horizontally on a surface, such as a wheelchair tray, ordinarily does not have to be made of as sturdy a material as one that will not rest on a surface when being used.

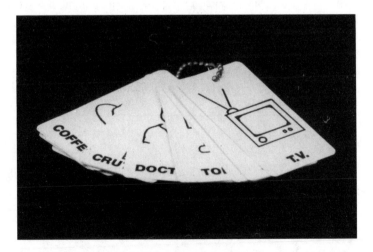

FIGURE 5–16 **A portable communication board consisting of cards held together by a keychain.**
Source: Courtesy of Ideas, Tempe, Arizona.

5. How easy to clean the board has to be: If a patient is likely to drool on or otherwise soil the board, it has to have an easily washable surface, such as that afforded by clear plastic contact paper.

6. Whether the board has to be transparent: This is sometimes necessary if an eyepointing response mode is to be used, as with the ETRAN and ETRAN-N boards (see Figures 5–17 and 5–18). A temporary transparent communication board, incidentally, can be fabricated by stretching a freezer bag over a bent wire coat hanger (King, 1990).

Size

Rectangular sheets of material used for fabricating communication boards can range in size from a few inches on the longest side (e.g., see Figure 5–16) to more than 18 inches on the longest side (e.g., see Figure 5–8). The optimum size for a particular client would be determined by several factors:

1. The number of symbol elements in the set being used: The greater the number, the larger the board would have to be.

2. The sizes of the symbol elements in the set being used: The larger they are, the larger the board would have to be.

3. The method to be used for indicating symbol elements: If symbol elements were to be indicated by a directed gaze, that is, eyepointing, rather than by pointing with a finger, there would have to be greater separation between elements and, hence, a larger board would be needed for a given number of elements.

4. How the board is to be mounted: If a communication board is to be used as a tray on a wheelchair, this places some restrictions on its minimum and maximum size.

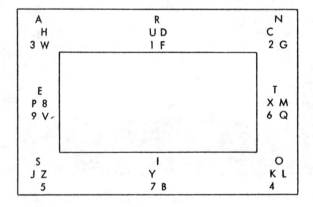

FIGURE 5–17 **ETRAN communication device.**
Source: Jack Eichler. Drawing courtesy of Trace Center, Madison, Wisconsin.

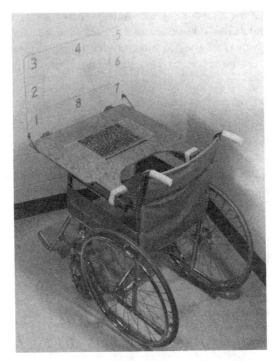

FIGURE 5–18   **ETRAN-N communication device attached to a wheelchair.**
Source: Courtesy of Trace Center, Madison, Wisconsin.

5. The degree of portability desired: If a communication board has to be portable, obviously it cannot be too large.
6. The maximum number of sheets of material that can be used: The greater this number, the smaller each can be.

Method of Reproducing Symbol Elements on the Board
Symbol elements can be reproduced on the board itself or on pieces of a material (usually paper or card stock) that can be attached to it. The latter frequently is done when symbol elements are introduced a few at a time or when the symbol elements on the board are to be updated periodically to meet the user's changing communication abilities and needs. (When this type of board is designed to be attached to a wheelchair as a laptray, the pieces of paper or card stock on which the symbols are reproduced can be sandwiched between the plywood base of the tray and the transparent Plexiglas sheet that covers it.)

Symbol elements can be printed and drawn with felt-tipped markers or lettering pens. Black ink can be used for all, or different color inks can be used to indicate a category to which each belongs (e.g., red for nouns and blue for verbs). If a symbol set includes letters of the alphabet (singly or in combination), they can be reproduced with a microcomputer. Rub-on or stick-on letters can also be used.

Photographs can be attached to a board with rubber cement. Braille message components can be embossed on pieces of paper and attached to a board in this same manner.

Mounting the Board

To be useful, a communication board must be positioned so that message components that are indicated by the user are visible to the person (or persons) with whom he or she is communicating. It is necessary that the full board be both visible to the user and compatible with his or her motoric ability to indicate message components on it. For many persons, and for most types of boards, a horizontal placement, such as a tabletop or laptray, is satisfactory. About the only type of board for which such a placement would never be satisfactory is a transparent plastic one, such as the ETRAN (Figure 5–17), ETRAN-N (Figure 5–18), and LC-ETRAN (Figure 5–19), on which message components are indicated by eyepointing (this type of board usually is mounted vertically).

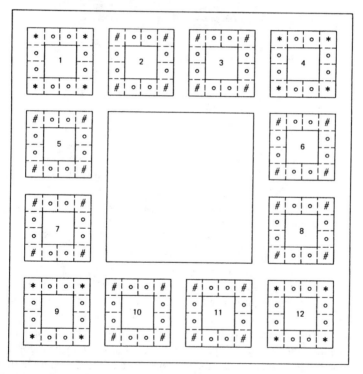

FIGURE 5–19 **The LC-ETRAN chart for encoding up to 144 message components on the basis of location and color.**
Source: van Tatenhove, 1986.

If a board cannot be used when positioned horizontally, some type of stand (or support mechanism) will be needed to position it at an angle at which it can be used. One type of device that may be usable is an overbed table. The angle of the table surface is adjustable on some of them. A communication board could be attached temporarily or permanently to the tabletop. If permanently attached, it could be sandwiched between the tabletop and a sheet of transparent Plexiglas the same size and shape. The communication board would then be available whenever the table was in place.

A camera tripod tilthead attached (by a bolt with a 1/4-20 thread) to some sort of supporting mechanism (e.g., a wheelchair frame) also could be used to position a communication board at a desired angle. A piece of plywood that was slightly larger than the communication board could be attached to the tilthead (by a piece of metal drilled and tapped with a 1/4-20 thread attached to the center of the plywood), and the communication board could be mounted on the plywood.

Board Surface (Covering)

The surface of a communication board may be covered to protect it. The two materials used most frequently for this purpose are transparent plastic contact paper and transparent Plexiglas. The first, of course, would only be usable on communication boards that were not designed to be modified. The second would be usable also on those that were not so designed. When used on a board designed to be modified, the plexiglas sheet could be hinged to the board by means of a wide piece of tape (such as furnace duct tape) on one edge; the Plexiglas sheet then could be raised whenever it was necessary to modify the symbol set on the board.

For further information on constructing and using communication boards, see Anderson (1980); Angelo & Goldstein, 1990; Feallock (1958); Fishman, Timler, & Yoder (1985); Glennen & Calculator, (1985); Goldberg & Fenton (n.d.); Gordon et al., (1985); Haight, 1992; Johnson, 1988; Mayer-Johnson, 1989; McDonald & Schultz (1973); McEwen & Karlan, 1988, 1989; Mizuko & Hahnstadt, 1992b; Poock & Blackstone (1992); Sayre (1963); Silverman, 1987c; Vanderheiden (1977); Vanderheiden & Grilley (1976); Vicker (1974); White & Chambers (1985); and Wu & Voda (1985).

Strategies for Indicating Message Components

Three types of strategies can be used to indicate message components on a communication board: scanning, encoding, and direct selection. These are also used with electronic gestural-assisted communication aids for the same purpose.

Scanning. The simplest of the three is *scanning*, as it demands less from the user motorically than the other two. Scanning strategies include "any technique (or aid) in which the selections are offered to the user by a person or display, and where the user selects the characters by responding to the person or display. Depending upon the aid, the user may respond by simply signalling when he sees the correct choice presented" (Vanderheiden & Grilley, 1976, p. 21).

A communication board that would be usable with a scanning response mode is illustrated in Figure 5–20. Its format is that of a rectangular, row-column matrix. Each of the 42 cells contains a message component—a letter of the alphabet, a digit, a mark of punctuation, or one or two words. (Of course, any of the other types of graphic symbol elements that were described in the first section of this chapter or a different size row-column matrix could have been used instead.) The scanning would be done by a person with whom the user wished to communicate. The person would point to a segment of the board consisting of one or more cells and would ask the user whether it contains the message component he or she wishes to transmit. If the answer was yes and the segment contained more than one cell, the person would point, in turn, to each of the cells in the segment and would ask whether it contained the message component. This process would continue until there was a yes response. The message segment in the cell for which there was a yes response would be noted; and if the message consisted of more than one message segment, the process outlined would be repeated. The board would be scanned once for each symbol element in the message. Thus, the number of scans for a message would be equal to the number of cells whose contents are needed to encode it.

The simplest type of scanning strategy would be to point to the individual cells in a matrix one after the other and ask for each whether it contains the message component the person wishes to transmit, continuing until he or she gives a yes response. Although any message can be transmitted by using this strategy, it is relatively time-

	1	2	3	4	5	6	7
1	NEW WORD	A	E	I	O	U	NO
2	YES	.	?	B	C	D	F
3	G	H	J	K	L	M	N
4	P	Q	R	S	T	V	W
5	X	Y	Z	1	2	3	4
6	5	6	7	8	9	0	END

FIGURE 5–20 **Representative alphabet communication board for scanning or encoding.**

consuming. A slightly more complex type of scanning strategy, two-step scanning, tends to be more efficient. With this strategy the board is divided into segments, each containing a number of cells (usually the same number of cells). A segment, for example, may be a row of cells. The person being communicated to would point to each of the segments (e.g., rows) one after the other and ask for each if it is in this segment. When the person doing the communicating gives a yes response, the person being communicated to points to the cells in that segment one after the other and asks for each, "Is it in this cell?" This process continues until a second yes response is received. This two-step process is repeated for each symbol element in (or segment of) a message.

For a person to use a communication board with a scanning response strategy, it is only necessary motorically that he or she be able to signal yes and no. There are a number of ways in which these can be signaled (see chapter 4). He or she also must be sufficiently intact visually, to identify the message components on the board; *conceptually*, to understand their meanings; and *auditorily* (or visually if the person can speechread and/or comprehend gestures), to understand the questions asked.

Although almost anyone can use a communication board with a scanning response strategy—even children as young as 4 years (Mizuko & Esser, 1991)—it is relatively slow. It can require for most symbol elements in a message a yes-no response for almost every cell on the communication board used. The other two response modes, encoding and direct selection, allow messages to be transmitted at a faster rate (the latter more so than the former).

The linear, row-column, and directed scanning strategies described earlier also can be used for interfacing clients with some dedicated electronic augmentative communication aids and microcomputers that have been programmed to function like them. Light or cursor movements are used instead of hand movements for indicating message components, and switch activations are used instead of yes-no responses for specifying those needed to communicate a message. Word prediction may be combined with scanning to reduce the number of switch activations needed to communicate a message (Horstmann & Levine, 1990). With one such strategy (Heckathorne, Voda, & Leibowitz, 1987; Horstmann & Levine, 1990) that can be used with a microcomputer-based system, after the first two letters of a word are selected, a list of the seven most likely ones are displayed and the appropriate one can be selected by scanning (assuming that it is one of the ones displayed). Only three scannings would be needed to communicate at least some of the multisyllabic words in a message, which should both speed up communication and be less fatiguing to the user.

Encoding. An *encoding* response strategy consists of "a technique . . . in which the desired choice is indicated by a pattern or code of input signals, where the pattern or code must be memorized or referred to on a chart" (Vanderheiden, 1976, p. 22). The simplest type of encoding scheme would consist of a large chart on which is printed a

a) Scanning or direct-selection communication board

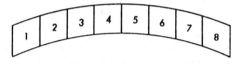

b) Direct-selection communication board

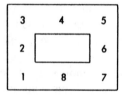

c) Eyepointing chart (ETRAN-N)

d) Electronic rotary pointer scanning device

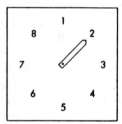

FIGURE 5–21   **Representative devices for encoding message components using two digits.**

series of messages a person might want to transmit (e.g., "I am hungry") that are numbered consecutively and a communication board of the type illustrated in Figure 5–20, with each cell containing one of the numbers that appears on the chart (the number of cells being equal to the number of messages on the chart).

A one-step or two-step scanning strategy could be used with the communication board to signal the number of messages on the chart the person wished to transmit. With this strategy only a single scan of a communication board is necessary to transmit a message. Of course, it has the limitation that only a relatively small number of predetermined messages could be transmitted using it. This limitation could be partly overcome by including a message on the chart similar to the following: "The message I want to communicate is not on the chart. Please use my other communication board." A communication board of the type illustrated in Figure 5–20 could be used with a one-step or two-step scanning response strategy to transmit the message. This type of system could be particularly useful for communication of basic needs in a hospital or nursing home.

A slightly more complex encoding strategy will transmit the message component in any cell on a communication board similar in format to that depicted in Figure 5–20 by means of two digits. The first digit would indicate the row number of the cell containing the component and the second the number of the column in which it appears. If there are 64 or fewer cells on the communication board (a maximum of eight rows and eight columns), the encoding device only has to display the digits from 1 to 8. Four devices that could be used to transmit a row-column, two-digit code are illustrated in Figure 5–21. The first (see Figure 5.21a), which is a two-row communication board, can be used with a one- or two-stage scanning response mode or a direct-selection response mode (i.e., the user points to the digits in some manner). The second (see Figure 5–21b), which is a single-row communication board, can be used with either a scanning or direct-selection response mode. It is particularly advantageous for the person who is able to move his hand laterally but not forward and backward well enough to indicate reliably (point to) message components arranged in rows. The third (see Figures 5–18 and 5–21c) is a transparent Plexiglas communication board known as the ETRAN-N (Vanderheiden, 1976), intended for use with an eyepointing response mode. The fourth (see Figure 5–21d) is an electronic rotary pointer scanning device that can be stopped at any digit by a switching mechanism activated by the user. These, of course, are not the only types of devices that could be used to transmit a two-digit code.

These two encoding strategies are indirect in the sense that they indicate messages (or message components) to be transmitted on a chart rather than transmitting them directly. There is a type of encoding strategy that will transmit a message directly. It is used with the ETRAN Eye Signaling System (see Figure 5–17) for spelling out messages, developed by Jack Eichler. The following description of the ETRAN system is taken from Eichler (1973):

General Arrangement

The sender and receiver sit facing each other four or five feet apart as in normal conversation. The chart stands upright midway between the two people permitting them to view each other through the large aperture at its center. The elevation of the chart should be adjusted so that the eyes of the sender appear to be at the center of the aperture as viewed by the receiver.... The chart faces the receiver. The sender reads backward through it.

Method

The sender spells out words, one letter at a time by glancing at one of the eight distinct areas on the chart. It is easy for the receiver to see which area has been selected by watching the sender's eyes. Some letters require a redirection of the sender's eyes from the selected area to one of the four corners of the chart. [This is explained in the paragraph below, on code.]

The sender's and receiver's eyes meet after each letter. The receiver should speak the letter while still watching the sender's eyes. This will permit any confirmation or correction that may be necessary. The receiver should then write the letter on his message paper and return his gaze to the sender which indicates he is ready for the next letter. Speed of transmission usually improves up to a letter per second as a receiver gains experience.

The Code

Each of the eight distinct areas on the chart has one letter elevated above the remainder of the group. Taken all together, the elevated letters are the eight most frequently used letters in the English language. They have been incorporated into the code in such a way as to require only one glance by the sender. He directs his eyes to one of the chart areas and shifts immediately back to the receiver in order to specify the elevated letter in that area.

The selection of all letters and digits other than the elevated ones requires the sender to move his eyes to one of the four corners of the chart after selecting an area group and before returning his gaze to the observer. A glance at the upper right hand *corner of the chart indicates the* upper right hand *symbol has been selected, and so on, matching the corner of the chart to the position of the symbol among the three or four symbols in the original area selected. The fact there has been a second glance rules out the elevated letter in the original area.*

The Sender

A patient starting out with the chart will be unfamiliar with the locations of the letters and will send false signals as he searches for the desired letter. If a patient wants to memorize the chart first, this can be done. However, the best way for him to become familiar with the chart is to begin using it. He will quickly learn all symbol locations, and the chart, from his standpoint, will become merely something on which to focus his eyes as he indicates the letters for the receiver.

The Receiver

Any adult, or child, who can read, will "catch on" to the eye signaling system in three or four minutes of total instruction and practice. Inexperi-

enced observers should always write the message as it is being transmitted and should always use the chart as described above. Members of the patient's family and any attendants who use the system daily will develop their own shortcuts and will probably communicate without the chart at times. As in copying any code, receivers must not be too quick in chopping off a multi-syllable word merely because its first letters constitute a word. Request confirmation from the sender in such cases or request he punctuate words as well as sentences.

Punctuation

The dot in the chart's lower, center group represents all punctuation marks. If the receiver's imagination does not meet the degree of exactness needed in certain messages, he and the sender should assign numbers to any special symbols required.

A user and receiver who are thoroughly familiar with the chart can dispense with it; the receiver can "read" the user's eye movements (Handicapped youth "talks" . . . , 1974).

The encoding strategies used to indicate message components on the ETRAN-N (Figure 5–18) and LC-ETRAN (Figure 5–19) charts, particularly the latter, are similar to those just outlined for the ETRAN chart. It is possible to use mirrors/prisms with these charts to compensate for some eye movement defects (see ten Kate & Hepp, 1989).

Direct Selection. *Direct selection,* the most efficient of the three strategies used to encode message components on a communication board, includes "any technique in which the desired choice is directly indicated by the user" (Vanderheiden & Grilley, 1976, p. 26). The user indicates the components of a message by pointing to them in the appropriate sequence. Because each gestural response indicates a message component, this strategy requires fewer movements to transmit a message than do encoding or scanning. Thus, it transmits messages faster and with less fatigue than either of the others.

A number of different gestures (or patterned movements) of the musculature of the extremities, head and neck, and face can be used to indicate message components. The three most frequently used types are hand (or finger) gestures; eye gestures, or directed gaze (Goossens & Crain, 1987); and head gestures used in conjunction with a headpointer or headstick (Jewell, 1989). The first is pointing with a finger or another part of the hand. This is the type used most often. The hand used does not have to be completely normal neuromuscularly. A person who lacks adequate finger control for pointing may be able to do so with his knuckle or another part of his hand.

A person who is unable to point with a part of his hand may be able to do so by directing his gaze, or eyepointing. Even severe quadriplegics may have sufficient control of the musculature of their eyes to indicate message components in this man-

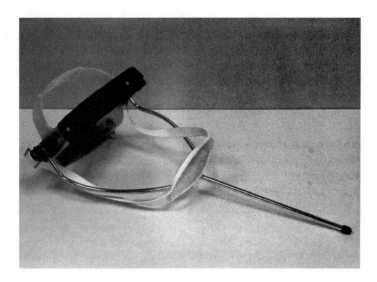

FIGURE 5–22   **A headstick.**

ner. An eyepointing response mode can be used with a transparent, vertically mounted board such as the ETRAN or ETRAN-N (see Figures 5–18 and 5–19) or with a standard communication board. For it to be usable with the latter, the message components on the board have to be fairly widely separated from each other.

Another strategy that can be used by someone unable to point with his hand is to point with a headstick (see Figures 5–22 and 5–23). Many quadriplegics have sufficient head control to use such a device. An occupational therapist who has worked with persons who have neuromuscular disorders should be able to fabricate one and teach the client how to use it (Jewell, 1989).

Preparing Instructions
Another consideration when fabricating a communication board is preparing instructions for its use. These instructions should be attached to the board, as persons who need to communicate with the patient may not know how to use the board. If the instructions are only a few sentences long, they usually can be attached to the front of the communication board. Otherwise, they can be attached to the back of it (with a note on the front indicating so).

What kinds of information should be included in these instructions? The answer to this question would partly depend on the type of response strategy the person used. A direct-selection response strategy, for example, ordinarily would require fewer instructions than would a scanning or encoding strategy. The following set of instructions, prepared for use with the board illustrated in Figure 5–21 with a scanning response strategy, is representative:

This letter-number board is used by _____ to communicate. He or she spells out the words in the message. Because _____ is unable to point to the letters and numbers on the board, the person with whom he (she) is communicating must do it for him (her). To communicate with _____, you should point to the squares in the order diagrammed on the next page:

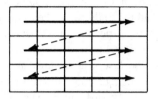

As you point to each square ask "THIS ONE?" and wait for a yes or no signal. _____ signals yes and no as follows:

_____

_____

_____ As he or she signals letters and numbers, print them with the attached pencil across the top of the board. _____ will indicate he (she) is finished by signaling the square in the lower right hand corner marked END.

FIGURE 5–23   **A headstick being used to indicate message components on a communication board.**
Source: McDonald, 1976.

The board for which these instructions were prepared was mounted with a blank space 3 inches high at the top, covered by transparent plastic contact paper. The message components signaled were printed in this space with a grease pencil.

With Whom Can Boards Be Used?

Communication boards have been used with all populations of severely communicatively impaired children and adults. Judging by the frequency of their use, they would appear to be relatively acceptable to persons in at least a segment of these populations. The speed at which messages can be transmitted with a communication board is determined in large part by the response strategy and symbol set used. The only neuromuscular requirement for using a communication board is being able somehow to signal yes or no. (Of course, a board can be used more efficiently if the user is sufficiently intact neuromuscularly to point to message components.)

Ordinarily it should take only a few minutes to teach the mechanics of using a communication board, so long as a method of indicating is selected that will not overtax the user's neuromuscular, sensory, and cognitive abilities. However, if he or she has to be taught to signal yes or no or to understand the symbol system used on the board, the time and energy investments required could be considerable; those necessary to teach a person to interpret messages transmitted by a communication board ordinarily would be nominal.

Are Boards Less Efficient Than Electronic Communication Devices?

Judging by the relatively large number of papers published in the AAC literature during the past 10 years dealing with the use of microcomputer-based and dedicated electronic communication devices for face-to-face communication and the relatively small number dealing with communication boards (see References section), it would seem reasonable to assume that the former make possible more efficient communication than do the latter. This is not necessarily the case, however. Haight (1992), for example, reported finding no greater efficiency during face-to-face communication when a client who had cerebral palsy communicated with a Light Talker (a dedicated electronic communication aid) than when she did so with a communication board.

Manipulable Symbols

A second type of nonelectronic gestural-assisted communication aid consists of sets of *manipulable symbols* that can be arranged by the user on a magnetic board, tabletop, or other surface in appropriate sequences for encoding and transmitting messages. Premack-type plastic symbols, such as Non-SLIP, are of this type. Any of the symbol sets described in the first section of this chapter (with the exception of Morse code and synthesized speech) also could be used with such aids by having the symbol elements or message components reproduced on individual pieces of a material such as cardboard, cloth, wood, Masonite, or Plexiglas.

The main advantage of this type of aid over that afforded by a communication board is that it makes fewer demands on a user's memory. He does not have to remember the part of a message he has already encoded, because he can see it. However, these aids do have several limitations when compared to those utilizing communication boards. First, they require better hand function. It is easier motorically to point to a message component than to pick up a small piece of material on which it is reproduced and place it in the appropriate location on a display. And second, the number of manipulable symbols that it would be practical for a person to have within reach probably could not exceed 75. If a larger set were used, it would be difficult to arrange them so that the user could easily locate and reach for the ones he or she needed. A communication board, on the other hand, can have as many as 400 symbols reproduced on it.

Manipulable symbols have been used with several populations of children and adults, including aphasics (Gardner et al., 1976; Glass, Gazzaniga, & Premack, 1973), autistic children (Premack & Premack, 1974), mentally retarded children (Premack & Premack, 1974; Carrier, 1974a, 1974b, 1976; Carrier & Peak, 1975), and cerebral palsied children (material on Slip-n-Slide communication board in Vanderheiden, 1976). For further information about manipulable symbol sets, see the section on Premack-type plastic word symbols in this chapter.

Drawn or Written Symbols

A third class of nonelectronic gestural-assisted communication strategies includes those in which symbols are *drawn or written*. Messages are transmitted in such systems by writing or drawing the symbols that encode them in the appropriate sequence on a piece of paper or other material (e.g., a Magic Slate).

The symbol set used most often is English or some other natural language. It is important to note that if a person is able to print or write English or another language, this will afford him or her a more flexible communication system than any of the others described in this book. It is desirable to develop as much as possible the ability of all severely communicatively impaired persons to communicate through writing.

Two other symbol sets can be used in this manner: Blissymbolics and Braille.

Is it possible for a person who has a neuromuscular disorder to learn to write or draw symbols that can be identified? The answer is yes, in some cases. A person who is hemiplegic on the dominant side can often be taught to write or draw with his nondominant hand. A person who has both hands affected (a quadriplegic or diplegic) may be able to use a mouth-held writing device (Gertenrich, 1966); or, through muscle training, positioning, or stabilization (or some combination of the three), it may be possible for him or her to improve the functioning of one hand sufficiently to use it for writing or drawing. An occupational therapist who is experienced in the area of neuromuscular disorders can often be helpful in teaching the use of a hand-held or mouth-held writing device.

ELECTRONIC GESTURAL-ASSISTED COMMUNICATION STRATEGIES

The hardware of all electronic gestural-assisted communication aids consists of three types of components: switching mechanisms, control electronics, and displays (see Figure 3–1). There are a number of switching mechanisms and displays that can be used in such aids. Also, there are a number of special features that can be incorporated into their control electronics. Representative switching mechanisms and displays are described in this section. The electronics that specific switching mechanisms to control specific displays also are described. The intent of this discussion is to provide the reader with a good enough understanding of the functioning of switching mechanisms, displays, and control electronics so that he or she would be able to design a system for a particular client and describe its components to the person who will be making the device. For information about components for such systems, see Brandenberg and Vanderheiden (1987a, 1987b, 1987c) and Vanderheiden, Snyder, & Kelso (1992).

Switching Mechanisms

The switching mechanism interfaces the client with the communication aid. The client's gestural manipulation of a switching mechanism indicates or reproduces on a display the components of messages he or she wishes to transmit.

All switching mechanisms perform two functions: (1) They connect (directly or by means of a metallic substance) the ends of two wires, thereby permitting an electric current to flow from one to the other, and (2) they separate the ends of the two wires (or cause the metallic substance to separate from one or both ends of them), thereby interrupting the flow of electric current between them. Almost all switching mechanisms have such a metallic substance in them. This substance functions in a manner similar to a drawbridge that connects the two shores of a river. When the drawbridge is down, the two shores are connected and traffic can flow from one to the other. When it is up, the two shores are not connected and traffic cannot flow between them.

The bridge function of switching mechanisms is illustrated in Figure 5–24. The circuit consists of a battery connected to a light bulb by means of two wires, one of which has been cut into two pieces. The piece of metal that could bridge the ends of these two pieces of wire in Figure 5–24a does not connect them; and the bulb, therefore, would not be lit. In Figure 5–24b, the piece of metal does bridge, or connect, the ends of these two wires, thereby permitting an electric current to flow from one to the other and causing the bulb to light.

The bridge function of a switching mechanism is illustrated further in Figure 5–25. The tilt switch in this figure consists of a small globule of mercury and the ends of two pieces of wire sealed in a glass bulb or envelope. The glass bulb in the illustration is tilted in a manner so that the globule of mercury does not bridge the ends of the two wires. This situation is thus comparable to that illustrated in Figure 5–24a. If the

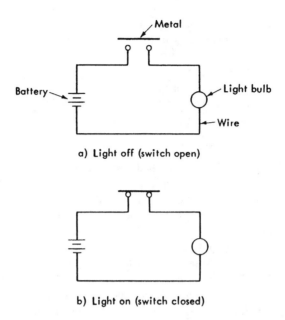

a) **Light off (switch open)**

b) **Light on (switch closed)**

FIGURE 5–24 **Open and closed switching mechanisms.**

glass bulb had been tilted upward so that the tip was pointed at twelve o'clock (rather than between seven o'clock and eight o'clock, as in the figure), the mercury globule would have bridged the two wire ends and the situation would have been comparable to that illustrated in Figure 5–24b.

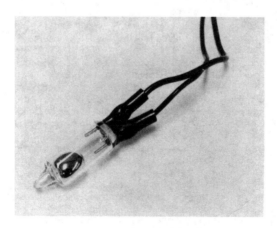

FIGURE 5–25 **Tilt switch in open position.**

Switching mechanisms that contain a bridge also contain a device for raising and lowering the bridge, which insulates the user from the electric current that flows when the bridge is lowered. There are a number of devices that can perform this function, and switches are categorized primarily on the basis of the type of device used for this purpose. In the following discussion we describe some of these switches. The scheme used to classify switches was adapted from Holt and Vanderheiden (1974) and Holt, Buelow, and Vanderheiden (1976).

Push Switches

Physical pressure applied directly by a patterned movement (gesture) of a body part (e.g., a finger) or indirectly by an implement controlled by a body movement (e.g., headstick) is used to either "lower the bridge" (turn on the switch) or "raise the bridge" (turn off the switch). The position of the bridge usually is maintained for as long as physical pressure is applied. With such switches, the bridge may be lowered or raised when pressure is applied.

Push switching mechanisms for controlling communication aids usually have three basic components: (1) a switch that can be activated by physical pressure, (2) a surface that will activate the switch when physical pressure is applied to it, and (3) some sort of housing for the switch and pressure surface. (In some such mechanisms the switch is activated by applying pressure to it directly.)

One type of switch that can be used in such mechanisms is a *lever microswitch* (Figure 5–26). These switches are relatively inexpensive (less than $2.00 in 1994) and

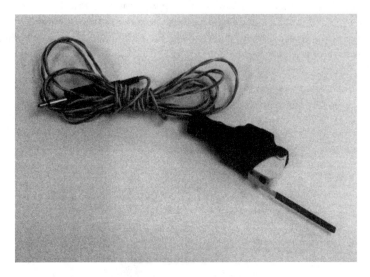

FIGURE 5–26   **Lever microswitch with cable.**

can be purchased at almost any store that sells electronic components (e.g., Radio Shack stores). They are activated by applying pressure to the lever and can be wired so that pressure applied to it will either "lower the bridge" or "raise the bridge." Because they can be mounted at any angle in space, they can be activated by downward pressure, upward pressure, lateral pressure, or pressure applied from any other angle.

The surfaces to which pressure can be applied to activate switches in push switching mechanisms are varied. *Push buttons* can be made in almost any shape and size (most are round or rectangular). They can be flush with the surface on which they are mounted, protrude outward from it, or be recessed. A recessed push button helps to prevent accidental activation.

Keyboards are made up of push button switches. They can be modified in several ways to make them more accessible to persons who are motor impaired. One way is to make the keys on them larger (Figure 5–27). Another is to mount a *keyguard* made from a sheet of plastic or metal that has a hole at the location of each key a fraction of an inch above it (Figure 5–28). The keyguard recesses the keys and helps to prevent their being activated accidentally.

Keyboards can also be modified by reducing the number of keys on them. *Reduced keyboards*, which contain fewer than 26 alphabetic keys, can be accessed and used by some motor-impaired persons more easily than conventional ones. Each key represents more than one character. When a key is activated, an automatic *disambiguation* process predicts which of the characters is the appropriate one based on linguis-

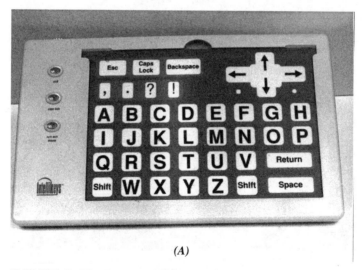

(A)

FIGURE 5–27 **Four large-key keyboards intended for augmentative communication with microcomputers.**

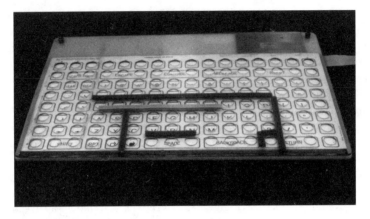

(B)

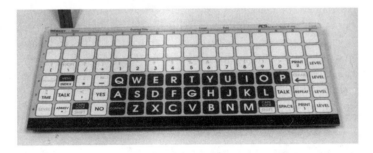

(C)

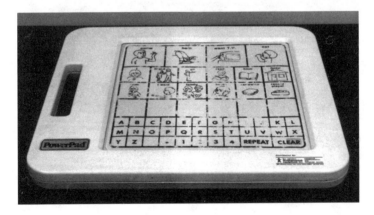

(D)

FIGURE 5–27 *Continued*

tic rules and what has already been typed (Arnott & Javed, 1992). This prediction is usually correct. If the prediction is incorrect, the user presses an error key. The disambiguation process then predicts the next most likely character. If it also is incorrect, the user continues to press the error key until the correct character is produced.

Also, keyboards can be made more accessible by reassigning the keys on them—changing their location (Chubon & Hester, 1988; Hurlburt & Ottenbacher, 1992). This can be done on microcomputers using memory resident keyboard utility software. Chubon and Hester (1988) have developed a keyboard configuration that appears to be more efficient (i.e., faster and less fatiguing) than the standard "qwerty" one for persons who use a single finger or a head- or mouthstick. The standard qwerty configuration was designed for typing with both hands (i.e., 10 fingers). Hurlburt and Ottenbacher (1992), after evaluating the performance of four adults with high-level spinal cord injuries with the qwerty and another keyboard configuration, concluded that previous experience with a particular configuration may be a more important factor in determining performance than is the specific configuration used.

Keyboard use can be made more rapid and less fatiguing by reducing the number of keystrokes needed to type a message (Higginbotham, 1990a, 1990b, 1992). Several strategies have been developed for doing this. Some utilize abbreviation codes for frequently used words that contain fewer letters than the words themselves (Higginbotham, 1992; Vanderheiden & Kelso, 1987). Others utilize software that predicts (and types) words after the first few letters have been keyboarded based on them and/or on the preceding words (Ricketts & Booth, 1993; Soede et al., 1989; Swiffin et al., 1987). For descriptions of keystroke-saving strategies, see Higginbotham (1992).

A type of switching mechanism that functions in much the same manner as a keyboard is a *graphics tablet*. These are devices that have a flat, smooth surface on which message components (letters, words, and/or drawings) are reproduced (see Figure 5–27d). The user generates a message component by touching (applying a little pressure to) the graphics tablet where it is reproduced. If the size of the tablet were 12 × 12 inches, and the message components were 1 × 1 inch or smaller, it would be possible to display more than 100 components on the tablet. For further information about the use of graphics tablets for augmentative communication, see Osguthorpe and Chang (1987, 1988).

Push plates are similar to push buttons except that they are larger (Figure 5–29) and thus do not require as good a level of motor functioning as do push buttons. Downward pressure applied anywhere on the plate will activate a switch. If they are pivoted at the center, push plates can be used in seesaw fashion to control two different switches (Figure 5–30).

Paddles have a pivoted arm that when pushed (Figure 5–31) or blown (Figure 5–32) up, down, to the side, or forward activates a switch. A paddle also can be used to activate two switches—pushing it to the right can activate one and pushing it to the left can activate the other (Figure 5–31). They can be of any size and shape a user can

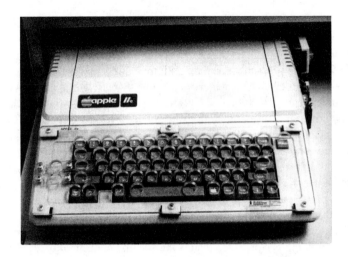

FIGURE 5–28   **A plastic keyguard mounted over a computer keyboard.**

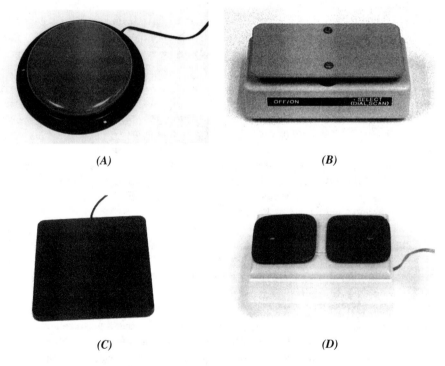

(A)   *(B)*

(C)   *(D)*

FIGURE 5–29   **Four push plate switching mechanisms.**

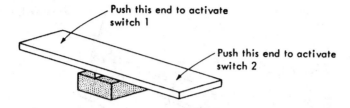

FIGURE 5–30 **Seesaw rocking lever for activating two microswitches.**
Source: Courtesy of Trace Center, Madison, Wisconsin.

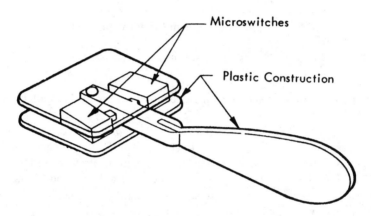

FIGURE 5–31 **Hand paddle for activating two microswitches.**
Source: Courtesy of Ontario Crippled Children's Centre, Toronto.

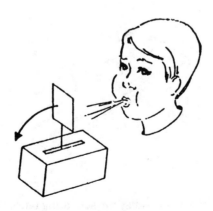

FIGURE 5–32 **Air paddle for activating one switch.**
Source: Courtesy of the Trace Center, Madison, Wisconsin.

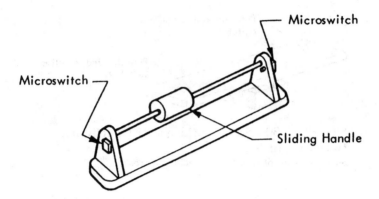

Microswitch

Microswitch

Sliding Handle

FIGURE 5–33 **Slide mechanism for activating two microswitches.**
Source: Courtesy of the Ontario Crippled Children's Centre, Ontario.

manipulate. A spring mechanism returns them to a neutral position after they have activated a switch.

Movement of a *sliding handle* (Figure 5–33) or *foot trolley* (Figure 5–34) along a slide, grove, or track may be used to activate a switch. These switches usually have two positions, one at each end of the slide, groove, or track. They can be fabricated so that sliding a handle or foot trolley to one end turns on a device and sliding it to the other turns the device off. Or they can be built so that sliding a handle or foot trolley to each end activates a different switch.

A *wobblestick* is a device that when pushed off center in any direction activates a single switch. Of the several types the most common is a rigid rod or shaft (Figure 5–35). Another type is a rubber ball that can be suspended from an electrical

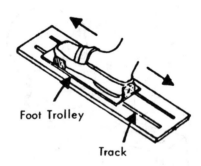

Foot Trolley

Track

FIGURE 5–34 **Foot trolley for activating one or two microswitches.**
Source: Courtesy of the Trace Center, Madison, Wisconsin.

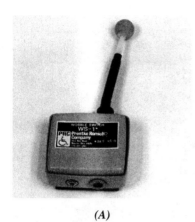

(A)

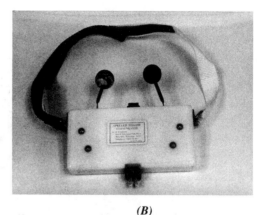

(B)

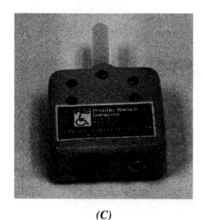

(C)

FIGURE 5–35   **Three wobblestick switching mechanisms. Switching mechanism C can be activated by tongue movement.**

cord (Figure 5–36). Pushing the ball off center (e.g., by moving the head) activates a single switch. A third type, known as a *leaf switch* (Figure 5–37), consists of a flexible, plastic-covered, spring-steel shaft that, when pushed, activates a single switch.

Joysticks are vertical devices that when pushed off center in a specific direction activate a particular switch (Figure 5–38). Joysticks used with communication aids are usually designed to activate two to eight switches, the ones illustrated in Figure 5–38 can activate up to four. Some use a gating scheme (Figure 5–38A), which helps to guide the stick to the desired switch.

With *pillows, pads,* and *squeeze bulbs,* pushing (or squeezing) a foam-padded or air-filled pillow, fabric, or rubber pad (see Figure 5–29C) or an air-filled bulb activates a single switch. These can be made in almost any size and shape.

Several pressure-sensitive switches have been designed that can be activated by movements of specific body parts. Examples are an air-filled bulb or a push button

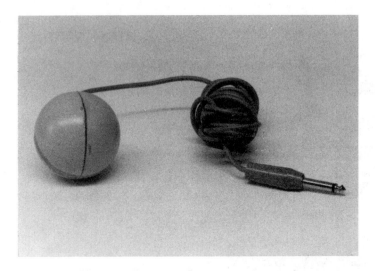

FIGURE 5–36 **A wobblestick consisting of a rubber ball containing a tip (mercury) switch. The ball is suspended; and moving it to the side with a part of the body (e.g., the head) activates the switch.**

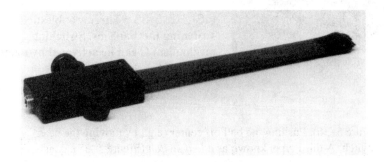

FIGURE 5–37 **A leaf switch.**

that is squeezed between the chin and the chest and a pressure-sensitive element molded into an artificial palate, which is activated by tongue pressure.

The switching mechanism must be mounted where the user can apply pressure to it. In most cases this is done by placing it on (or attaching it to) a tabletop or wheelchair. Mounting devices are available that can position a switching mechanism at almost any location in space (Figure 5–39).

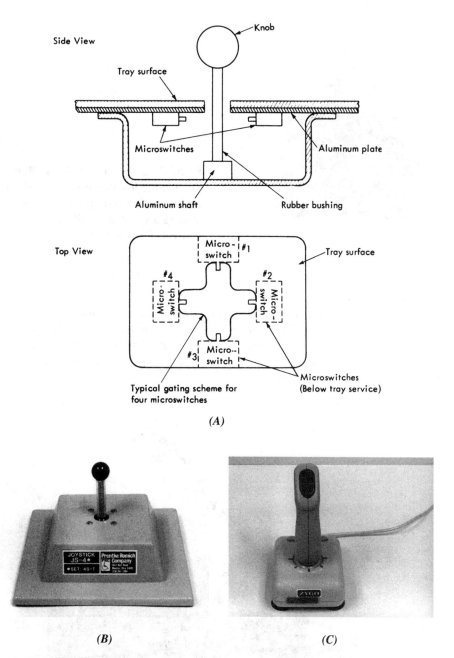

FIGURE 5–38 **Joysticks. (A) Joystick with gating for four microswitches. (B and C) These joysticks control four switches and were designed for augmentative communication.**
Drawing A Courtesy of Ontario Crippled Children's Centre.

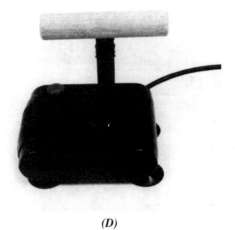

FIGURE 5–38 **(D) This standard videogame joystick was adapted for augmentative communication by adding a wooden handle. It also controls four switches.**

(D)

Position Switches

A change of position (orientation) in space of the switch mechanism by a patterned movement (or gesture) of a body part such as an arm is used to lower the bridge (turn on the switch) or raise the bridge (turn the switch off). The position of the bridge is maintained for as long as the body part remains at the same position in space.

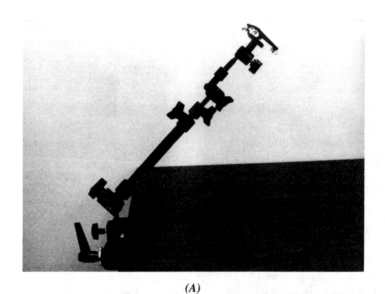

(A)

FIGURE 5–39 **A switch positioning device (A) with a switch attached (B).**

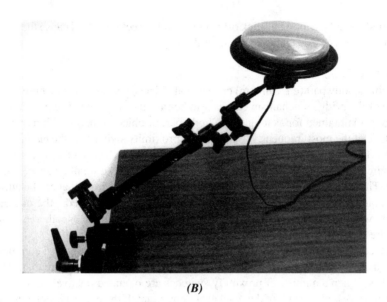

(B)

FIGURE 5–39 *Continued*

Position switches, also known as *tip or tilt* switches, usually consist of a small globule of mercury and two wire ends in a glass envelope (Figure 5–25). They can be attached to an arm or other body part that can be moved enough in space to change the position of the mercury globule. Particular patterned movements of this body part (Figure 5–40) are used to position the mercury in the glass envelope to bridge the two wire ends.

Mercury position switches can be activated also by wobblesticks (Figures 5–35 and 5–36). Pushing the stick off center causes the mercury to bridge the two wire ends. It may be necessary to use three or more mercury switches in such a device,

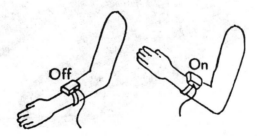

FIGURE 5–40 **Tip (or tilt) switch attached to the arm.**
Source: Courtesy of the Trace Center, Madison, Wisconsin.

mounted so that pushing the stick off center in any direction would cause the mercury to bridge the wire ends in at least one of them.

Proximity Switches

Bringing a body part (e.g., an arm) or a special object (e.g., a magnet) within a certain range of the bridge mechanism causes it to be raised or lowered. The position of the bridge is maintained for as long as the body part or object remains within this range.

One of the most frequently used types of proximity switches is the *magnetic reed* switch. This consists of two wirelike pieces of metal (reeds), each of which is attached to a wire end, that are mounted directly over the other with a small air space between them. The one on the bottom has on it a piece of metal (e.g., iron) that can be attracted by a magnet. If a magnet is placed over (on top of) the two reeds, the one on the bottom will be drawn upward and come into contact with the top one, thereby "bridging" the two wires and activating the switch.

Reed proximity switches have been used in several gestural-assisted communication aids. The switching mechanism in the aid in Figure 5–41 uses more than 80 such switches. When a number of proximity switches are mounted relatively close to each other, the size and strength of the magnet are important. If the magnet is either too large or too strong, it may activate more than one switch at a time. The reed switches are covered by a sheet of Formica plastic on which a symbol is reproduced above each switch. The magnet need not be in direct contact with a switch to activate it.

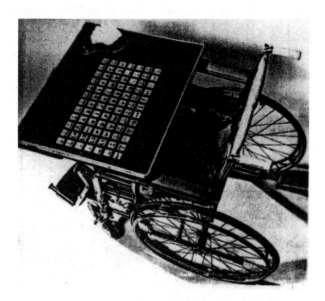

FIGURE 5–41   **Multiple proximity switch control for display.**
Source: Courtesy of the Trace Center, Madison, Wisconsin.

Pneumatic Switches

Blowing into or sucking on the end of a tube changes the air pressure in it, thereby activating a pressure-sensitive device (transducer) that either lowers the bridge (turns on a switch) or raises the bridge (turns off a switch). These sometimes are referred to as *sip and puff* or *suck and blow* switches. Only very small pressure changes are needed to activate the pressure transducers in them. Their use is illustrated in Figure 5–42.

Pneumatic switches can be activated in another way. A squeeze bulb or air-filled pillow can be attached to one by means of a piece of rubber tubing. Squeezing or pressing the bulb or pillow with some part of the body activates the transducer, which changes the position of the bridge. The air paddle (see Figure 5–32) can also be classified as a pneumatic switch because it is activated by blowing.

Touch Switches

Touching a metal surface (contact) on a glove to a metal contact plate (Figure 5–43) lowers the bridge, turning on the switch. The person is the mechanism used for raising and lowering the bridge. Touching the metal contact plate with the metal contact surface on the glove is equivalent to bringing the two wire ends (Figure 5–24) together. An electric current would pass through the person when the contact was made if it were not for the insulating property of the glove. This would, of course, be dangerous.

Touch switches can be activated by a part of the body other than a hand. A mental contact could, for example, be mounted on a sock (which adequately insulated the person from an electric shock), and touching the foot with the sock to a contact plate would lower the bridge (turn on the switch).

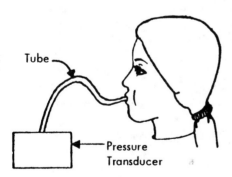

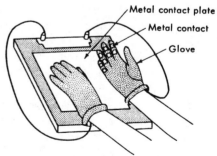

FIGURE 5–42 **Pneumatic ("suck and puff") device for activating one switch.**
Source: Courtesy of the Trace Center, Madison, Wisconsin.

FIGURE 5–43 **Touch switch with contacts on a glove.**
Source: Courtesy of the Trace Center, Madison, Wisconsin.

Sound-Controlled Switches

Sound-controlled switches are activated by sound energy that is transduced, or converted, into electrical energy by a microphone. The sound may be generated by a device (whistle, tone generator) or by the vocal tract (cough, hum, prolonged vowel). If the sound is generated by the vocal tract, the microphone can be placed near the user's mouth or attached to the throat by means of a disk of tape that is sticky on both sides. (Microphones that are intended to be attached to the throat usually are about the size of a nickel in diameter.)

With a microcomputer-based augmentative communication system, a *speech recognition device* (which contains a microphone) can be programmed so that only a particular sound or syllable produced by a particular person at a particular intensity will activate it. It may also be possible to program such a device to discriminate between several user-produced speech sounds (or syllables or words), thereby creating a multiswitch switching mechanism (Coleman & Meyers, 1991; Fried-Oken, 1985; Noyes & Frankish, 1992; Zimmer et al., 1991). Furthermore, it appears likely that a speech recognition device of this type on a microcomputer with artificial intelligence software could be used to generate spoken and/or printed message components (see Sy & Deller, 1989).

If a throat microphone is not used, there will be no physical contact between the user and the communication system. This eliminates the possibility of the user receiving an electric shock if the system malfunctions.

Light-Controlled Switches

Light-controlled switches are activated by directing a beam of light at a photoelectric cell (transducer) or by interrupting a light beam that is directed at such a device. With the first of these, the beam from a light source that is attached to the user's head (or some other body part) is directed to a spot on a device in front of the user (Figure 5–44). He or she can see where the beam is directed on the device and maneuver it to the desired location. A large number of switches can be activated by such a device. See Smith, Christiaansen et al. (1989) for a description of the use of this type of switching mechanism with a microcomputer.)

With the second approach, a beam of light that is directed at a photoelectric cell is interrupted by an object or a part of the body (e.g., a hand) passing between the light source and the photoelectric cell. This type of switching mechanism is used in some alarm systems and on some automatic elevator doors.

With both of these approaches, there is no physical connection between the user and the communication system.

Eye Closure Switches

Eye closure switches, which some writers classify as light controlled, are activated by the difference in the amount of infrared radiation (light) reflected by an open and a closed eye (Grattan, Palmer, & Mason, 1987). The radiation level is measured by a small device that is aimed at the eye and can be attached to an eyeglass frame. Cir-

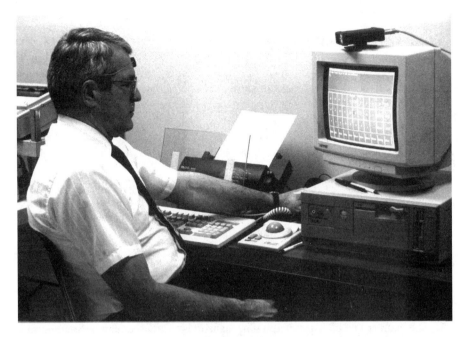

FIGURE 5-44   **A head-mounted light-activated switching mechanism.**

cuitry is built into these switches that makes them insensitive to short, involuntary eyeblinks. They can be used with scanning communication aids (Grattan, Palmer, & Mason, 1987; Kilgallon, Roberts, & Miller, 1987).

Several attempts have been made to develop more sophisticated devices of this type, ones that uses small changes in gaze to activate a series of switches. There have even been attempts to create eye position–controlled keyboards (see ten Kate & van Nifterick, 1988).

For further information about the switching mechanisms described in this section, as well as others, see Blackstone (1986), Brandenberg and Vanderheiden (1987b), Einis & Bailey (1990), Fried-Oken (1985), Grattan and Palmer (1984), Harwin and Jackson (1986, 1990), Holt, Buelow, and Vanderheiden (1976), Radwin, Vanderheiden, and Lin (1990), Rubin and Stark (1984), Stassen, Soede, and Bakker (1982), and ten Kate et al. (1985).

Selecting a Switching Mechanism

A number of switching mechanisms have been described. What factors should be considered when deciding which mechanism to use with a particular person? The five criteria listed here are intended as guidelines.

1. The *least sophisticated* (least complex) switching mechanism that will meet the user's communication needs should be selected, other things being equal. The more complex a switching mechanism, the more likely it is to malfunction. If both a push-button and a voice-operated switching mechanism would equally meet a person's needs, the push button probably should be selected.

2. A switching mechanism that requires a *gesture that does not have to be learned* (developed) is preferable to one requiring a gesture that does have to be learned, other things being equal. Obviously, if the user can make the gesture required to activate the switching mechanism, he or she can begin to learn to use it immediately.

3. The *least energy-consuming* switching mechanism that will meet the user's communication needs should be selected, other things being equal. Some switching mechanisms require more effort than others to activate. A person is apt to limit use of a switching mechanism (and, hence, a communication device) if using it is fatiguing.

4. The switching mechanism selected for a person should be one that does *not interfere much* with his or her ongoing activities, other things being equal. One that requires something to be attached to the body (e.g., a head-mounted light source) is more likely to interfere than is one that does not.

5. The manner in which a switching mechanism is to be used may be an important consideration in its selection. Some switching mechanisms (e.g., push buttons) are easier to activate in a *sustained manner*—for more than a few seconds—than are others (e.g., suck or puff switches). Rotary scanning displays sometimes require a switch to be activated in this manner.

6. The speed at which messages can be encoded is also an important selection criterion. Message encoding is more rapid with some switching mechanisms than with others (Szeto, Allen, & Littrell, 1993).

Displays

All electronic gestural-assisted communication aids have at least one display. The elements of the symbol set (message components) used may be

> All reproduced on the display, with those needed to encode a message somehow indicated in the appropriate sequence.

> Printed by the display on a piece of paper, on the surface of a cathode-ray tube (as on a television set or computer monitor screen), or on an illuminated alphanumeric display panel (e.g., a single-line liquid-crystal display of the type used on electronic calculators).

> Signaled by means of a noise, light, or vibration code (e.g., Morse code) generated by the display.

> Transmitted as speech.

All of these elements, of course, are not usable with every symbol set.

Some representative displays that are used in gestural-assisted communication aids are described here. For further information about these and other types of displays, see the multivolume *Rehabilitation Resource Book* series (Brandenberg & Vanderheiden, 1987a, 1987b, 1987c) and Vanderheiden, Snyder, & Kelso (1992).

Noise, Light, or Vibration Generators

These devices produce a noise, light, or vibration pattern when a switch is activated in a particular manner. The bursts of noise, light, or vibration emitted by them transmit messages in a code, such as Morse code (Figure 4–3). They can be activated by any of the switching mechanisms described in this section.

The device of this type that probably has been used most frequently in gestural-assisted communication aids is a battery-operated, transistor, code audio-oscillator that in 1994 could be purchased from a Radio Shack or similar store for less than $15 (Figure 5–45). It emits a clear, crisp tone through a built-in speaker for as long as the switch is turned on. The switching mechanism is attached to the device by two wires. It is housed in a small plastic case that could be attached to a vertical surface, such as the side of a wheelchair, by double-sided tape.

Almost any child or adult who uses a communication board could benefit from this type of audio-oscillator and a switching mechanism attached to his or her wheelchair, bed, or both. Such persons, when they want something, can get the attention of others in the same room or elsewhere by activating a switch. Once the user has someone's attention, he or she can use their communication board to indicate what is

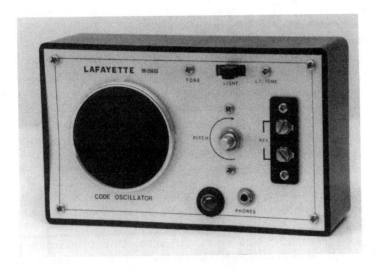

FIGURE 5–45   **Code oscillator alerting device.**

wanted. Without such an aid, a communication board user may have no reliable means of alerting people in the immediate environment when he or she wants to communicate. Coded messages can also be transmitted by a device that produces a vibration and light pattern when activated.

Rotary Scanning Displays

Rotary scanning displays (Figure 5–21d) have a pointer (similar to a clock hand) that is attached to the shaft of an electric motor. The pointer and motor are mounted at the center of a sheet of material, such as Plexiglas. Symbol elements (message components) are attached to this sheet around its perimeter. The motor (and thus the pointer) can be started and stopped with almost any type of switching mechanism. With some displays of this type, the pointer will revolve in only one direction; with others, it can revolve both clockwise and counterclockwise. The speed of rotation of the pointer can be fixed or variable. If the speed is variable, it may be fixed by an internal adjustment, or it may be under the control of the user (e.g., the farther off center the person pushes a wobblestick, the faster the speed of rotation). The sheet of material on which the motor and pointer are mounted can be of almost any size; the larger the sheet, the greater the number of symbols that can be mounted on it. The power source for the motor may be batteries, or the unit may have to be plugged into an electrical outlet.

The main limitation of a rotary scanning display is that only a limited number of symbol elements (message components) can be mounted on it if it is to be kept relatively small, because they only can be mounted at the edges. The type that is described next can utilize the entire board for displaying symbols.

Rectangular Matrix Displays

Rectangular matrix displays have a rectangular surface that is divided (or partitioned) into rows and columns (Figure 5–46). The maximum number of symbol elements (message components) that can be displayed on them is equal to the number of cells in the resulting matrix, or the product of the number of rows times the number of columns. (If a matrix had 3 rows and 5 columns, this number would be 15.)

Only one symbol element would appear in each matrix cell. It could be printed or drawn directly on the display, or it could be attached to it. Any of the symbol sets mentioned in the first section of this chapter except for Braille, Morse code, and Premack-type plastic symbols can be used with this type of display.

Displays of this type contain a mechanism that makes it possible for a single cell selected by the user to stand out for longer than a predetermined period of time. This can be done in several ways, including the following:

1. By placing a miniature "bulb" in the corner of each cell on the display board and lighting the "bulb" in the cell containing the message component to be transmitted for longer than a predetermined period of time (Figure 5–47).
2. By placing a miniature bulb behind each cell on the display board (the display board being either transparent or translucent plastic) and lighting the bulb behind the cell containing the message component to be transmitted for longer than a predetermined period of time.

a) Linear scanning

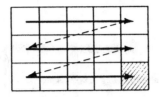

b) Row-column scanning

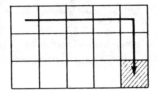

c) Directed scanning

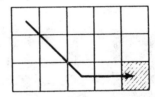

FIGURE 5–46 **Representative scanning approaches for indicating message components with an electronic rectangular matrix display.**

A user can light a bulb longer than a predetermined period of time by manipulating a switching mechanism when the bulb is lit in that cell.

Most rectangular matrix displays use a *scanning* strategy for indicating (transmitting) message components. Bulbs are lit in a pattern that may be partly controllable by the user, each for the same predetermined period of time. The user activates a switch when the bulb is lit in the cell containing the message component to be transmitted. This causes the bulb to remain lit for longer than it would if the scanning process were continuing. After a certain period of time, or after the user activates the switching mechanism in a particular way, the scanning process begins again, permitting another message component to be transmitted. The user repeats this process until all the components of the message have been transmitted.

Several scanning strategies can be used with this type display for indicating (transmitting) message components. Three of these are illustrated in Figure 5–46. The message component the user wishes to transmit in these illustrations is in the cell at the lower right-hand corner of the display.

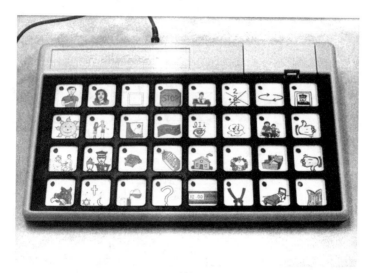

(A)

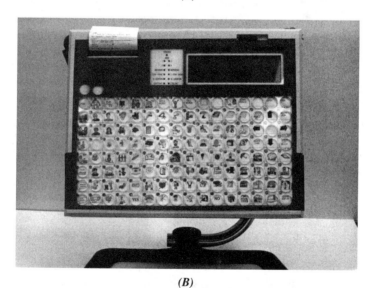

(B)

FIGURE 5–47 **Two communication devices with rectangular matrix displays. A miniature "bulb" is in the upper left corner of each cell in both devices.**

With a *regular linear scanning strategy* (Figure 5–46a), the bulbs in the top row of cells are lit, one after the other, after the user activates (presses) a switch. If the message component the user wants to transmit is not in the top row, the bulb in the first cell of the second row lights after that in the last cell of the first row went off. This process continues until the user activates the switch a second time, causing the light in the cell that was on to remain lit. Rather than the user activating the switch twice, the user may "hold down" the switch until the light in the cell containing the message component is lit. The user would then release the switch, thereby causing it to remain lit. This method is sometimes is called an *inverse linear scanning strategy* (Angelo, 1992).

A third possibility—a *step linear scanning strategy* (Angelo, 1992)—is for the user to activate the switch repeatedly to advance the light from cell to cell. When the cell is reached that contains the message component, the user stops activating the switch. Lights on the board (Figure 5–46a) then go on and off 14 times before going on in the cell that contains the message component the user wants to transmit. A display that uses this type of scanning mode can be controlled by almost any kind of switching mechanism.

With a *row-column strategy* (Figure 5–46b), the bulbs in the top row of cells are lit, one after the other, until the one in the column containing the message component is lit. The user then activates the switching mechanism, thereby causing the scanning to proceed downward until the bulb in the cell containing the message component is lit. The user then activates the switching mechanism a second time, causing the light in this cell to remain lit. The user may have to activate the switching mechanism a third time to prepare the display for signaling the next message component (i.e., causing the bulb in the first cell of the top row to be lit), or this may occur automatically after a predetermined number of seconds.

The inverse scanning strategy can also be used. The user "holds down" the switch until the light in the top row of the column containing the message component is lit. He or she then releases the switch and activates it again, thereby causing the scanning to proceed downward. When the light in the cell containing the message component is lit, the user releases the switch. Lights on the board go on and off six times before going on in the cell containing the message component the user wants to transmit.

With a *directed scanning strategy* (Figure 5–46c), the bulbs in the cells are lit, one after the other, that lie in the shortest path to the one containing the message component the user wishes to transmit. The path can be vertical, horizontal, angular, or combinations of the three. The light would go on and off four times before going on in the cell containing the message component the user wanted to transmit. Displays using this type of scanning mode usually are controlled by joysticks (Figure 5–38).

Rectangular matrix displays can be fabricated that have a relatively large number of cells. Devices containing more than 300 cells have been built.

Rectangular matrix displays must be positioned where they can be seen easily by both the user and the person(s) with whom he or she is communicating. A special device sometimes is used for this purpose (Figure 5–48).

Microcomputers can be programmed to simulate rectangular matrix displays on

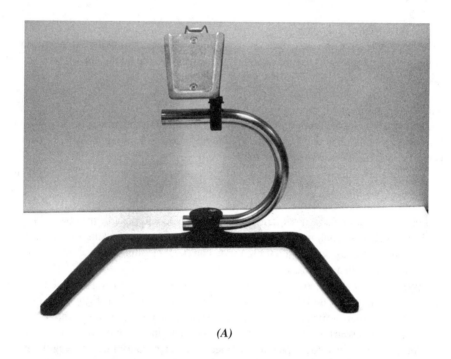

(A)

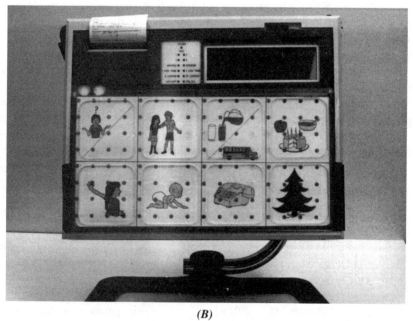

(B)

FIGURE 5–48   **A device for positioning rectangular matrix displays (A), with one such display mounted. (B).**

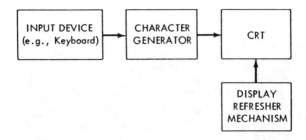

FIGURE 5–49   **Components of a CRT display.**

a monitor screen (Angelo, 1992; Korabic, Silverman, & Rosa, 1987; Newman, Sparrow, & Hospod, 1989; Treviranus & Tannock, 1987). Linear, row-column, or directed scanning strategies can be used for indicating message components. Various types of switching mechanisms can be used for controlling the computer and, thereby, the scanning process. Microcomputer-based augmentative communication systems are dealt with elsewhere in this chapter.

CRT (Cathode-Ray Tube) Displays

CRT displays can be television sets or computer monitors. Messages are displayed on a screen—a cathode-ray tube. Although they usually do so character (letter or digit) by character, they can also display messages in larger units (words, phrases, or sentences). Because these devices are almost always used in communication aids that have desktop microcomputers in their control electronics, they usually have an editing capability that allows the user to insert or delete characters. This capability can be used to correct errors arising from such sources as accidentally activating the switching mechanism and for editing messages or responses that would be necessary if the device were used for schoolwork. Graphic symbols—including Blissymbolics—can also be displayed on them.

CRT displays can be used alone or in conjunction with a printing device such as a strip printer or a computer printer. When they are used with printers, messages usually are formulated and edited on the CRT display. The advantage of doing so is that it is easier to correct errors and do other types of editing on a screen than on a piece of paper.

CRT displays, when in use, are positioned so that they can be seen by both the user and those with whom he or she is communicating.

Augmentative communication aids containing CRT displays must have the following four components: an input device, such as a keyboard; a character generator; a CRT terminal; and a display refreshing mechanism. These components are diagrammed in Figure 5–49. Activation of an input device (which contains a switching mechanism such as a keyboard) causes letters, digits, or larger language units to be generated by the character generator and displayed on the CRT terminal. To keep the message on the CRT terminal from fading out, a mechanism continuously refreshes the characters on it. The editing function of the CRT display is controlled by the input device.

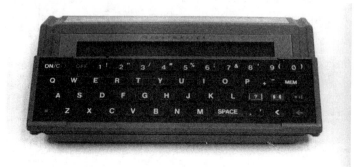

(A)

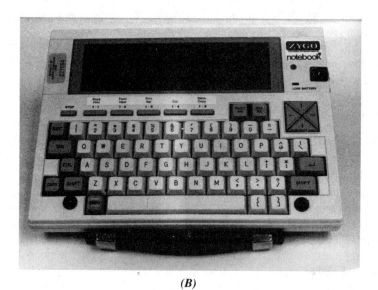

(B)

FIGURE 5–50 **Two representative communication devices with an LED/LCD display above the keyboard.**

LED and LCD Displays

LED (light-emitting diode) and LCD (liquid-crystal display) displays print out a message character by character (or in larger units) on a panel (Figure 5–50). The panel may display a single line of text or a number of lines.

The characters on an LED display are outlined in light by miniature transistors, called light-emitting diodes, that are arranged in rows and columns on the panel. This type of display was used on most electronic calculators manufactured during the 1970s. A representative arrangement of LEDs on such a panel is illustrated in

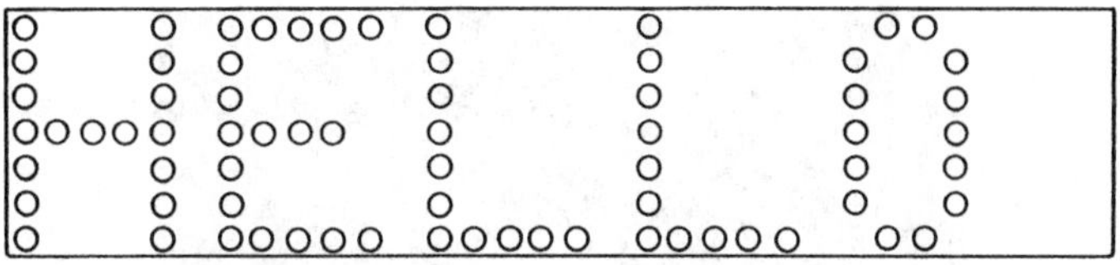

```
○     ○  ○○○○○  ○       ○              ○ ○
○     ○  ○      ○       ○          ○       ○
○     ○  ○      ○       ○          ○       ○
○○ ○○○○  ○○○○○  ○       ○          ○       ○
○     ○  ○      ○       ○          ○       ○
○     ○  ○      ○       ○          ○       ○
○     ○  ○○○○○  ○○○○○   ○○○○ ○       ○ ○
```

FIGURE 5–51   **A representative LED display, consisting of 231 light-emitting diodes arranged in a 7 × 33 matrix.**

Figure 5–51. This display panel has on it 231 LEDs, arranged in 7 rows and 33 columns. A panel of this size, incidentally, was used in a gestural-assisted communication aid referred to as the "Talking Brooch" (Newell & Brumfitt, 1974) because it was pinned to the user's clothing.

Any letter or digit can be outlined by causing certain of the diodes to emit light. These panels usually display a single row of characters and can be fabricated in almost any length. Although they can be controlled most efficiently by a keyboard, other types of switching mechanisms can also be used to activate the character generator.

Messages can be printed out in two ways on LED displays. First, a display can be filled with words, erased, filled again (if a message was not completed), erased, and so on, until a message is transmitted completely. Second, the characters in a message can be made to move across the display relatively smoothly from right to left in a manner similar to the "newscasts" on some buildings. This second approach was used with the LED display of the "Talking Brooch" communication aid. Only five characters were visible on this display at any one time. The manner in which each new character gradually moved from the right-hand end of the display, displacing those already present, is illustrated in Figure 5–52. The characters ceased moving when all of them in a message had been displayed.

Liquid-crystal displays provide the same types of readouts as do LEDs and can be used in place of them. They are the type used on most electronic calculators and laptop computers. The characters on LCDs usually are formed from combinations of short vertical and horizontal lines as illustrated here:

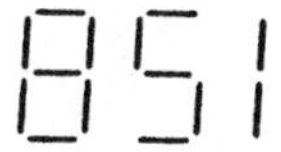

LCDs use less current than do LED displays, so batteries last longer. Also, significantly reduce the size of portable communication aids because they can be made thinner than LED displays.

Strip (Line) Printer Displays

Strip printers print messages made up of letters, digits, and punctuation marks on narrow strips of paper (usually heat sensitive) that are only wide enough to reproduce

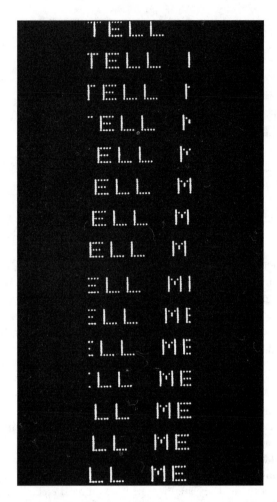

FIGURE 5–52   **Illustration of the floating
display of the "Talking Brooch".**
Source: From Copeland, 1974.

a single line of characters (Figure 5–53). The paper, which is approximately the same
width as telegraph ticker tape, is fed into the printer in rolls. (The rolls may be in
cassettes, which facilitates loading them into the printer.) The length of a paper strip
on which a message is printed is determined by the number of characters in the
message. The strip can be of any length that does not exceed that of the paper in the
device. If it is desired to save a message, the printed strip can be cut into pieces and
attached to a sheet of paper (as is done with telegrams). Although strip printers can be

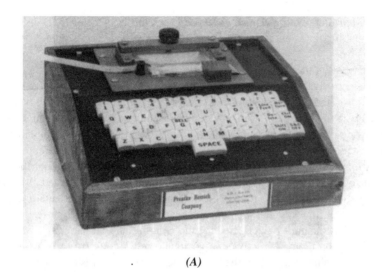

(A)

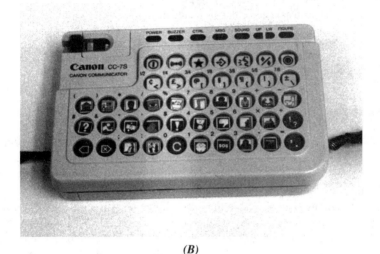

(B)

FIGURE 5–53 **Two communication devices with strip printers. The strip printer in B is in the upper left corner.**

controlled by almost any type of switching mechanism, keyboards are the most efficient for the purpose.

Strip printers are frequently used as displays in portable gestural-assisted communication devices because they are usually smaller than other types of devices that can print, and they can be battery operated. Messages can be "typewritten" directly with a strip printer, or they can be composed on a CRT, LED, or LCD display with editing capability and sent to a strip printer after they have been edited.

Electric Typewriters

Modified electric typewriters (particularly those manufactured by IBM) have been used as gestural-assisted communication aids. There are several ways in which typewriters can be adapted to make them usable by persons who have a neuromuscular disorder.

A device can be added that enables the user to insert paper in rolls instead of sheets. It is unnecessary with such a device for the user to have adequate control of the upper extremities to insert sheets of paper into the machines, although he or she would, of course, require assistance when a new roll of paper was needed. A keyguard can be mounted over the keys to help prevent them from being accidentally activated (Figure 5–28). With a keyguard in place, the user's fingers rest on it instead of on the keys. Thus, keys cannot be activated by the weight and extraneous movements of fingers resting on them. To activate a particular key, the user inserts a finger or a device (such as a headstick) into the hole in the keyguard that is over that key.

Small, battery-operated electronic typewriters (which became available during the 1980s) can be used as wheelchair-mounted gestural-assisted communication aids. These devices could be purchased in 1994 for less than $150. Because almost all have an LCD display built in, they can be used "conversationally" for asking and answering questions as well as for written communication. If necessary, a keyguard can be fabricated from a piece of Plexiglas and mounted over the keyboard.

Teletypewriters

Similar in function to electric typewriters, teletypewriters differ from them in two ways: (1) They print messages on a roll of paper, and (2) characters are printed in response to a coded electrical signal that can be generated by either a second teletypewriter, a TDD (Telecommunication Device for the Deaf), or a computer connected to it by a telephone line.

A teletypewriter is installed in the user's home or office. He or she transmits a message, which will be printed by another teletypewriter, TDD, or computer by dialing a telephone number at which one has been installed on the telephone line (e.g., the police department in some cities). The person called can respond by typing a message on his or her device, which will be printed by the user's teletypewriter. This same type of communication is possible using two microcomputers if they have telephone modems (see Silverman, 1987).

Computer Printers

Microcomputer-based augmentative communication aids usually have a printer as one of their components. There are several types that can be used in such aids. One type that has been used in portable battery-operated ones—the strip printer—was described earlier in this section. Used most often are *dot-matrix* printers.

Dot-matrix printers form characters from a matrix of dots (Figure 5–54). Some

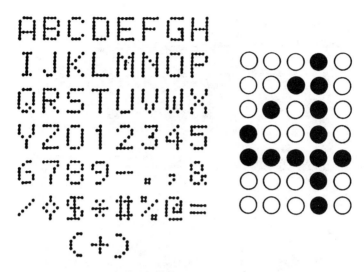

FIGURE 5–54 **Letters, numerals, and symbols reproduced by a dot-matrix printer.**

printers can use larger matrices than others; the larger the matrix used, the less obvious the dot structure of the characters. The matrix may be sufficiently large to make the characters appear almost solid; such characters are referred to as "near letter quality." They can be used for printing both text and graphics.

Speech Generators (Synthesizers)
Speech generators produce speech by playing recorded speech segments (Record-player "voice" . . . , 1977) or by generating (synthesizing) them using a computer (Microprocessor-based voice synthesizer . . . , 1977). Communication systems that use the latter strategy may be dedicated—that is, intended specifically for augmenting communication—or microcomputers with speech synthesizers. Four representative systems of the dedicated type are illustrated in Figure 5–55.

Some speech-generating communication aids utilize picture symbols (e.g., Picsyms) or letter sequences as codes for words and phrases (Haight et al., 1992). For example, the code for the word "time" could be a picture of a clock, and the code for the phrase "Let's eat" could be LE. There is some evidence that people are able to recall letter sequences more accurately than picture symbols for encoding messages (Light et al., 1990; Light & Lindsay, 1992).

Speech synthesizers are available for almost all microcomputers. With appropriate software and special switching mechanisms, microcomputer-based speech-generating communication aids can be made to function in a manner similar to dedicated ones. For further information about microcomputer-based communication devices, see Silverman (1987).

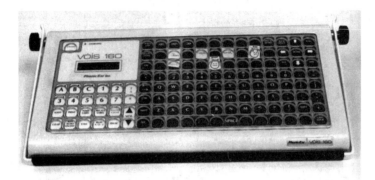

(A)

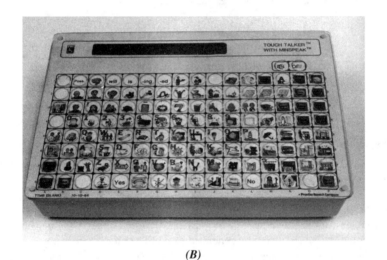

(B)

FIGURE 5–55 **Four speech-generating devices.**

Augmentative communication aids that can generate speech should be particularly useful to severely communicatively impaired persons who have normal hearing for communicating by telephone.

For further information about the use of synthesized speech for augmentative communication, see the following papers and their reference lists: Baker (1986); Dahl & Galyas, 1990; Damper (1982, 1986a, 1986b); Damper et al. (1987); Deliege, Speth-Lemmens, and Waterham (1989); Dowden, Yorkston, and Stoel-Gammon (1987); Eulenberg and Rosenfeld (1982); Frecks & Beukelman, 1990; Freedman, 1992; Frumkin (1987); Ghisler, 1990; Heckathorne, Voda, and Leibowitz (1987); King

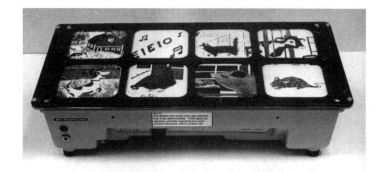

(C)

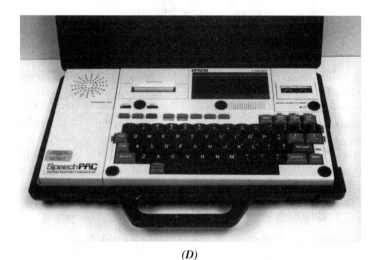

(D)

FIGURE 5–55 *Continued*

(1983); Mirenda and Beukelman (1987); Montgomery (1982); Silverman (1987); St Louis, 1990; Vanderheiden and Kelso (1987); Venkatagiri, 1994; and Westman, Bowen, and Crary (1987).

Selecting a Display

A number of displays have been described. What factors should be considered when deciding which display to use for a particular person? The six criteria suggested here are intended as guidelines.

1. *Need for portability.* If a communication aid has to be portable, there will be limits on its maximum size and weight. Also, it is highly desirable that the device can operate on batteries. Rotary scanning displays, rectangular matrix displays, LED displays, LCD displays, strip printers, small-screen (four or five inch) battery-operated television sets, speech-generating devices, and code oscillators usually can be used in such aids because they can be made relatively small and light in weight and powered from batteries.
2. *Need for editing capability.* If it is important for the user to be able to edit the messages he or she has formulated, a microcomputer with word processing software and a CRT display or multiline LCD display alone or in conjunction with a printer (strip or computer) probably would be the best choice.
3. *Need for a record of messages transmitted.* If an aid is intended to be used for written as well as "conversational" communication, it should contain a strip printer, computer printer, typewriter, or teletypewriter.
4. *Need for telephone communication capability.* If the user needs to be able to communicate by telephone without using a telecommunication relay service (see chapter 8), a code generator, a teletypewriter, a microcomputer with modem, or a speech generator can be used. The speech generator is the most flexible because it can be used to communicate on any telephone.
5. *The symbol set used.* Rotary scanning displays, rectangular matrix displays, and CRT displays tend to be more practical than other types for visual symbol sets not consisting of letters and digits (e.g., photographs, drawings, and Blissymbols).
6. *Motivation to learn Morse code.* An audio code oscillator (with an appropriate switching mechanism) can provide an inexpensive, flexible, portable communication aid if the user and those with whom he or she communicates are willing to learn Morse code. It can be used to communicate by telephone. A permanent record can be made of messages transmitted by tape-recording the audio code signals. For schoolwork or business communication, the signals can be recorded on a dictating machine and transcribed by someone who knows Morse code or who is willing to consult a code chart.

It should be evident from the discussion that gestural-assisted communication aids are likely to require more than one type of display to meet users' communication needs adequately. When selecting components for these aids, therefore, it probably is safest to assume that more than one type of display will be needed now or in the future, unless there is evidence to the contrary.

Control Electronics

The control electronics interface the switching mechanism with the display(s). They make it possible to indicate or generate message components on a display by activating a switching mechanism in a particular manner and to do so reliably. The control electronics of a gestural-assisted communication aid perform two or more of the following functions:

1. Connecting the switching mechanism to the display
2. Supplying electric power to the display and to other components requiring it
3. Transforming a user's activations of the switching mechanism into a form that will control the display
4. "Remembering" the components of a message until a user wishes to display them
5. Preventing the switching mechanism from being activated accidentally

The control electronics of all such systems perform the first two functions. The third and fourth functions, when needed, can be performed by a microcomputer. The microcomputer may be a commercially available unit (e.g., Macintosh or IBM Personal Computer) or a device built into a dedicated communication system. The fifth can be performed by a microcomputer or by a separate device. Some components used to perform these functions are described briefly in the following paragraphs.

Connecting the Switching Mechanism to the Display
Connection usually is done with electric cables. The cables contain a number of insulated electric wires, and the number of wires in a cable is positively related to the number of switches in the switching mechanism. There are at least two wires for each switch. The wires in a cable are color-coded to identify them. Communication aids with a computer or delay circuit in the control electronics, or with more than one display, usually have more than one cable. One cable, for example, may connect the switching mechanism to the computer and a second connects the computer to the display.

The cables used to connect the components of a communication device should be adequately shielded from electrical radiation sources in the environment, such as fluorescent lamps and CB radios. The shielding is built into the cable. If shielding is inadequate, these extraneous, environmental energy sources may interfere with the functioning of the device. Such interference is particularly apt to occur when inadequately shielded cables are used that are relatively long.

When it is necessary (or desirable) for a display to be located at a distance from the user and it would be dangerous (or undesirable) to use an electric cable to connect the switching mechanism to the control electronics (e.g, a microcomputer) and/or to the display, another approach may be usable. An example of a situation in which the use of a cable may not be desirable would be a classroom in which a large CRT display was located where it could be seen by the teacher and the members of the class and in which the user was seated at a desk or in a wheelchair on which was mounted a keyboard-type switching mechanism. The user could participate in class discussions by printing his or her comments on the CRT display. With this approach, the switching mechanism probably would be connected to the display by low-power radio signals. The switching mechanism is used to activate a radio transmitter that is located next to it. The resulting signals are transmitted to a radio receiver that is located next to the display and is connected to it.

Supplying Electric Power

All the displays used in electronic gestural-assisted communication aids require electric power to function. The same is true of microcomputers and other devices containing electronic circuits that are used in these systems. The power source can be batteries or an electric outlet.

Batteries differ with regard to their voltage, the electrochemical process by which they generate their power, and whether they are rechargeable. They are made in a number of voltages. If batteries are connected in series (the positive terminal of one contacting the negative terminal of the next), the resulting voltage will be the sum of the individual voltages. Thus, four 1.5-volt batteries connected in series will generate 6 volts. There is no theoretical limit to the number of batteries that can be combined in series, but there is obviously a practical limit.

Several types of chemical processes can be used in a battery to generate electric energy. The process used partly determines the length of time a battery will continue to deliver its nominal (specified) voltage. Among the types that tend to deliver their nominal voltages the longest are alkaline batteries. Although they are more expensive than most other types of nonrechargeable batteries, their relatively long life makes them desirable for use in communication aids; they have been reported to last as much as 10 times longer than conventional batteries.

Such types of batteries have to be replaced when they no longer generate their nominal voltage. There is a type of battery, however, that can be recharged, by plugging the unit in which it is mounted into an electric outlet for a specified number of hours. If these batteries are used in a communication aid, they can be recharged at night while the user is sleeping. An auxiliary battery pack can be included in the system if it is apt to require more power during the day than can be supplied by a single set of batteries. Although the initial cost of rechargeable batteries is more expensive than that of disposable ones, they tend to cost less over their lifetime.

If the power source for a communication aid is from an electric outlet, it is important to determine whether the outlets to be used will provide the voltage required by the aid. If they do not, an adapter will have to be used. This would be particularly important to check if some of the components of the aid were manufactured outside of the United States and not intended for export.

Transforming a User's Activations

Transforming a user's activations of a switching mechanism into a form that can control a display is done ordinarily with a special device, the switching mechanism being connected to its input and the display to its output (Figure 5–56). In some cases the device is a computer (Figure 5–57). Gestural-assisted communication aids that have a computer as a component in their control electronics include those that use a

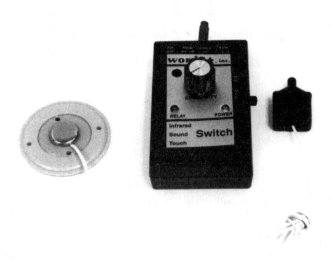

FIGURE 5-56   **A device for transforming switch activations into a form that can control a display.**

Morse code input, use a scanning response mode controlled by a single switch, or contain a speech synthesizer.

Computer systems have two types of components: hardware and software. The hardware includes the mechanical and electric components of the system and the software the instructions that control the functioning of the hardware.

The hardware of a microcomputer system consists of four units: input, central processing unit (microprocessor), output, and memory (Figure 5-57). Input is a switching mechanism (e.g., a keyboard) through which instructions and data are entered into the central processing unit (microprocessor). The microprocessor manipulates the data as specified by the instructions and stores the processed data in memory. The processed data are retrieved from memory and used to control an output device—a printer, a CRT display, or a speech synthesizer. For further information about hardware components of microcomputer-based augmentative communication aids, see Brandenberg and Vanderheiden (1987a, 1987b, 1987c); Fairhurst and Stephanidis (1985, 1988, 1989); Foulds (1982); Seamone (1982); Silverman (1987); and Smith et al. (1989).

The software of a microcomputer system consists of sets of instructions, or pro-

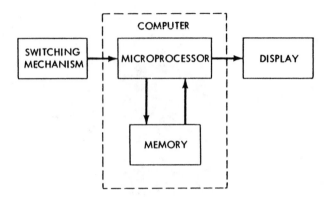

FIGURE 5–57 **Installation of a computer in a gestural-assisted communication aid.**

grams, that tells the computer's microprocessor how to perform desired functions. A program may be written in a single computer language or in several.

Adaptive hardware and software is available for persons who are too severely impaired to access microcomputers in the usual way. There are several computer databases and books from which information about such hardware and software can be obtained (see Casali & Williges, 1990; Mizuko, 1993).

Microcomputer systems are available that would be adequate for many augmentative communication applications for less than $500. One such system, which utilizes the Radio Shack Color Computer, can be assembled for less than $250 (Korabic, Silverman, and Rosa, 1987). Apple II microcomputers (particularly the IIc and IIe models) are often available used for less than $500 and can be easily adapted for use as augmentative communication aids.

"Remembering" the Components of a Message

A microcomputer can be programmed to store some or all of the components of a message (phonemes, letters, digits, punctuation marks, words, phrases, etc.) in memory from which they can be retrieved and displayed whenever the user wishes. A microcomputer also can be programmed to display message components that have been encoded (assigned a number) and stored in memory. The user would input the digit code of the message component that he or she wanted displayed and the microprocessor would retrieve that component from memory and display it.

Preventing the Switching Mechanism from Being Activated Accidentally

If a user of a gestural-assisted communication aid has a neuromuscular disorder, he may accidentally activate a switching mechanism because of involuntary movement or poor motor control. This is particularly apt to be a problem in aids that use a keyboard-type switching mechanism because the individual switches tend to be close to each other.

A microcomputer can be programmed so that the gesture used to activate a switch—pressing, sucking, phonating, or tilting the arm—has to be maintained for a predetermined amount of time (e.g., 3 seconds) before the switch will activate. Its duration would be positively related to the degree of disturbance in the control of the musculature used to perform the gesture; the greater the disturbance, the longer the gesture would have to be maintained. This delay time, of course, should be kept as short as a user's neuromuscular functioning will allow.

▶ 6

Neuro-Assisted Strategies

Almost all severely communicatively impaired children and adults can learn to communicate by the use of one or more gestural strategies (see chapter 4), gestural-assisted strategies (see chapter 5), or a combination of the two. A few, however, are so involved motorically that they either are unable gesturally to activate a switching mechanism reliably or cannot do so without becoming unduly fatigued. At least some of these persons may be able to use a microprocessor-based communication aid in the manner described in this chapter. Doing so, however, should be viewed as a last resort because the communication aids in this category have several limitations when compared to comparable ones controlled gesturally:

1. The switching mechanisms of these aids tend to *cost more.*
2. These aids tend to *transmit messages at a slower rate.*
3. These aids are *more likely to malfunction* because they tend to be more complex electronically.
4. It is necessary with these aids to *attach something to the user* (surface electrodes). The only gestural-assisted ones for which this is necessary are those that use a headstick or a tip/tilt switch.
5. The state of the art for these aids is *not as highly developed,* and the literature describing them is relatively small.

These aids differ from gestural-assisted ones in only one way: They are activated, or controlled, by electrical signals generated by the body rather than by muscle gestures or movements. Users of a neuro-assisted aid activate it by willfully varying in an agreed upon manner an aspect (or attribute) of some electrical signals emanating from their bodies. They may, for example, vary the intensity or frequency of such signals. A change in the frequency or intensity of a particular set of electrical signals emanating from a user's body can be detected by electrodes attached to the skin at a particular location. This location is determined by the type of electrical activity used to control, or activate, the system. If it is brain waves, the electrodes are mounted on the user's head; if it is muscle action potentials, they usually are attached to the skin over the muscle group (or groups) whose activity level(s) is (are) being used to control the device.

Theoretically, any electrical signals generated by the body can be used to control a communication aid as long as

The user can learn willfully reliably to vary an aspect of it (e.g., its intensity or frequency) in an agreed-upon manner

Learning to do this would not be detrimental to the user's health

The aspect of the signal varied can be monitored by electrodes attached to the person

Two types of biological electrical signals capable of being partially brought under voluntary control through biofeedback techniques are muscle action potentials and brain waves. (Biofeedback techniques are dealt with later in this chapter.) Both can be monitored by electrodes attached to the skin (surface electrodes), and both can be controlled well enough by some persons (with no reported detrimental effects on their health) to activate reliably, or control, an electric typewriter, teletypewriter, or microcomputer (Combs, 1969; Dewan, 1966; LaCourse & Hludik, 1990; Nishikawa et al., 1984; Rice & Combs, 1972; Torok, 1974; Writing made possible . . . , 1976).

The remainder of this chapter deals with the use of muscle action potentials and brain waves to control communication aids. Although the literature in this area is limited, there is a relatively large literature dealing with control by biofeedback techniques. Both the instrumentation and teaching techniques that are used in EMG and EEG biofeedback research (for monitoring and modifying muscle action potentials and brain waves, respectively) probably has been adapted for controlling microprocessor-based communication aids.

MUSCLE ACTION POTENTIALS

Muscle action potentials are electrical signals that are associated with the contraction of muscle fibers. They do not arise from the contraction itself but from the electrical signals conducted along the axons of lower motor neurons (anterior horn cells) to the muscle fibers they innervate, which causes them to contract. The process by which they arise can be summarized as follows:

The striated muscle of man is composed functionally of motor units in which the axons of single motor (anterior horn) cells innervate many muscle fibers. Hundreds of muscle fibers may be innervated by a single axon. All of the fibers innervated by a single motor unit respond immediately in an "all-or-none" pattern to adequate stimulation. The interactions of many motor units can produce relatively smooth motor performance. Increased motor power results from activation of a greater number of motor units or from repeated activation of a given number of motor units. The action potential of a muscle consists of the sum of the action potentials of many motor units. The action potential of normal muscle fibers originates at the motor end plates and is triggered by an incoming nerve impulse at the myoneural junction. It then spreads along muscle fibers, exciting contraction. (Chusid & McDonald, 1960, p. 209)

Note particularly that (1) when normal muscle is at rest, there are no action potentials, and when it is in a state of contraction, there are action potentials; and (2) the greater the number of motor units (in a muscle) that are activated, the greater the magnitude of the action potential. Both phenomena have been utilized in the control of communication aids.

A muscle's action potential can be detected by surface electrodes attached to the skin. (They can also be detected by needle electrodes, but these are not practical for use with communication aids because they have to be inserted into the muscle.) A surface electrode consists of a small metal disk (sometimes silver) to which an insulated electric wire has been soldered (see Figure 6–1). This wire usually has a male connector attached to its other end so that it can be plugged into, or interfaced with, an amplifier. These electrodes usually are used in pairs and are attached to the skin over the muscle being monitored, approximately 1 inch apart. A third, or ground, electrode also may be used.

Switching mechanisms that utilize muscle action potentials are called myoswitches. Some myoswitches utilize more than one set of electrodes. LaCourse

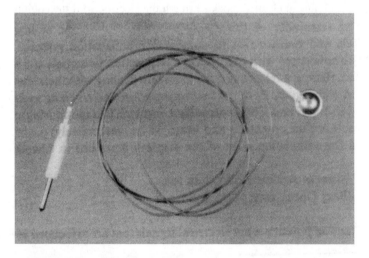

FIGURE 6–1 **Surface electrode, with insulated electric wire and connectors attached.**

and Hludik (1990), for example, describe a myoswitch that utilizes four sets of electrodes to detect vertical and horizontal eye movements.

Care must be taken in attaching surface electrodes to the skin. According to Smorto and Basmajian,

> *It is extremely important in applying surface electrodes to ensure that the electric insulation between the muscle and the electrode is reduced to a minimum. Since a poor contact must be avoided, continued pressure is obviously important. Fortunately, the pressure provided by the adhesive strips used for securing the electrodes is usually adequate. Electrical contact is greatly improved by the use of a saline "electrode jelly"; this is retained between the electrode and the skin by making the silver disk of the electrode slightly concave on the aspect to be applied to the skin. The dead surface layer of the skin along with its protective oils must be removed to lower the electrical resistance to practical levels of about 3,000 ohms. This is best done by light abrasion of the skin at the site chosen for electrode application. In recent years we have found that it is best produced by "rubbing in" those types of electrode jelly that have abrasive included in their formula. (1977, pp. 10–11)*

Muscle action potentials are very weak electrical signals, and thus have to be amplified to activate a display (e.g., a light or tone generator) and trigger a switching mechanism (e.g., a relay). An amplifier intended for low-level bioelectric signals is used for this purpose (see Figure 6–2). It should contain isolation and filtering circuits in addition to those circuits required for amplification. Isolation circuits prevent the user from receiving an electric shock (through the electrodes) if the equipment malfunctions. High-pass and low-pass filtering circuits restrict the frequency range of signals the unit will detect to that within which muscle action potentials fall. Without these filtering circuits, the unit may respond to other bioelectric signals as well, such as those associated with heart activity.

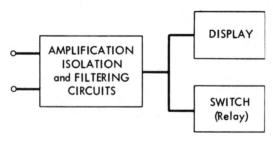

FIGURE 6–2 **Components of a myoswitch.**

After the muscle action potentials are amplified, they can be used to activate a display and a switching mechanism (see Figure 6–2). The purpose of the display, which can be an oscilloscope (or a microcomputer programmed to mimic one), a meter, a light, or a sound generator, is to make the user aware of the pattern of muscle action potentials detected by the electrodes so that he or she can learn to produce them to activate the communication aid.

Considerable evidence in the biofeedback literature suggests that if a covert bioelectric process (such as the generation of muscle action potentials) can be made overt, a person is likely to be able to gain some degree of voluntary control over it. Such a process can be made overt in several ways:

1. Displaying it on an oscilloscope screen (or on the monitor of a computer system programmed to mimic an oscilloscope)
2. Having it cause a light to go on when it is the appropriate magnitude
3. Having it cause a light to increase in brightness as it increases in magnitude
4. Having it cause a sound to be generated when it is the appropriate magnitude
5. Having it cause a sound to increase in volume as it increases in magnitude
6. Having it cause a sound to increase in pitch as it increases in magnitude
7. Having it cause the needle on a meter to move in a particular direction

Accordingly, the user would be instructed to look at or listen to the display and attempt to cause one of the following to occur:

1. An increase in the height of the electrical signals displayed on the oscilloscope or monitor screen
2. A light to turn on (or off)
3. A light to increase in brightness
4. A sound to be generated
5. A sound to increase in volume
6. A sound to increase in pitch
7. The needle on a meter to move in a particular direction

The user would know when he or she observed one of these occurring that he or she had been successful in varying the bioelectric signal in the manner necessary for controlling the communication aid. The user may not be aware consciously of specifically what he or she did to vary the signal (awareness of the control process on this level usually is not essential). He or she would practice until changes in light, tone, needle position, or waveform occurred whenever the user wished. Then the user would be ready to use the bioelectric signal to activate the switching mechanism of a communication aid.

Amplified muscle action potentials that will activate a display can also be used to activate a switching mechanism (Figure 6–2). Switching mechanisms that can be activated in this manner are likely to contain one of three electrical components: a relay, a solenoid, or an integrated circuit.

A relay has three parts that allow it to function as a switch: two strips of metal that serve as electrical contacts and an electromagnet (see Figure 6–3). The two metal strips metal are mounted perpendicular to each other so that their ends are slightly separated when the electromagnet mounted beneath the horizontal one is not energized. When the electromagnet is energized (by a signal abstracted from the amplified muscle action potentials), it pulls the horizontal strip downward, causing its end to contact that of the vertical one. This "closes the bridge" (see Figure 5–24) or activates the switch. The electromagnet would not be energized until the muscle action potentials were of sufficient magnitude to cause a display to function in one of the ways described in this section.

A solenoid consists of an electromagnet and a pivoted metal strip, or arm, that is mounted in close proximity to it (Figure 6–3). When the electromagnet is energized, the part of the arm that is in close proximity to it is pulled toward it. This causes the end of the arm to move a fraction of an inch. If a push switch such as a lever microswitch (see chapter 5) is mounted slightly below the arm, the arm will depress it when the electromagnet is energized.

Integrated circuits are more likely to be used in myoswitches than are solenoids or relays. They tend to be more reliable because they have no moving parts. Also, the

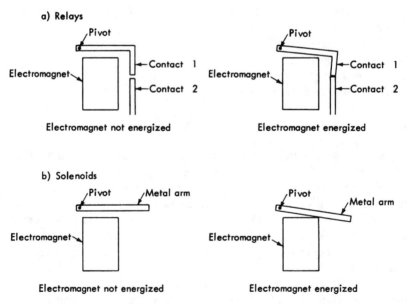

FIGURE 6–3   **Function of the electromagnets in relays and solenoids.**

time it takes for a myoswitch with an integrated circuit to be ready to be activated again is shorter than it is for one containing a solenoid or relay.

Myoswitches that can be used to control communication aids are available commercially. The one illustrated in Figure 6–4 can monitor muscle action potentials with surface electrodes at either one or two sites. When monitored at only one site, it functions as a single-switch switching mechanism.

There are two basic types of muscle action potential patterns that have been used to control neuro-assisted communication systems. One is an increase in magnitude when a user wishes to activate a switch followed by a decrease. A myoswitch used in this manner can perform any of the functions of a switching mechanism containing a single switch.

The second type consists of alternating periods of increase and decrease that correspond to patterns of dots and dashes in Morse code (see Table 4–3). These patterns can be produced in several ways. A relatively short muscle contraction can stand for a dot and a longer one for a dash. It is crucial that the dots do not overlap the dashes (with regard to duration of contraction). Another way that these patterns can be produced is to use a unit containing two myoswitches (see Figure 6–4). Each

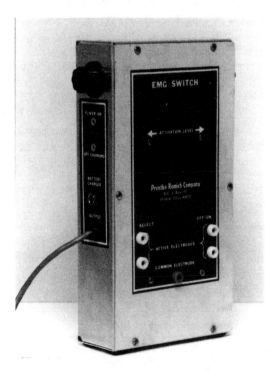

FIGURE 6–4 **A myoswitch.**

monitors the activity of a different muscle (e.g., one on the right arm and one on the left arm). The user would contract one muscle when he wished to produce a dot and the other to produce a dash. The resulting Morse code pattern could be translated into English by a computer and the message displayed on a monitor or printed out.

What factors should be considered when deciding whether a particular muscle (or muscles) can be used for activating a myoswitch? There are several:

1. The ease with which the muscle (or muscles) can be contracted: The greater the ease, the more usable the muscle for the purpose.
2. Whether or not the muscle contracts involuntarily: If a muscle contracts involuntarily because of a neuromuscular disorder, it may activate the aid, thereby interfering with message transmission.
3. The ease with which electrodes can be attached to the skin without interfering with ongoing or daily activities: Some electrode locations are likely to interfere more with such activities than are others.
4. The electrical resistance of the skin: There are some locations on the body at which it is easier to lower the resistance of the skin to an acceptable level than it is at others.
5. The closeness of the muscle to the skin: The closer the muscle to the skin, the more successful one is likely to be in monitoring its action potentials by surface electrodes.

It is desirable, but not essential, that the muscle(s) used to activate a myoswitch function normally. If a person can contract some of the fibers in a muscle whenever he or she wishes to, and none of the fibers in it contract involuntarily, it may be usable for activating a microswitch.

All the symbol sets described in chapter 5 that are usable with electronic gestural-assisted communication aids are also usable with communication aids that are controlled by myoswitches. Also, the components of the control electronics for gestural-assisted communication aids are usable with the type described here.

For further information about communication aids that can be controlled by muscle action potentials, see Combs (1969), Dewan (1966), LaCourse & Hludik (1990), Nishikawa et al. (1984), Rice and Combs (1972), Torok (1974), and Writing made possible . . . (1966). Also, the literature on electromyography biofeedback and, in physical medicine and physical therapy, on the use of muscle action potentials to control such devices as wheelchairs provide useful information about designing and fabricating myoswitches and teaching people how to use them.

BRAIN WAVES

There is some suggestion in the literature (Dewan, 1966) that the *alpha rhythm in the brain*, as detected by surface electrodes attached to the scalp over the occipital lobe, can be controlled sufficiently well to generate a Morse code pattern that can be used to spell out messages on a CRT display (computer monitor). Alpha rhythm can be enhanced or reduced to form dots and dashes by controlling eye function (Dewan, 1966; Mulholland & Evans, 1965). According to Dewan,

> *if the subject becomes alert or focuses his eyes with his eyes open (or, with practice, even with them closed) this rhythm tends to disappear, whereas it tends to be enhanced when the subject relaxes with his eyes closed and with minimal concentration or "visualization." Recently, T. Mulholland and the present author independently noticed that eye position can also play an important role, the upward position tending to enhance alpha activity. (1966, p. 349)*

Dewan trained three persons (who were normal neurologically) to send alpha dots and dashes "by altering their eye position, focusing muscles, and in some cases, by opening and closing the eyes" (1966, p. 349) accurately enough to type out messages character by character on a teletypewriter. The time need for sending each character was more than 30 seconds. He was able to rule out the possibility that the EEG Morse code actually was being sent by neck muscle contractions.

The biofeedback training procedures used would be the same as those for EMG biofeedback.

A second possibility for utilizing brain waves to interface a client with an augmentative communication device is through changes in the P300 component of the event-related brain potential (ERP). When persons are assigned a task that requires them to determine to which of two possible categories each item in a series belongs, and one of the items occurs rarely, these rare items will elicit an ERP with an enhanced positive-going component with a latency of about 300 milliseconds, labeled the P300 (Farwell & Donchin, 1988). Such a series could consist of the letters of the alphabet. They could be displayed in rows and columns on a computer monitor screen. The cursor could be programmed to move from one to the other after a specified number of seconds (linear scanning strategy). The user would assign each letter indicated by the cursor to one of two categories: the next letter in the message or not the next letter in the message. The first would be the category containing the rare item—the appropriate letter. Mentally assigning a letter to this category would result in a change in brain waves (in P300), which, when detected, would function like any other kind of single-switch switching mechanism—that is, cause the letter to be selected. Farwell and Donchin (1988) have described instrumentation that can be used to detect P300 and have reported data on its applicability for augmentative communication.

A third possibility for utilizing brain waves is through the phenomenon known as *alpha band asymmetry*. Alpha brain wave power tends to be less in the left hemisphere of the cerebral cortex than in the right during the performance of verbal tasks and less in the right than in the left during the performance of spatial tasks, including nonmotor ones (Keirn & Aunon, 1990). An example of a nonmotor verbal task would be mentally composing a letter to a friend, and an example of a nonmotor spatial one would be visualizing a geometric figure being rotated in space. Two sets of electrodes—one over the left cerebral hemisphere and one over the right—would be used to detect hemispheric changes in alpha brain wave power. To control a single-switch scanning communication aid, the client could do a brief verbal task to turn the switch "on" and a brief spatial one to turn it "off." Keirn and Aunon (1990) have reported data suggesting that it may be possible to interface a client with a communication device in this way.

The components of an EEG switch are similar to those of a myoswitch (see Figure 6–2). Similar types of surface electrodes, displays, electronic circuits, and switching mechanisms are used. Because it appears that messages can be transmitted at a faster rate by EMG than by EEG (Dewan, 1966; Farwell & Donchin, 1988), the former probably would be preferable in most instances.

▶ 7

Assessment Procedures

Many communication strategies have been described that can be used to augment speech and other communication abilities. This chapter provides guidelines for selecting from among them the one (or ones) most likely to be optimal for a particular client. The optimal communication strategy for a person is the one that would come closest to meeting his or her communication needs at a relatively low cost. Cost refers here not only to the expense of purchasing and maintaining components (switching mechanisms, displays, etc.) but also to the time investments required of both client and clinician.

In assessing an optimal augmentative communication strategy, seven questions need to be answered:

1. What is the cause of the person's communicative disorder?
2. How does the person currently communicate?
3. What are the person's communication needs?
4. How well does the person perform the communication activities needed in his or her environment?
5. What is the person's inner, receptive, and expressive language status?
6. Of the augmentative communication strategies, which would the person be able to use?
7. Of the usable strategies, which would be optimal for meeting the person's communication needs?

Types of information are indicated that usually have to be obtained to answer these questions. They can be gathered through observation and interviewing informants in the clinical setting and/or in the client's natural environment—home or school (Kangas & Allen, 1992). Those mentioned, of course, are not the only ones that ever would be needed for this purpose. They are, however, ones that would be needed to answer these questions for almost all severely communicatively impaired children and adults.

WHAT IS THE CAUSE OF THE DISORDER?

At the start, it is important to know the nature of the condition responsible for the person being severely communicatively impaired. Certain aspects of this information, including those listed here, could influence the choice of a communication strategy.

Whether the condition is progressive. If a person has a progressive neurological condition, it would be important to consider how long he or she would be likely to be able to use each of the various strategies that could be selected. Ideally, a strategy (or strategies) should be selected that the client can use for a relatively long period of time.

The impact of the condition on the functioning of the musculature of the extremities, trunk, face, and neck. If the musculature of one or both upper extremities functions normally, a manual gestural strategy might be considered. And if some trunk muscle groups function normally, they might be usable for activating a switching mechanism.

The impact of the condition on cognitive and sensory functioning. If either cognitive or sensory functioning is disturbed, this, of course, can influence both the choice of a symbol set and the approach used to indicate (or generate) message components.

The permanence of the impact of the condition on speech. If the impact on speech is temporary (which could be the case for a person seen shortly after a stroke before there has been much opportunity for spontaneous recovery), a different strategy might initially be selected than if the impact were likely to be permanent.

The prognosis for ambulation. If a person is likely to be confined to a bed or wheelchair, some strategies (e.g., a large communication board) tend to be more practical than if he or she is likely to be ambulatory.

Whether there is litigation pending. If the condition resulted from trauma and there is litigation pending, this could reduce a person's motivation to learn to communicate more effectively.

The stage at which the person is in the grieving process. If the person is very depressed and the depression is not directly related to his or her inability to communicate, it may be difficult to get the person to use any augmentative communication strategy.

Information about a client's condition and its impact on his or her motor, sensory, and cognitive functioning can be obtained from the physician and from the physical and occupational therapists if he or she is receiving or has received these services. It also can often be obtained from those who are taking care of the client (e.g., nurses and family members).

HOW DOES THE PERSON CURRENTLY COMMUNICATE?

Almost all severely communicatively impaired persons have some ability to communicate. Their communication may be limited to yes and no gestures to answer questions, or it may be limited to eye gaze, changes in body orientation, contact gestures such as giving and showing, and/or making "upset" kinds of noises (McLean et al., 1991; Romski, Sevcik, Reumann, & Pate, 1989). These strategies, of course, are similar to how an infant communicates.

The information about how a client currently communicates can suggest possible communication strategies. For example, if the client were using mime (pantomime) or a nonstandard manual gestural code, it probably would be possible to teach him or her to use Amer-Ind or Ameslan. In addition, it can indicate whether there is a need to augment his or her speech and gestural communication (which is usually the case), or whether this is so severely impaired that a communication strategy is needed to serve as an alternative to or substitute. This information also provides a baseline for assessing the impact of intervention with a particular strategy on a person's ability to communicate.

The clinician should investigate both speech and nonspeech channels when attempting to determine how a person communicates. Nonspeech channels include nonverbal (gestural) aspects of oral communication—writing, typing, and other strategies described in chapters 4, 5, and 6. It is conceivable that a person being evaluated has been taught to use a strategy described in these chapters or has learned to use it on his or her own. The kinds of information that are needed to describe how a child or adult communicates are the following:

The person's use of speech. The focus here is on the person's ability to use words, word approximations, and other vocal sounds (including inflection patterns) for communication. If the person uses word approximations or sounds generated by the vocal tract that are intelligible to others, these can be considered to be part of his or her speech communication.

The person's use of writing. It is important to determine how well the person can encode and transmit messages by writing or printing with a pen or pencil. If the person is hemiplegic on the dominant side, his or her ability to write with both right and left hands should be evaluated.

The person's ability to type. It would be particularly important to determine how well the person could type if he or she was unable to print or write intelligibly. If the person has access to a microcomputer with word processing software, it also would be important to determine how well he or she can use the keyboard.

The person's ability to communicate by gesture. Of interest here would be face and body gestures that accompany attempts at speech, pointing to desired objects, mime (pantomime), and use of the gestural strategies described in chapter 4. Some severely speech-impaired persons (including young children) develop their own gestural communication to compensate for the impairment (Thal & Tobias, 1992). It is particularly important to determine whether the person has reliable yes and no gestures, and if so, what those gestures are.

The person's ability to understand speech and to read. The focus here is on how well the person does these at home and elsewhere.

The person's comprehension of gesture. The focus here is on gestures that most people can understand, such as facial and body gestures accompanying speech, shaking the head yes and no, shrugging the shoulders, and simple mime.

The person's knowledge of Morse code. It would only be important to determine this if the client were so involved motorically that a strategy might be considered in which Morse code is used for generating message components. He or she might have learned it in Boy Scouts, or in the army, or while meeting the requirements for an FCC ham radio license.

In addition to determining how the person communicates, it is also important to determine how often he or she attempts to do so in various ways. If the person does not attempt to communicate very often, this could have one of several implications with regard to a willingness to use augmentative communication.

First, attempting to communicate often could indicate that the person probably would use augmentative communication. This is particularly likely to be the case if the reason for his or her not communicating often is being unsuccessful doing so or finding it too fatiguing. Second, not attempting to communicate very often could indicate that the person would be unwilling to accept augmentative communication. It could have this implication if he or she is not communicating often because of depression. If the person's depression is specifically related to not being able to communicate, it is unlikely to interfere with the acceptance of augmentative communication. If, however, it is primarily related to the person's reaction to the condition that caused him or her to become severely communicatively impaired or something else other than not being able to communicate, it may have to be decreased or eliminated before the client would be willing to use any communication strategy.

A person may not be communicating much because he or she has relatively little need or opportunity to communicate. This is likely to be so if the person lives alone or is a resident of an institution such as a nursing home or a facility for the mentally retarded. By increasing his or her need and opportunity to communicate, there is a greater likelihood that he or she will use augmentative communication.

Finally, in addition to determining how and how often the person communicates, it is important to determine what messages he or she is able to communicate and by what means (Smith, 1991). What words and ideas has the person been successful in communicating by speech, gesture, or a combination of the two? Persons with whom he or she communicates frequently should be asked to make a list of the words and ideas he or she has communicated to them and to indicate how it was done.

WHAT ARE THE PERSON'S COMMUNICATION NEEDS?

A client's communication needs are determined primarily through interviews with informants who are involved in the person's life: parents and other family members, friends, teachers, employers, and care staff (Beukelman & Garrett, 1988). The person may also be consulted when determining them. These communication needs can range from being able to communicate a few basic desires to the staff in a hospital or nursing home to being able to function as a professional, including using a telephone and a microcomputer with word processing software.

It is necessary to consider face-to-face communication, telephone communication, and written communication when defining a person's communication needs. Some persons will require augmentative communication strategies for all three, and others will require them for only one or two. A single strategy may be usable for two or three of them (e.g., one containing a microcomputer), or a different strategy may be used for each.

When defining a client's communication needs (i.e., developing a communication needs statement), the clinician must take into consideration the comprehension abilities of the persons with whom the client will have to communicate. If, for example, the client needs to be able to communicate with young children, an aid for face-to-face communication that generated speech would be more appropriate than would one that generated printed English.

HOW WELL DOES THE PERSON PERFORM THE COMMUNICATION ACTIVITIES NEEDED IN HIS OR HER ENVIRONMENT?

The ultimate goal of intervention with augmentative communication is to meet a person's functional communication needs—those in his or her environment (Frattali & Lynch, 1989). This goal is fully attainable in some cases, and in others it can only be approached.

The clinician should make a judgment concerning the extent to which the person's communication ability meets his or her communication needs. A person is encountered occasionally who, though limited in ability to communicate, can communicate well enough to meet those needs. Such a person probably would not be a good candidate for augmentative communication. You, of course, would have to be confident that a person's communication ability was adequate for meeting his or her needs before ruling out augmentative communication on this basis. And you would want to reevaluate such a person if his or her communication abilities and/or needs changed.

This question should be answered as objectively as possible both prior to and following intervention through use of a functional assessment (see Beukelman, Yorkston, & Lossing, 1984; Frattali & Lynch, 1989). The differences between the pre- and postintervention answers can be used to document the impact of the intervention on the client.

WHAT IS THE PERSON'S INNER, RECEPTIVE, AND EXPRESSIVE LANGUAGE STATUS?

Inner Language Status

A person's inner language status is partly a function of his or her ability to make sense out of the sensory environment (Myklebust, 1954). If a person does not abstract the units of experience (e.g., objects) that are symbolized by words, gestures, and the like, he or she will not understand those symbols or be able to use them. He or she also will be unable to learn other symbols for them (e.g., Blissymbols).

Inner language can be partly evaluated by determining the extent to which a person is aware of how things are organized in the environment. For example, for a child whose use of the upper extremities is reasonably good, the following objects can be arranged randomly on a table in front of him or her: a dollhouse table, four chairs that will fit around it, and a doll family that can be positioned to sit in the chairs. If with little hesitation the child places the chairs around the table and attempts to seat the dolls in the chairs, this would suggest that inner language functioning is at least at a 2-year-old level (Weber, 1972).

Receptive Language Status

To determine a person's receptive language status, it is necessary to assess his or her ability to understand speech and nonverbal (gestural) communication and to read. If a person experiences difficulty understanding speech because of a hearing loss, auditory agnosia, or receptive aphasia, this can interfere with the use of any augmentative communication strategy described in this book. The extent to which it is likely to interfere is partly a function of the type and severity of the auditory impairment. Of course, even with a severe auditory impairment (e.g., deafness), it is still possible to gain some benefit from augmentative communication.

A number of tests and parts of tests can be used to estimate how well a person understands speech (see Roth & Cassatt-James, 1989). Almost all aphasia tests contain items usable for this purpose. Also, there are a number of tests intended for assessing child language (e.g., the Peabody Picture Vocabulary Test; see Dunn & Dunn, 1981) that contain such items.

Either a rotary or a rectangular matrix display with a scanning response mode can be used to assess the speech comprehension of persons who are unable to point, through the use of a multiple-choice format. The rectangular matrix display can be a dedicated one or it can be simulated by a microcomputer on a monitor screen. A set of stimuli consisting of photographs, drawings, words, or other symbols (see chapter 5) can be mounted temporarily on one of these displays. The person being tested can indicate the member of the set he or she thinks is the correct response by manipulating a switching mechanism. If the Peabody Picture Vocabulary Test were administered in this manner, the four drawings presented for each stimulus word would be mounted temporarily on the display, one set at a time, and the person would indicate the drawing he or she thought illustrated a particular one by manipulating a switching mechanism. This approach could also be used for assessing reading ability and, possibly, comprehension of gestures.

Persons who have difficulty understanding nonverbal or gestural communication are also likely to have difficulty learning to use augmentative communication strategies, particularly the gestural type described in chapter 4. A person's ability to understand gestural communication can be better than, the same as, or worse than his or her ability to understand speech. It would tend to be better than speech for the deaf and the same as or worse than speech for some brain-damaged persons (Duffy, Duffy, & Pearson, 1975).

Procedures for assessing comprehension of gestures are not as well standardized as are those for evaluating speech comprehension. One task for the purpose would be instructing the person by mime (pantomime) to manipulate some objects (e.g., put a ball in the cup). An appropriate response would suggest that the gestural instructions were understood. It, of course, is important before using a mime to make certain that a "normal" person of the examinee's age can understand it, particularly if the examinee is a child.

Persons who have difficulty reading English may still be able to use an English language symbol set (see chapter 5). Whether they can would depend on several factors, including their ability to read English, the prognosis for improving this ability, and their communication needs.

There are a number of achievement tests for determining how well a child can read. Items that can be used for determining reading level in adults are included in most aphasia tests. If items have a multiple-choice response format, they can be adapted for severely motorically impaired persons by temporarily mounting the possible responses on a rotary scanning display or rectangular matrix display (see chapter 5). Such test adaptations, however, may affect test performance (Bristow & Fristoe, 1987).

Expressive Language Status

Expressive language includes the abilities to speak, to communicate by gestures, and to write. Knowing a person's speech level is important because no matter what augmentative strategy is selected, he or she is always encouraged to use speech along with the strategy. A person's speech level also influences the choice of a communication strategy. If a person has some usable speech, he or she may not require as flexible a strategy as would be needed otherwise. There are items for determining speech level in almost all aphasia tests and in tests of children's language development.

A person's ability and willingness to communicate by gesture can influence the choice of a communication strategy. If a person uses gesture, it suggests that he or she finds communicating with it acceptable. Consequently, the person is less likely to resist learning a formal gestural system (e.g., Ameslan or Amer-Ind) than would otherwise be the case. Items that can be adapted for evaluating a person's ability to communicate by gesture can be found in several language tests, including the Parson's Language Sample (Spradlin, 1963), the Illinois Test of Psycholinguistic Abilities (Kirk, McCarthy, & Kirk, 1968), the Let's Talk Inventory for Adolescents (Sutton, 1989), and the Porch Test of Communicative Ability (Porch, 1971).

Communicating by writing can partially compensate for the inability to communicate by speech. All severely communicatively impaired persons (except possibly preschool children and adults who have very limited communication needs) should be provided with a strategy for generating printed messages if they are unable to write. Such a strategy may involve the use of a microcomputer with word processing software (Berninger & Gans, 1986). Items for assessing an adult's writing ability can be found on most aphasia tests. A child's writing ability can be assessed by standardized achievement tests.

For further information about assessing the language competence and performance of persons who are severely communicatively impaired, see Nelson (1992).

OF THE AUGMENTATIVE COMMUNICATION STRATEGIES, WHICH WOULD THE PERSON BE ABLE TO USE?

When selecting an augmentative communication strategy for a child or adult, initially all existing types should be considered. Doing so maximizes the probability that at least one strategy will be identified that the person could use. It also maximizes the probability that the communication strategy that will be optimal will be among those identified.

Three general aspects of functioning should be considered when attempting to determine whether a person could use a particular strategy: motor, sensory, and cognitive. Approaches are described in this section for evaluating each to determine whether it is sufficiently intact for use with a particular communication strategy.

Motor Functioning

It is necessary to evaluate motor functioning if the person has or is suspected of having an apraxia or a neuromuscular disorder. A person's motor status is one of the primary determinants of the communication strategies he or she can use. The less impaired a person is motorically, the greater the number of strategies and the more efficient the strategies he or she would be able to use. Almost any message can be transmitted faster and with less energy drain by a manual gestural strategy such as Ameslan or Amer-Ind (see chapter 4) than by an aid controlled by a myoswitch (see chapter 6).

There are two basic approaches that can be used for evaluating motor functioning. One is to attempt to elicit all overt bodily movements that could be used for augmentative communication. Because almost any movement could be used for this purpose, the functioning of almost the entire motor system would have to be evaluated, including that of the four extremities, the trunk, and the face and neck. Such an evaluation could take a great deal of time.

The alternative approach is to attempt to elicit only certain overt bodily movements that could be used for augmentative communication. Selection of this subset of movements could be based on a series of assumptions:

1. If a person does not have (or is not suspected of having) an apraxia or a neuromuscular disorder, it is unnecessary to evaluate motor functioning.
2. The muscle groups that are most desirable to use for augmentative communication are those of the upper extremities. Thus, these are the muscle groups to be evaluated first. If the functioning of the musculature of one or both upper extremities appears normal or adequate for a communication strategy that would meet the person's needs, further evaluation of muscle functioning is unnecessary.
3. The musculature of the face or neck is the most desirable for augmentative communication after the upper extremities. Thus, these muscle groups are evaluated second. If the functioning of a portion of this musculature appears adequate, further evaluation of muscle functioning is unnecessary.
4. The musculature of the lower extremities or trunk (particularly the latter) is almost always the least desirable for augmentative communication. One exception might be a person in a wheelchair who has the ability to control a switching mechanism, particularly a keyboard, with a foot. Thus, this musculature is usually evaluated last.

Note that with this approach it is necessary to assess all overt bodily movements only when the musculature of the upper extremities, face, and neck appears inadequate for a communication strategy that will meet the person's needs.

Several factors should be considered when assessing the adequacy of a particular gesture (or movement) for interfacing a person with (or allowing him or her to use) a particular communication strategy:

The *accuracy* with which it can be produced

The *speed* with which it can be produced

The *force* (pressure) it can exert

The presence of *hyperactive stretch reflexes* and other abnormal reflexes associated with spasticity

The presence of *tremor* or other involuntary movement

The extent to which doing it *fatigues* the person

The greater the potential accuracy, speed, and force of the movement and the less it tends to tire the client, the more useful it will be for interfacing him or her with a communication strategy. In contrast, hyperactive stretch reflexes or involuntary movement can reduce its usefulness.

Two approaches can be used to assess the adequacy of a particular muscle gesture for a particular communication strategy. The first, or direct, approach, is to have the person use the gesture in the context of the strategy. To determine the person's ability to produce a particular hand gesture necessary for Amer-Ind or Ameslan, he or she would be asked to imitate an Amer-Ind or Ameslan sign containing that gesture. To evaluate the person's ability to produce the gesture needed for activating a particular switching mechanism, he or she could be observed while attempting to activate that switching mechanism. For further information about this approach in the context of motor requirements for producing manual signs, see McEwen and Lloyd (1990).

Although the direct method provides highly reliable information about the adequacy of a particular gesture for a particular communication strategy, it has several limitations. First, it might not be possible to have all or even most of the communication aids available that the person could use. Few clinical facilities can afford to keep on hand the hardware for the variety of communication aids that might be needed by their clients. A second limitation is that it may be more time- and energy-consuming than necessary. Several communication strategies that a person could use may require the same gesture; a given gesture, for example, may be usable for activating more than one switching mechanism.

The second approach that can be used to determine the adequacy of particular muscle gestures for a particular communication strategy is systematically evaluating the gestures that could be used for the purpose. The examinee is asked to imitate these gestures, and their adequacy is described. The assumption is made that if the examinee can produce the gesture (or gestures) required to use a particular communication strategy, he or she will be able to use that strategy. With this approach, then, the adequacy of a person's gestures is inferred rather than observed (as in the direct approach). Such inferences can usually be made quite reliably if the examiner is acquainted with the motor requirements of the communication strategies being considered. This approach tends to be more practical than the direct method because a great deal of hardware is not necessary.

A procedure for systematically implementing the inferred approach is outlined in this section. The primary source for our discussion of gestures is Daniels and Worthingham's *Muscle Testing* (1986). This book contains detailed descriptions and drawings of each gesture.

The gestures evaluated are divided into two groups: upper extremities and face and neck. Each gesture, if possible, should be evaluated first against gravity. If the person is unable to produce the gesture normally under this condition, it is then evaluated with gravity eliminated. A gesture that can be performed reasonably well with gravity eliminated but not against gravity can be used for some purposes in interfacing a person with a communication aid.

For persons who are so severely impaired motorically that they are unable to produce the needed gestures even with gravity eliminated, the examiner should note whether there is any evidence of muscle contraction when they attempt to produce each gesture. If there is contraction under this condition, the gesture might be usable for activating a myoswitch (see chapter 6).

Gestures Involving the Upper Extremities

Twenty-seven gestures are described in this section. Each should be evaluated for accuracy, speed, force, presence of abnormal reflexes, presence of involuntary movement, and fatigue level for both right and left extremities.

1. *Scapular abduction and upward rotation.* To test against gravity, the person lies on his back with the arm being evaluated flexed to 90 degrees with slight abduction and the elbow in extension. He attempts to move the arm upward by abducting the scapula. To test without gravity, the person sits with the arm being evaluated, resting on a table, flexed to 90 degrees. He attempts to move the arm forward by abducting the scapula.

2. *Scapular elevation.* To test against gravity, the person sits, with his arms at his sides, and attempts to raise his shoulders as high as possible. To test without gravity, the person lies on his stomach with his forehead touching the surface on which he is lying and his shoulders supported by the examiner. He attempts to move his shoulders toward his ears. (Obviously, a person would not lie on his stomach to communicate. This posture is only used for testing.)

3. *Scapular adduction.* To test against gravity, the person lies on his stomach, with the arm being evaluated abducted to 90 degrees and laterally rotated and with the elbow flexed to a right angle. The examiner stabilizes his thorax. He attempts to raise the arm in horizontal abduction. To test without gravity, the person sits with the arm being evaluated resting on a table, midway between flexion and abduction. The examiner stabilizes his thorax. He attempts to abduct the arm horizontally and, if successful, adducts the scapula.

4. *Scapular depression and adduction.* To test against gravity, the person lies on his stomach, with his forehead resting on the surface on which he is lying and with the arm being tested extended overhead. The patient attempts to raise the arm and move scapula upward.

5. *Shoulder flexion to 90 degrees.* To test against gravity, the person sits, with the arm being tested at his side and with the elbow slightly flexed. The examiner stabilizes his scapula. He attempts to flex (raise) his arm to 90 degrees. To test without gravity, the person lies on the side not being tested, with the arm being tested at his side and the elbow slightly flexed. The examiner stabilizes his scapula. He attempts to bring his arm forward to 90 degrees of flexion.

6. *Shoulder extension.* To test against gravity, the person lies on his stomach, with the arm being tested medially rotated and adducted (at side). The examiner stabilizes his scapula. He attempts to extend (raise) the arm. To test without gravity, the person lies on the side not being tested, with the arm being tested flexed (at his side) and resting on a smooth board. The examiner stabilizes his scapula. He attempts to extend the arm (i.e., to slide it backward on the surface of the board).

7. *Shoulder abduction to 90 degrees.* To test against gravity, the person sits, with the arm being tested at his side in midposition between medial and lateral rotation and the elbow slightly flexed. The examiner stabilizes his scapula. He attempts to abduct (raise) the arm to 90 degrees. To test without gravity, the person lies on his back, with the arm being tested at his side in midposition between medial and lateral rotation. The examiner stabilizes his scapula. He attempts to abduct the arm to 90 degrees.

8. *Shoulder horizontal abduction.* To test against gravity, the person lies on his stomach, with the shoulder being tested abducted to 90 degrees, the upper arm resting on the surface on which he is lying and the lower arm hanging vertically over the edge. The examiner stabilizes his scapula. He attempts to abduct (raise) the upper arm. To test without gravity, the person sits with the arm being tested supported (e.g., on a tabletop) in a position of 90 degrees of flexion. The examiner stabilizes his scapula. He attempts to horizontally abduct the arm (i.e., move it backward on the surface).

9. *Shoulder horizontal adduction.* To test against gravity, the person lies on his back, with the arm being tested abducted to 90 degrees. He attempts to adduct the arm (i.e., move it toward the midline of the body). To test without gravity, the person sits with the arm being tested resting on a table in 90 degrees of abduction. The examiner stabilizes his trunk. He attempts to bring the arm forward.

10. *Shoulder lateral rotation.* To test against gravity, the person lies on his stomach, with the shoulder being tested abducted to 90 degrees, upper arm resting on the surface on which he is lying and the lower arm hanging vertically over the edge. The examiner stabilizes the scapula. He attempts to swing his lower arm forward and upward and to laterally rotate his shoulder. To test without gravity, the person lies on his stomach with the entire arm being tested hanging over the surface on which he is lying in medially rotated position. The examiner stabilizes his scapula. He attempts to laterally rotate the arm.

11. *Shoulder medial rotation.* To test against gravity, the person lies on his stomach with the shoulder being tested abducted to 90 degrees, upper arm supported on the surface on which he is lying, and the lower arm hanging vertically over the edge. The examiner stabilizes the scapula. He attempts to swing his lower arm backward and upward and medially rotate the shoulder. To test without gravity, the person lies on his stomach with the arm of the extremity being tested hanging over the edge of the surface on which he is lying in lateral rotation. The examiner stabilizes the scapula. He attempts to medially rotate the arm.

12. *Elbow flexion.* To test against gravity, the person sits, with the arm being tested at his side and forearm supinated. The examiner stabilizes his upper arm. He attempts to flex the elbow. To test without gravity, the person lies on his back, with the shoulder of the extremity being tested abducted to 90 degrees and laterally rotated. The examiner stabilizes his upper arm. He attempts to flex the elbow by sliding his forearm along the table.

13. *Elbow extension.* To test against gravity, the person lies on his back, with the shoulder of the extremity being tested flexed to 90 degrees and the elbow flexed. The examiner stabilizes his arm. He attempts to extend the elbow. To test without gravity, the person lies on his back, with the arm being tested abducted to 90 degrees and laterally rotated, with the elbow flexed. The examiner stabilizes his arm. He attempts to extend the elbow by sliding his forearm along the table.

14. *Forearm supination.* The person sits, with the arm being tested at his side, elbow flexed to 90 degrees, and forearm pronated. The examiner stabilizes his arm. He attempts to supinate the forearm.

15. *Forearm pronation.* The person sits, with the arm being tested at his side, elbow flexed to 90 degrees, and forearm supinated. The examiner stabilizes his arm. He attempts to pronate the forearm.

16. *Wrist flexion.* The person sits, with the forearm of the extremity being tested resting on a table supinated. The examiner stabilizes his forearm. He attempts to flex the wrist.

17. *Wrist extension.* The person sits, with the forearm of the extremity being tested resting on a table pronated. The examiner stabilizes his forearm. He attempts to extend the wrist.

18. *Flexion of metacarpophalangeal joints of fingers.* The person sits with the hand of the extremity being tested resting on a surface. The examiner stabilizes his metacarpals. He attempts to flex the fingers (all four together) at their metacarpophalangeal joints, keeping the interphalangeal joints extended.

19. *Flexion of interphalangeal joints of fingers.* To test flexion of the proximal interphalangeal joints, the person sits, with the hand of the extremity being tested resting (on a table) on the dorsal surface, palm upward with wrist and fingers extended. The examiner stabilizes the proximal phalanx of the finger being tested. The person attempts to flex the middle phalanx of this finger. To test flexion of the distal interphalangeal joints, the person sits, with the hand of the extremity being tested resting palm upward on a table with fingers extended. The examiner stabilizes the middle phalanx of the finger being tested. The person attempts to flex the distal phalanx of this finger.

20. *Extension of metacarpophalangeal joints of fingers.* The person sits, with the arm being tested resting on a table, with the hand supported by the examiner, wrist in midposition, fingers flexed. The examiner stabilizes his metacarpals. He attempts to extend the proximal row of phalanges (all four) with the interphalangeal joints partially flexed.

21. *Finger abduction.* The person sits, with the hand being tested supported by the examiner, palm downward with fingers adducted. The examiner stabilizes his metacarpals. He attempts to abduct the fingers.

22. *Finger adduction.* The person sits, with the hand being tested supported by the examiner, palm downward, fingers abducted. He attempts to adduct the fingers.

23. *Flexion of joints of thumb.* To test flexion of the metacarpophalangeal joint of a thumb, the person sits, with the hand being tested resting palm upward on a table. The examiner stabilizes the first metacarpal of his thumb. He attempts to flex the first phalanx of the thumb. To test flexion of the interphalangeal joint of a thumb, the person sits, with the hand being tested resting palm upward on a table. The examiner stabilizes the first phalanx of his thumb. He attempts to flex the distal phalanx of the thumb.

24. *Extension of joints of thumb.* To test extension of the metacarpophalangeal joint of a thumb, the person sits, with the hand being tested resting on a table. The examiner stabilizes the first metacarpal of his thumb. He attempts to extend the first phalanx of the thumb. To test extension of the interphalangeal joint of a thumb, the person sits, with the hand being tested resting on a table on the ulnar border. The examiner stabilizes the first phalanx of his thumb. He attempts to extend the distal phalanx of the thumb.

25. *Thumb abduction.* The person sits, with the hand being tested supported by the examiner. The examiner stabilizes the four metacarpals of the fingers and the wrist of this hand. He attempts to abduct the thumb by raising it vertically.

26. *Thumb adduction.* The person sits, with the hand being tested supported by the examiner. The examiner stabilizes the medial four metacarpals of the fingers of this hand. He attempts to adduct the thumb.

27. *Opposition of the thumb and fifth finger.* The person sits, with the hand being tested resting palm upward on a table. He attempts to bring the palmar surfaces of the distal phalanges of the thumb and fifth finger together.

Gestures Involving the Face and Neck
Fourteen gestures are described in this section. Again, each should be evaluated for accuracy, speed, force, presence of abnormal reflexes, presence of involuntary movement, and fatigue level.

1. *Neck flexion.* The person lies on his back. The examiner stabilizes his lower thorax. He attempts to flex the cervical spine (neck).
2. *Neck extension.* The person lies on the table on his stomach, with his head over the edge (neck in flexion). The examiner stabilizes the upper thoracic area and scapulae. He attempts to extend the cervical spine (neck).
3. *Moving head from side to side.* The person sits on a chair. The examiner stabilizes his shoulders. He attempts to turn his head to one side and then to the opposite side.
4. *Raise eyebrows.* The person, while in a sitting position, attempts to raise his eyebrows, which, if successful, forms horizontal wrinkles in the forehead.
5. *Close eyes.* The person, while in a sitting position, attempts to close both eyes tightly.

6. *Direct gaze to the right.* The person, while in a sitting position, attempts to move his eyes to the right.

7. *Direct gaze to the left.* The person, while in a sitting position, attempts to move his eyes to the left.

8. *Compress lips.* The person, while in a sitting position, attempts to approximate and compress his lips.

9. *Smile.* The person, while in a sitting position, attempts to raise the lateral angle of the mouth upward and lateralward.

10. *Suck.* The person, while in a sitting position, attempts to suck water through a straw.

11. *Blow.* The person, while in a sitting position, attempts to blow out a candle or a match.

12. *Phonate.* The person, while in a sitting or lying position, attempts to produce a speech or a nonspeech sound (e.g., a sustained vowel or a voluntary cough).

13. *Extend and retract tongue.* The person, while in a sitting position, attempts to protrude his tongue between the central incisors and then retract it.

14. *Close jaws.* The person, while in a sitting position, attempts to close his jaws tightly.

Implications of Motor Functioning Data

The results of a motor assessment are relevant when you are attempting to identify gestural, gestural-assisted, and neuro-assisted communication strategies that would be possible for a person to use. Some implications that the results have for this purpose are indicated here.

1. If the musculature of one upper extremity functioned essentially normally, the person would have the motor capability for learning a manual gestural strategy such as Amer-Ind. If the musculature of both upper extremities functioned normally, he or she probably would have the motor capability for learning any of the gestural strategies described in chapter 4.

2. If the musculature of an upper extremity functioned sufficiently well that a person could touch with a finger (or another part of the hand) any point on a communication board, he or she would have the motor capability to use one with a direct-selection response mode (see chapter 5).

3. If a person can produce certain gestures with an upper extremity reasonably normally (see Table 7–1), he or she probably has the motor capability for activating certain switching mechanisms that can interface him or her with an electronic gestural-assisted communication aid (see chapter 5). The person should be able to activate a switching mechanism that is marked with an X in Table 7–1 with the gesture indicated; he or she may be able to activate that marked with a ? with this gesture. The switching mechanisms listed in Table 7–1, of course, may not be the only ones that can be activated by a particular gesture, and there may be a switching mechanism in

TABLE 7–1 **Switching Mechanisms Activated by Particular Gestures of the Upper Extremities**

Switch Type	Scapular Abduction and Upward Rotation	Scapular Elevation	Scapular Adduction	Scapular Depression	Shoulder Flexion to 90°
Pushbutton					
Push plate					?
Paddle					
Sliding handle or foot trolley					
Wobblestick					?
Pillow, pad, or squeeze bulb	?	?	?	?	?
Tip, or tilt, switch					X
Magnetic reed switch					
Suck or blow switch					
Touch switch					
Sound-controlled switch					
Light-controlled switch				X	
Myoswitch		?	?	?	?
(location of electrodes)	Over serratus anterior	Over trapezius (superior fibers)	Over trapezius (middle fibers)	Over trapezius (lower fibers)	Over deltoideus (anterior fibers)

Switch Type	Shoulder Extension	Shoulder Abduction to 90°	Shoulder Horizontal Abduction	Shoulder Horizontal Abduction	Shoulder Lateral Rotation
Pushbutton					
Push plate	?		?	?	?
Paddle	?		X	?	
Sliding handle or foot trolley			?	?	
Wobblestick	?	?	X	X	
Pillow, pad, or squeeze bulb	X	?	X	X	X
Tip, or tilt, switch		X	?		?
Magnetic reed switch			?	?	
Suck or blow switch					
Touch switch	X	?	?		X
Sound-controlled switch					
Light-controlled switch	?	X	?	?	?
Myoswitch (location of electrodes)	Over latissimus dorsi	Over deltoideus	Over deltoideus (posterior fibers)	Over pectoralis major	Over infraspinatus

Continued

TABLE 7-1 *Continued*

Switch Type	Shoulder Medial Rotation	Elbow Flexion	Elbow Extension	Forearm Supination	Forearm Pronation
Pushbutton					
Push plate	?		X	?	?
Paddle			X		
Sliding handle or foot trolley					
Wobblestick			X		
Pillow, pad, or squeeze bulb	X	X	X	X	X
Tip, or tilt, switch	?	X	X	?	?
Magnetic reed switch					
Suck or blow switch					
Touch switch	X		X	X	X
Sound-controlled switch					
Light-controlled switch		?	X		
Myoswitch	?	?	?	?	?
(location of electrodes)	Over subscapularis	Over biceps brachii	Over triceps brachii	Over biceps brachii	Over pronator teres

Switch Type	Wrist Flexion	Wrist Extension	Flexion of Metacarpophalangeal Joints of Fingers	Flexion of Interphalangeal Joints of Fingers
Pushbutton			?	
Push plate	X	X		
Paddle	X	?		
Sliding handle or foot trolley				
Wobblestick		X		
Pillow, pad, or squeeze bulb	X	X	X	?
Tip, or tilt, switch				
Magnetic reed switch	?	?		
Suck or blow switch				
Touch switch	X	X	?	X
Sound-controlled switch				
Light-controlled switch				
Myoswitch	?	?		?
(location of electrodes)	Over flexor carpi radalis	Over extensor carpi radialis longus		Over flexor digitorum superficialis

Continued

TABLE 7-1 *Continued*

Switch Type	Extension of Metacarpophalangeal Joints of Fingers	Finger Abduction	Finger Finger Adduction	Flexion of Joints of Thumb
Pushbutton		?	?	?
Push plate		?		
Paddle				
Sliding handle or foot trolley				
Wobblestick				?
Pillow, pad, or squeeze bulb		?	?	
Tip, or tilt, switch				
Magnetic reed switch		?		
Suck or blow switch				
Touch switch		?	X	X
Sound-controlled switch				
Light-controlled switch				
Myoswitch	?			?
(location of electrodes)	Over extensor digitorum communis			Over flexor pollicis

Switch Type	Extension of Joints of Thumb	Thumb Abduction	Thumb Adduction	Opposition of Thumb and Fifth Finger
Pushbutton		?	?	
Push plate		?		
Paddle				
Sliding handle or foot trolley				
Wobblestick				
Pillow, pad, or squeeze bulb		?	?	?
Tip, or tilt, switch				
Magnetic reed switch				
Suck or blow switch				
Touch switch		?	X	X
Sound-controlled switch				
Light-controlled switch				
Myoswitch	?	?	?	
(location of electrodes)	Over extensor pollicis	Over abductor pollicis	Over adductor pollicis	

187

this table not marked with an X or ? for a particular gesture that can be activated with it. All the switching mechanisms in the table are described in chapter 5.

4. If the musculature of the neck functioned essentially normally, the person probably would have the motor capability for using a communication board with a direct-selection response mode, indicating message components with a headstick (see chapter 5).

5. If the musculature of the mandible and neck functioned essentially normally, the person probably would have the motor capability for using a communication board with a direct-selection response mode, indicating message components with a mouth-stick (see chapter 5).

6. If the musculature of the eyes functioned normally, the person probably would have the motor capability for using a communication board, such as the ETRAN or ETRAN-N, with a direct-selection or encoding response mode, indicating message components by directing gaze, or eyepointing (see chapter 5).

7. If the person can produce certain gestures with the face or neck (see Table 7–2) reasonably normally, he or she probably has the motor capability for activating certain switching mechanisms that can be used to interface him or her with an electronic gestural-assisted communication aid. (See comment 3 for information relevant to interpreting Table 7–2.)

8. If the person can produce certain gestures with the upper extremities (see Table 7–1) or face and neck (see Table 7–2) at least partially, he or she may have the motor capacity for activating a myoswitch that can be used to interface him or her with an electronic microcomputer-based aid (see chapter 6). Electrode placements that may be usable for activating a myoswitch are indicated in Tables 7–1 and 7–2.

Sensory Functioning

The degree of intactness of a person's auditory, visual, and tactile-kinesthetic-proprioceptive systems partially determines the augmentative communication strategies it is possible for him or her to use. If a person has difficulty understanding speech, his or her ability to benefit from any of the communication strategies described in chapter 4, 5, or 6 may be reduced unless the auditory problem can be compensated for visually (as could be done by transmitting messages in manual sign or by improving his or her ability to speechread).

If a person has difficulty understanding visual symbols (words or Blissymbols), there are many gestural-assisted and neuro-assisted communication strategies he or she will be unable to use unless the visual problem can be compensated for by tactile or auditory means. The reason, of course, is that if a person cannot understand the visual symbols on a display, he or she would have difficulty using them to encode messages.

With a communication board it is sometimes possible to compensate for a visual deficit by making it possible to identify visual message components by Braille (see chapter 5). The Braille equivalent of each visual message component would appear

TABLE 7-2 **Switching Mechanisms Activated by Particular Gestures of the Face and Neck**

Switch Type	Neck Flexion	Neck Extension	Moving Head from Side to Side	Raise Eyebrows	Close Eyes
Pushbutton	With headstick				
Push plate	With headstick				
Paddle					
Sliding handle or foot trolley					
Wobblestick					
Pillow, pad, or squeeze bulb	X	X			
Tip, or tilt, switch					
Magnetic reed switch			With headstick		
Suck or blow switch					
Touch switch	X		With headstick		
Sound-controlled switch					
Light-controlled switch					
Myoswitch (location of electrodes)	? Over sternocleido-mastoideus	? Over trapezius (superior fibers)	X	? Over occipitofrontalis	X*

*Small light sources in an eyeglass frame shine on the white of the eye. If the eye is open a different amount of light is reflected than if it is closed.

Continued

189

TABLE 7–2 *Continued*

Switch Type	Direct Gaze to Right	Direct Gaze to Left	Compress Lips	Smile	Suck
Pushbutton					
Push plate					
Paddle					
Sliding handle or foot trolley					
Wobblestick					
Pillow, pad, or squeeze bulb			?		
Tip, or tilt, switch					
Magnetic reed switch					
Suck or blow switch					X
Touch switch			?		
Sound-controlled switch					
Light-controlled switch	X†	X†			
Myoswitch			?	?	
(location of electrodes)			Over orbicularis oris	Over zygomaticus major	

†Small light sources in an eyeglass frame shine on the eye. If gaze is directed, a different amount of light is reflected than if it isn't.

Switch Type	Blow	Extend and Retract Tongue	Phonate	Close Jaws
Pushbutton				With mouthstick
Push plate		?		With mouthstick
Paddle				
Sliding handle or foot trolley				
Wobblestick				
Pillow, pad, or squeeze bulb		?		?
Tip, or tilt, switch				
Magnetic reed switch				
Suck or blow switch	X			
Touch switch				
Sound-controlled switch	X		X	?
Light-controlled switch				
Myoswitch	?			?
(location of electrodes)	Over buccinator			Over temporalis

below it. A user could locate the components of a message by scanning the board with his or her fingertips.

With a microcomputer-based aid, it may be possible to compensate partially for a visual deficit by having message components "spoken" (by a speech synthesizer) as they are displayed on the monitor screen. This strategy should be particularly useful for persons who use a scanning response mode. As the cursor points to a message component on the screen (e.g., a letter), it is "spoken" by the speech synthesizer.

A disturbance in a person's use of tactile, kinesthetic, or proprioceptive sensation could have a detrimental effect on his or her ability to use gestural and possibly gestural-assisted communication strategies. It can impede the person's ability to produce muscle gestures needed for implementing them. A given deficit of this type would tend to affect a person's use of some strategies more than others. The more precise (or refined) the gestures needed to implement a strategy, the greater the probable impact of such a disability.

Information relevant to auditory, visual, and tactile-kinesthetic-proprioceptive functioning that can influence decisions about communication strategies is discussed in this section.

Audition

It is necessary to determine whether the person has a hearing loss, and if so, how much it interferes with speech comprehension. If the person is experiencing some difficulty understanding speech, perhaps this can be at least partly compensated for by a hearing aid and/or by auditory training and speechreading instruction. The status of hearing can be determined by audiometric testing.

It is also necessary to determine whether the person has auditory agnosia (or any other auditory perceptual or memory problem) or receptive aphasia, and if so, how much it interferes with speech comprehension. Most aphasia tests contain items that are usable for this purpose.

Vision

It is necessary to determine whether the person has a loss of visual acuity or a visual-field problem, and if so, how much it would interfere with reading, typing, indicating message components on a communication board, or activating an electronic switching mechanism. Although it would be best for the client's vision to be evaluated by an ophthalmologist or an optometrist, there are simple tests that can be used to screen for visual acuity and visual-field problems. A chart containing letters and other symbols of different sizes can be used to screen visual acuity; and moving the tip of the finger laterally through the visual field (upper and lower halves separately) can be used to screen for visual-field disturbances such as homonymous hemianopsia.

It is also necessary to determine whether the person manifests visual agnosia (or other visual perceptual or memory problems) or dyslexia, and if so, how much it would interfere with reading, typing, indicating message components on a communication board, or activating an electronic switching mechanism. Most aphasia tests contain items that can be used for evaluating these areas.

Tactile-Kinesthetic-Proprioceptive Functioning

It is necessary to determine whether there are disturbances in any of these areas that could interfere with manual signing, writing, typing, indicating message components on a communication board, or activating electronic switching mechanisms. A neurological examination should provide the necessary information. Of course, if the person could perform these activities normally, it would be safe to assume that tactile-kinesthetic-proprioceptive functioning is adequate.

Cognitive Functioning

Any disturbance in the person's ability to solve problems and see relationships can influence the choice of a communication strategy. Children diagnosed as mentally retarded and adults having such conditions as Alzheimer's disease, cerebral arteriosclerosis, or Huntington's chorea show this type of disturbance.

A disturbance in cognitive functioning can influence the choice of a symbol set in several ways. First, it can make it difficult or impossible for a person to use relatively abstract symbols, those that are not pictographic. He or she would be likely to experience far more difficulty using English words than photographs and drawings. And second, it can influence the size of the symbol set the person can manage and the complexity of its syntax. Because a disturbance in cognitive functioning is almost always accompanied by a learning deficit, a person so affected probably would be unable to learn as many symbols (message components) and as many ways of combining them as would his or her cognitively normal peer.

A standardized intelligence test can be used to assess cognitive functioning. One that is relatively "language free," such as the Leiter International Performance Scale (Arthur, 1952), is preferable because it assesses cognitive ability relatively independently of receptive and expressive oral language ability. Many severely communicatively impaired children and adults have a language deficit; if a relatively language-free test of cognitive functioning is not used, they may appear to have a severe cognitive deficit when, in fact, they do not have one.

How high a level of cognitive functioning is necessary to learn how to use a particular augmentative communication strategy? There have been several attempts (e.g., Kangas & Lloyd, 1988b; Owens & House, 1984; Shane & Bashir, 1980) based on the work of Piaget and others to develop criteria for predicting whether a severely communicatively impaired person has a sufficiently high level of cognitive readiness (i.e., has the cognitive prerequisites needed) for doing so. The accuracy of decisions based on these criteria for individual clients would be uncertain for at least two reasons. First, the validity of these criteria has not been established empirically—that is, sufficient data have not been reported to establish that persons who do not meet these criteria are incapable of learning to use particular augmentative communication strategies. And second, it is often extremely difficult, if not impossible, to establish the level of cognitive functioning of such persons with a sufficiently high level of reliability to rule out trying to teach the use of an augmentative strategy.

Perhaps the best way to determine whether a severely communicatively impaired client has a sufficiently high level of cognitive readiness to learn to use a particular strategy is to try to teach him or her to use it. If after a relatively short period of diagnostic therapy there is evidence that he or she can learn to use the strategy, this would indicate that there is an adequate level of cognitive readiness for doing so. The consequences of not teaching the use of an augmentative strategy to a client who was incorrectly judged on the basis of such criteria to have an inadequate level of cognitive readiness would be more serious than would trying to teach its use and discovering after a short period of therapy that his or her level of cognitive readiness was insufficient for learning it!

For further information about the implications of cognitive functioning for augmentative communication intervention, see Light and Lindsay (1991a).

OF THE USABLE STRATEGIES, WHICH WOULD BE OPTIMAL FOR MEETING THE PERSON'S COMMUNICATION NEEDS?

Once the communication strategies that it would be possible for the person to use have been identified, the next task would be to select the strategy that would be optimal for meeting his or her communication needs. That strategy would be optimal that came closest to allowing the client to meet these needs at a relatively low cost. Cost here refers not only to the expense of acquiring and maintaining necessary hardware but also to the time and energy investment required to learn to use the strategy.

Judging by the literature since the mid-1980s, there appears to be a bias toward electronic aids (particularly speech-generating ones). Communication boards tend to be regarded as being inferior to them. This is unfortunate because communication boards can do a better job of facilitating communication for some persons in some situations. As Michael Williams, a long-term user of both speech-generating electronic aids and conversation boards has commented (1991, p. 134):

> *As I mentioned earlier, I am not particularly keen on electronic communication in general. For me, it is a lot harder to use than a simple spelling board with a cooperative conversational partner. I spell quickly and accurately on a small, laminated, paper letter board I carry at my side. I am habituated to this method of communication, so I often do not use any of my three electronic voice-output aids.*

A worksheet that can be useful when attempting to identify the optimal strategy for a person is reproduced in Table 7–3. Various types of augmentative communication strategies are listed in the first column of this table. (Gestural-assisted and neuro-assisted communication strategies are not listed individually.) A "yes" or "no" would be recorded beside each strategy (column 2) to indicate whether the person should be able to use it (based on the results of the evaluation outlined in this chapter). For those strategies that are usable, a "grade" is assigned for each selection criterion (column 3, numbers 1 to 8). In the grading system used, A signifies excellent, B good, C satisfactory, and F unsatisfactory. The criteria on which each strategy is graded are the following:

1. The extent to which the strategy would allow the person to meet his or her communication needs.
2. The cost of components (i.e., hardware) and their maintenance; the higher this cost, the lower the grade.
3. The length of time it would probably take the person to learn to use the strategy well enough to meet his or her communication needs; the longer this time period, the lower the grade.
4. The portability of the aid (if one is used); the more portable the aid, the higher the grade.

TABLE 7–3 **Data Summary Worksheet for Identifying the Optimal Strategy for Meeting a Person's Communication Needs**

Name _____ Date _____ Examiner _____

Strategy	Could Person Use It?	Selection Criteria 1 2 3 4 5 6 7 8
Pantomime		
Amer-Ind		
Ameslan		
Left-hand manual alphabet		
Limited manual strategies		
Gestures for yes and no		
Eye-blink encoding		
Gestural Morse code		
Pointing		
Direct-selection communication board		
Encoding communication board		
Scanning communication board		
Direct-selection electronic aid		
Encoding electronic aid		
Scanning electronic aid		

A "grade" is assigned to each criterion for each strategy a person could use (which would be marked "yes" in the second column). In the grading system A signifies excellent, B good, C satisfactory, and F unsatisfactory. The selection criteria are described in the text.

5. The extent to which using the strategy is likely to interfere with ongoing activity (e.g., that involving the use of the hands); the greater the probable interference, the lower the grade.
6. The intelligibility of messages communicated by it to untrained observers; the higher their intelligibility, the higher the grade.
7. The amount of training likely to be necessary to learn to interpret messages communicated by it; the more training necessary, the lower the grade.
8. The acceptability of the strategy to users and interpreters; the more acceptable the strategy, the higher the grade.

The optimal strategy for a person (which may utilize more than one symbol set or aid) can be inferred from the grades assigned to the strategies he or she probably would be able to use. It would be the one that came closest to meeting his or her communication needs and would

Be acceptable to the client and those in his or her environment

Be highly intelligible to observers who were not trained (or were only minimally trained) to interpret messages transmitted by it

Interfere little, if at all, with the client's ongoing activities

Be sufficiently portable for the client's needs

Not take a great deal of time to learn to use

Not exceed available funding to purchase and maintain

For further information about the decision-making process in selecting augmentative communication strategies and devices for clients, see the following: Bolling (1985), Coleman, Cook, and Meyers (1980), Jones et al. (1990), Light (1989b), Lombardino and Langley (1989), Napper, Robey, and McAfee (1989), Owens and House (1984), Reichle and Karlan (1985), Rosen and Goodenough-Trepagnier (1983), Shane and Bashir (1980), Woltosz (1988b), and Yorkston and Karlan (1986).

SCREENING BEFORE ASSESSMENT

One of the challenges in this field is identifying persons who are severely communicatively impaired and thus should be assessed to determine if they could benefit from augmentative communication intervention. Several approaches have been used for doing so, including encouraging referrals from physicians and other health-care professionals, giving talks to lay and professional groups (particularly ones to which their caregivers are likely to belong), and screening populations that would be expected to contain them. One population for which such screening is being done in the United States (in part, because it is mandated by federal law) is residents of nursing homes (see Lubinski & Frattali, 1993).

INTERVENTION BEFORE ASSESSMENT?

It is not always possible to assess a client fully before beginning intervention. This is often the case with children who lack a reliable means of communication (Goossens', 1989). In such cases intervention has to begin with little or no knowledge of the client's level of cognitive development, ability to understand speech, literacy, hearing acuity, and vision. Once a reliable means of communication is established—even if it is a limited one consisting of signals for yes and no—it should be possible to complete the assessment. The additional information may enable the clinician to do an even better job of augmenting the client's communication.

▶ 8

Intervention Issues

Once the strategy that comes closest to being optimal for a person is identified, the next step is intervention. Service delivery in augmentative communication has a number of aspects (see Zellhofer & Beukelman, 1992, for an overview). Many have already been discussed. This chapter is devoted primarily to intervention issues that have not been dealt with elsewhere in the book, including

Candidacy requirements

Enhancing communicative competence

Professional ethics and client rights

Integrating AAC instruction into regular education settings

Putting together an interdisciplinary team

Enhancing "appearance of normality"

Defining intervention goals

Gaining acceptance for augmentative communication from potential users, caregivers, and those with whom they communicate

Generating motivation for communication

Increasing awareness of the nature of communication

Need for a diagnostic trial before a communication aid is purchased

Wheelchair positioning

Facilitated communication

Selecting a lexicon

Maximizing speed of message transmission

Clues for making "20 questions" more efficient

Periodically reassessing communication needs

Funding communication aid components

Telecommunication

Gaining administrative support for the use of augmentative intervention programs

Training persons in a user's environment to function as facilitators

Introduction cards and other methods for training persons in a user's environment to interpret messages transmitted by augmentative communication

Enhancing interaction between augmentative communication users and others

Emotional aspects of intervention

Assessing the impact of augmentative intervention programs on users

Preventive maintenance for communication aids

Utilizing microcomputer-based communication aids for recreation and education

Utilizing microcomputer-based communication aids for environmental control

Literacy learning

Vocational rehabilitation and employment rights

Lekoteks and toy libraries

Switch training

Advocacy

CANDIDACY REQUIREMENTS

In the past, severely communicatively impaired persons were excluded from augmentative communication intervention for several reasons. One was that they did not have certain prerequisites—for example, a particular cognitive level (Bodine & Beukelman, 1991). Another was their clinician's not being convinced that their natural speech would be inadequate for meeting their present and future communication needs (Bodine & Beukelman, 1991). The latter judgment would be based in part on predictions of clients' future speech performance (see Nishimura et al., 1987, for information about making such predictions for autistic children). Unfortunately, clinicians do not agree on the factors to consider when making this judgment (see Bodine & Beukelman, 1991).

Currently, the trend is to deemphasize candidacy requirements, to utilize a "try and see" rather than a "wait and see" approach (McGregor et al., 1992; Romski & Sevcik, 1988a; Swerissen, 1990). It appears to be generally accepted that almost any severely communicatively impaired child or adult can benefit to some degree from augmentative communication intervention.

ENHANCING COMMUNICATIVE COMPETENCE

Persons who use augmentative communication are not necessarily communicatively competent with it (Beukelman, 1991; McGuire, Wegner, & Molineaux, 1992; O'Keefe & Camarata, 1988; O'Keefe & Dattilo, 1990, 1992). Light (1989b, p. 137) has stated that communicative competence

> *is a relative and dynamic, interpersonal construct based on functionality of communication, adequacy of communication, and sufficiency of knowledge, judgment, and skill in four interrelated areas: linguistic competence, operational competence, social competence, and strategic competence.*

Functionality of communication implies having access to the message components (symbols) necessary for meeting one's communication needs. A symbol set that doesn't enable a person to express emotions, for example, would lack functionality. Adequacy of communication implies doing so well enough to meet one's communication needs. A person's communication ability could be quite limited but still adequate for meeting those needs.

To be communicatively competent, users must have sufficient linguistic, operational, social, and strategic competence. Linguistic competence involves an adequate mastery of the symbol set (or sets) being used. Operational competence implies proficiency in the use of the augmentative strategy or aid(s). Social competence implies having the necessary knowledge, judgment, and skill to know when and how to use communication to manipulate the environment. And strategic competence is achieved when users have the knowledge, skill, and judgment needed to make the best of what they "do know and can do" (Light, 1989b, p. 141).

In the past the emphasis in AAC intervention was often on linguistic and operational competence. Often the result was that although a person knew a strategy or had an aid that would enable him or her to better meet communication needs, this did not happen because the strategy or aid was being underutilized (Calculator, 1988c). To augment significantly a client's communication ability in the real world, AAC intervention must also focus on enhancing his or her social and strategic competence. Some strategies for enhancing them have been suggested (see Calculator, 1988c).

PROFESSIONAL ETHICS AND CLIENT RIGHTS

Practitioners must observe the fundamental rules of ethical conduct (see Romich & Zangari, 1989, for a "think piece" on this issue). For speech-language pathologists and audiologists, these rules are specified in the Code of Ethics of the American Speech-Language-Hearing Association.

Practitioners must also be sensitive to clients' individual rights. The following statement of the American Speech-Language-Hearing Association (1991b, p. 12) mentions some of them:

> *The speech-language pathologist and audiologist should recognize and hold paramount the interests and rights of the individual using the AAC system by being sensitive to individual cultural and linguistic needs. Individuals using an AAC system should be an integral part of the service delivery process. The individual's interests should be a primary consideration in the selection and implementation of a communication system. Opinions of the individual, family and caregivers need to be sought and considered when providing new or updating existing families and caregivers equipment and services.*

For further discussion of this issue, see National Joint Committee for the Communicative Needs of Persons with Severe Disabilities (1992) and McLean (1993).

INTEGRATING AAC INSTRUCTION INTO REGULAR EDUCATION SETTINGS

Many children who are severely communicatively impaired are educated in regular education settings. AAC services that target functional, educationally relevant outcomes can contribute significantly to the successful integration of these children (Calculator, 1991; Calculator & Hicks, 1987; Calculator & Jorgensen, 1990, 1991; Loeding, Zangari, & Lloyd, 1990; Phipps & Soper, 1992; Rowland, 1990). The following checklist of practices for providing AAC services target these outcomes (Calculator & Jorgensen, 1991, p. 208):

1. Educational priorities should be established collaboratively with parents, advocates, and other team members (as opposed to discipline-referenced priorities).
2. Observation, assessment, and intervention should occur in the natural settings in which individuals spend their time.
3. Functional skills should be taught systematically throughout the day, rather than at designated times.
4. Anyone coming in contact with the augmented communicator is a potential instructor of communication skills.
5. The effectiveness of intervention procedures should be evaluated relative to individuals' performances in their natural settings.
6. Educational plans specify desired communication behaviors relative to clusters of skills associated with the effective performance of a broader skill or activity.

Practices 2 through 5 also are appropriate for adult AAC intervention programs.

PUTTING TOGETHER AN INTERDISCIPLINARY TEAM

Most severely communicatively impaired persons require the services of more than one profession to achieve their potential. The interdisciplinary team assembled for the rehabilitation (or habilitation) of such a person may include a representative from any or all of the following professions: audiology, clinical psychology, education, engineering, medicine, nursing, occupational therapy, optometry, physical therapy, social work, speech-language pathology, and vocational counseling. The client and his or her significant others and primary caregivers (if these are other than family members) are also essential team members (Berry, 1987). In most cases the role of assembling a team for augmenting a client's communication and coordinating its activities would be assumed by a speech-language pathologist (Competencies for speech-language pathologists . . . , 1988). Obviously it is important that there be good communication between team members so they can reinforce behaviors that others are developing.

ENHANCING "APPEARANCE OF NORMALITY"

When selecting an augmentative communication strategy or aid for a person, the probable impact of alternatives on his or her "appearance of normality" should be considered. It is hoped the aid or strategy selected will not only be unlikely to reduce such appearance but also to enhance it.

There is considerable anecdotal evidence from autobiographies and other sources that persons who are severely communicatively impaired tend to be regarded as less intelligent than they actually are (Basil, 1992; Creech, 1980, 1984, 1988a, 1988b, 1990a, 1990b, 1990c; Creech et al., 1988; Creech & Viggiano, 1981; Kissick, 1984; Smith-Lewis & Ford, 1987; Viggiano, 1981, 1982). The choice of communication strategy can affect this judgment (Gorenflo & Gorenflo, 1991). For example, severely dysarthric adults who use high-quality computer-generated speech to communicate probably will be viewed as more intelligent than those who do so using their own speech if it is difficult to understand. And children who communicate using Blissymbols probably will tend to be viewed as more intelligent than those who do so using photographs and line drawings.

The perceived communicative competence of persons who are severely communicatively impaired also influences their "appearance of normality." Obviously, the more competent they are as communicators, the more normal they will appear to be. A number of variables have been hypothesized to influence perceptions of communicative competence, including the following: the length of the user's message, the grammatical completeness of the user's message, the intelligibility of the message, the rate and accuracy of message delivery, the pragmatic skills of the user, and the ability of the person being communicated with to develop effective compensatory strategies for facilitating communication (Bedrosian et al., 1992; Hoag & Bedrosian, 1992). However, very little research has been reported on how they influence the perception of communicative competence.

DEFINING INTERVENTION GOALS

One of the first tasks in an augmentative communication intervention program is formulating long-term and short-term goals. These specify the competencies the client has to develop in order to achieve the ultimate goal of learning to communicate well enough to meet his or her communication needs. The specific goals for a particular client would be determined by a number of factors, including the strategy that is to be used, his or her communication needs, and his or her motor, sensory, cognitive, and emotional status.

There are many competencies that clients may have to develop (or improve) to reach (or at least approach) their potential for communication. Among them are the following:

- Making the gestures necessary for activating a particular switch
- Learning the meanings of particular symbols
- Initiating communication and keeping conversations going
- Transmitting messages more rapidly
- Getting help by telephone in an emergency
- Using a microcomputer with a word processing program well enough to do school assignments
- Increasing the desire to communicate
- Increasing speech intelligibility
- Being willing and able to communicate both positive feelings (e.g., love) and negative feelings (e.g., anger)
- Training persons with whom the client interacts to interpret the symbols he or she uses

For further information on intervention goals, see Beukelman (1988), Blackstone (1986), Gillette (1992), Gregory (1992), and Kraat (1986).

GAINING ACCEPTANCE FOR AUGMENTATIVE COMMUNICATION

A necessary prerequisite for successful intervention with any augmentative communication strategy is its acceptance by the user, the user's caregivers, and those with whom he or she communicates. A potential user's reservations about a strategy tends to cause the strategy to be used less than it would otherwise, thereby reducing its potential for benefiting him or her. And if caregivers and persons with whom he or she communicates have similar reservations, they are likely to communicate their feelings to the user verbally, nonverbally, or both. Obviously, any negative reactions to attempts to use augmentative communication are likely to discourage its future use (as they would be response-contingent adversive reinforcers) and thereby reduce its potential for benefiting the user.

It is reasonable to assume that potential users, their caregivers, and those with whom they communicate will have some reservations about intervention with augmentative communication. Such reservations could arise from several sources:

The clinician has given up on improving (or developing) the person's speech.

Intervention with augmentative communication will reduce the person's motivation to improve his or her speech.

Using augmentative communication will call adverse attention to the person—that is, make him or her appear abnormal (Allaire et al., 1991).

The person is a "failure" if he or she has to communicate by means of an augmentative strategy.

Intervention with such a strategy will not significantly improve the person's ability to communicate.

Speech, though defective, is adequate for communication (Allaire et al., 1991).

The person is not ready for augmentative communication (Allaire et al., 1991).

Augmentative communication is not as adequate as normal communication (Beukelman & Yorkston, 1989).

In the following discussions, strategies are outlined for dealing with each of these reservations.

The Clinician Has Given Up

One of the most common causes of resistance to the use of augmentative communication is the belief held by the family of a potential user (particularly that of a child) or by the user himself that the clinician has given up on improving or developing speech. Here are two arguments that may be useful in dealing with this belief:

1. The clinician will continue to work on speech. However, it is unlikely that the person's speech will be adequate to meet his or her communication needs in the near future. The person needs a way to meet these needs now. He or she will be encouraged to use speech along with the augmentative strategy (i.e., to use total communication). If the person's speech improves, he or she will be encouraged to rely more on it and less on the augmentative strategy.

2. Learning and using an augmentative strategy seems to facilitate speech production in some severely communicatively impaired children and adults (see Table 2–2). Intervention with these strategies, therefore, can be viewed as speech therapy.

Augmentative Communication Will Reduce Motivation to Improve Speech

There is considerable evidence (see Table 2–2) that intervention with augmentative communication is highly unlikely to reduce verbal output. If such intervention does have an impact on verbal output (which it appears to do in at least a third of cases), it is to increase it.

Augmentative Communication Calls Adverse Attention to the User (i.e., Makes Him or Her Appear More Abnormal)

A person's attitude toward using augmentative communication probably is the main determiner of how "listeners" will react. If the person has an objective attitude, using it is unlikely to call adverse attention to him or her. An objective attitude in this context would be one of both intellectual and emotional acceptance of having to use augmentative communication. If the person is embarrassed, ashamed, or uncomfortable about having to use it, he or she is likely to communicate this attitude to "listeners," which in turn will tend to make them uncomfortable. In such instances, use of augmentative communication would call adverse attention to the person, not because of reactions to it, per se, but because of reactions to his or her signals about being uncomfortable with it.

Approaches for developing an objective attitude toward use of augmentative communication are essentially the same as those for developing an objective attitude toward wearing a hearing aid. Some people refuse to wear a hearing aid because they feel that it calls adverse attention to them. Suggestions in the audiology literature on gaining acceptance for a hearing aid probably would be applicable for developing an objective attitude toward using augmentative communication.

The Person Is a "Failure"

If the person and/or those with whom he or she communicates believe that he or she should be able to learn to communicate by speech and that the augmentative strategy should be a last resort, the strategy may be rejected because using it implies failure. The attitude of the clinician toward the strategy can have a profound impact on that of the person and those with whom he or she communicates. If the clinician views it as a last resort, they probably will do so also. A clinician is less likely to communicate such an attitude if he or she has a communication rather than a speech orientation (see chapter 1).

Intervention Will Not Significantly Improve Ability to Communicate

There is a high probability that intervention with augmentative communication will significantly improve a severely communicatively impaired child's or adult's ability to communicate. The outcome research summarized in Table 2–1 should be useful for convincing a potential user and his or her family that it could facilitate communication.

One successful strategy is getting clients and their families to agree to a trial period of therapy (e.g., 10 weeks) in which the client receives both traditional speech therapy and instruction in augmentative communication. If they want the augmentative program to be terminated at the end of the period, the clinician will do so. The client really has nothing to lose because he or she will continue to receive traditional speech therapy during this period. The client's ability to communicate, it is hoped, will improve significantly during this period and permission will be given for the program to continue.

Speech, Though Defective, Is Adequate

Some severely communicatively impaired persons (particularly those who have dysarthria) and their caregivers prefer speech that has relatively low unintelligibility to augmentative communication. A caregiver may be able to understand most of what the person says because of having had considerable experience doing so. A caregiver may even serve as the person's interpreter in much the same way as an interpreter for the deaf speaks (voices) what is being signed and a foreign-language interpreter translates and speaks in English what is being said in another language. A caregiver doing so would be functioning as a speech-generating communication aid.

It should be pointed out that while this strategy may enable the person to communicate efficiently with caregivers and with others when caregivers are present, it will not enable the person to do so at other times. It would be unrealistic for caregivers to assume that they will always be there when the person wants to communicate. The person's ability to communicate, therefore, needs to be augmented to enable him or her to do so efficiently in all situations.

The Person Is Not Ready for Augmentative Communication

If the severely communicatively impaired person is a child, caregivers may assume that he or she does not yet possess certain cognitive and other prerequisite abilities needed for learning an augmentative communication technique. Because the child is severely communicatively impaired, it may not be possible to determine with a high degree of certainty whether he or she has them. This should be explained to caregivers, and a short trial period of therapy should be recommended during which an attempt will be made to teach a technique that the child should be able to learn if he or she has these prerequisites. The best way to determine whether a person is capable of learning an augmentative communication technique is to attempt to teach it to him or her. If the person can learn the technique, he or she obviously possesses the prerequisites needed for doing so.

When seeking acceptance for augmentative communication intervention it can be helpful to give caregivers and/or potential users a handout that both describes and promotes it. Information from the "Augmentative and Alternative Communication" segment of the "Let's Talk" article in the June–July, 1992 issue of *Asha* can be incorporated into the handout.

Augmentative Communication Is Not as Adequate as Normal Communication

Persons who have become severely communicatively impaired after being normal speakers may resist using augmentative communication because it does not enable them to communicate as efficiently as they did previously (Beukelman & Yorkston, 1989). Rather than comparing their communication ability enhanced by augmentative communication with what it is without it, they compare their communication ability with it to what their ability was before their becoming severely communicatively impaired. Viewed from this perspective, augmentative communication will almost always be considered inadequate.

Becoming severely communicatively impaired is a significant loss. Consequently, it triggers the grieving process (see Clark, 1990; Tanner, 1980). At the initial stages of this process, it is normal for the person to be at least a little unhappy with what augmentative communication has to offer. However, by the time he or she reaches the final stage (i.e., acceptance), resistance to using augmentative communication should lessen considerably. If the person remains highly resistant to doing so for this reason, and it has been several years since he or she became severely communicatively impaired, he or she may have become fixated at some point in the grieving process and could require counseling in order to progress through it.

Some clients who reject augmentative communication for this reason can be helped by getting them to view their communication situation as one of challenge rather than of handicap. Anyone who has an intact speech mechanism should be able to communicate effectively. However, it is a real challenge to do so having one that is severely impaired. The situation here is somewhat similar to one encountered when playing poker. It isn't difficult to win a hand if you have an ace high full house, but it is a real challenge to do so if you have only a pair.

GENERATING MOTIVATION

A lack of motivation for (interest in) communication can arise from any of the following sources, singly or in combination:

Having everything done for one (i.e., not being expected to make decisions)

Having little or no opportunity to communicate (i.e., limited opportunity for interpersonal relationships)

Not understanding the benefits of communicating (i.e., how gratification can come from it)

Not wanting to communicate (because of depression, withdrawal, pending litigation, or some other reason)

Feeling one can communicate well enough (i.e., assuming that learning the strategy would have no advantage)

Reacting negatively to the augmentative strategies or devices that have been made available

How one would deal with a motivation problem would, of course, depend on its source. Several strategies are outlined in this section that may be helpful.

A child or adult who was not expected to make decisions probably would have little motivation to communicate. If a person has a difficult time communicating, it tends to take less time for the family or the staff at the institution to anticipate his or her needs rather than wait for them to be communicated. Anticipating needs rather than waiting for them to be communicated is particularly likely to occur in hospitals, nursing homes, and institutions for the mentally retarded. Persons in such institutions may, in fact, be discouraged from attempting to communicate because it makes client care more time-consuming for the staff. If a person were to sense that those with whom he interacted responded negatively to his attempts at communication, he or she probably would make fewer attempts to communicate, which would be likely to result in a vicious circle: Reduced attempts to communicate would lead to reduced practice in communicating, which in turn would lead to lack of improvement (or regression) in communication ability, which in turn would lead to discouragement of attempts to communicate, and so on (see Figure 8–1).

Lack of motivation to communicate resulting from not being encouraged to make decisions can be dealt with, in part, by expecting the person to participate in decision making to the extent allowed by his or her communication ability. If the person is able to understand speech reasonably well and signal yes and no, he or she can be expected to indicate choices by answering questions. By explaining the serious consequences of the person not being encouraged to communicate to those responsible for his or her care, it should be possible to obtain at least their partial cooperation.

Sometimes a person may not feel a need to improve his or her communication because he or she doesn't have much opportunity to communicate. This is particularly so for persons over the age of 65 who live alone and have limited opportunity for interpersonal relationships. Such persons can be motivated to improve their ability to communicate by increasing their opportunities for interpersonal relationships (e.g., by getting them involved with groups such as "golden age" clubs) or by convincing

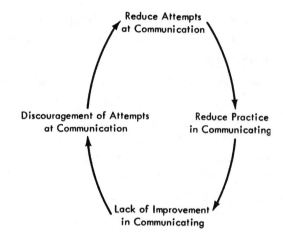

FIGURE 8–1 **Vicious circle resulting from discouragement of attempts at communication.**

them that even with their present opportunities for interpersonal relationships it would be advantageous for them to be able to communicate more effectively, or both of these.

One way to increase the opportunities for communication, particularly for persons in residential settings (e.g., institutions for the mentally retarded), is to use peer tutoring (Hooper & Bowler, 1991). Clients who know how to use a particular augmentative strategy or device tutor those who are learning to use it, under the direction of a clinician. This approach provides both tutors and learners with opportunities for communication. Hooper and Bowler (1991) have reported some success using peer tutoring to encourage the use of manual signs by mentally retarded adults outside of the therapy room.

A third reason why a person (particularly a child) may not be motivated to learn to communicate better is that he or she may be unaware of the benefits from doing so. The person may not be aware that communicating better would give him or her more options and greater control. Strategies for increasing awareness of the nature of communication and of the benefits that can be derived from it are described in the next section.

Still another reason is that he or she either does not enjoy communicating or feels that it would be disadvantageous to learn to do it better. Naturally, persons who are depressed or withdrawn do not tend to be highly motivated to communicate. Most, if not all, adults shortly after becoming severely communicatively impaired will evince depression as a part of the grieving process (Clark, 1990; Tanner, 1980). The depression is apt to persist for those who are unable to find something to give their life meaning (Frankl, 1985). Also, persons whose communicative disorders resulted from trauma and who are in the process of suing the parties responsible for injuring them probably will not be highly motivated to learn to communicate better until the litigation process in which they are involved has been completed. The approach used to motivate such persons would, of course, depend on the reason(s) why they do not choose to communicate better.

A person may not be motivated to learn an augmentative strategy because he or she can communicate well enough to meet his or her communication needs. A person's communication needs may be quite limited (and are likely to continue being so in the future), and his or her communication ability, though severely impaired, is adequate for meeting them.

Finally, a person may resist learning and using an augmentative strategy because he or she simply does not like it. One reason could be a lack of compatibility between the available lexicon and his or her communication style (Iacono, 1991, 1992). Another could be a reaction to the strategy itself. One of my adult clients who was capable of communicating by writing on a pad of paper refused to do so in most situations for more than six months because it made him feel uncomfortable. He continued trying to communicate by speaking even though his speech was less than 10 percent intelligible.

INCREASING AWARENESS OF THE NATURE OF COMMUNICATION

Before persons are capable of communicating with any strategy, they have to understand how being able to communicate would permit them to manipulate (or control to some extent) their environment (Romski, Sevcik, & Pate, 1988). If a person is taught a communication strategy and is unaware of how to use it to manipulate his or her environment (e.g., for making requests; see Wacker et al., 1988), knowing the strategy will not make the person a more effective communicator. Although adults who have little or no speech because of dysarthria, verbal apraxia, dysphonia, or glossectomy are likely to understand the nature of communication, children who are severely communicatively impaired because of mental retardation, childhood autism, congenital aphasia, or dysarthria may not understand this process if they have not been made aware of it (Schweigert & Rowland, 1992). Hence, increasing awareness of the nature of communication is a necessary component of an intervention program for many severely communicatively impaired persons, particularly children.

Understanding communication as a process requires several kinds of awareness, including the awareness that gestures, sounds, printed (visual) configurations, and switch activations (see Schweigert, 1988, 1989) can represent, or symbolize, objects and events; and transmission of an appropriate symbol (or sequence of symbols) at an appropriate time can cause a desired event to occur.

Developing Awareness That Gestures, Sounds, and Printed Configurations Can Symbolize Objects and Events

An initial step in any augmentative communication intervention program is making certain the client realizes that gestures, sounds (both speech and other), and printed configurations (words, Blissymbols, drawings, manipulatable tokens, etc.) can represent objects and events. To develop this awareness, he or she must be able to do the following (Carrier & Peak, 1975, pp. 6–7):

1. Discriminate among the various members of the symbol set
2. Discriminate among various classes of environmental stimuli that call for different symbolic responses
3. Discriminate among various sequential arrangements of stimuli (declarative sentences, interrogative sentences, etc.)
4. Associate symbols and environmental stimuli (meanings), and
5. Associate sequential arrangements and meanings

The client has to be able to discriminate among the various gestures, sounds, and printed configurations that are being used as symbols (i.e., the various members of the symbol set). Strategies for developing such awareness for a symbol set consisting of manipulatable tokens are included in the Non-SLIP Program (Carrier & Peak, 1975). These strategies are adaptable for other types of symbol sets.

The client also has to be able to discriminate among the various classes of objects or events ("units of experience") that can be represented by the symbols in the set he or she will be using. To do this, the client must be aware of both how they are similar and how they differ. Specifically, he or she must be aware of the attribute(s) on the basis of which individual objects and events are assignable to a class (or category) that can be represented by a given symbol. An apple, a peanut, a hamburger, and ice cream, for example, all have the attribute of being edible. They are thus assignable to a class (or category) that can be represented by a symbol such as the word "food," a gesture in which a finger is pointed to the mouth or to a drawing of someone eating. The client also must be able to discriminate objects and events for which the use of the symbol would be appropriate from those for which it would be inappropriate (because they do not possess the attribute, or attributes, necessary for assignment to the category symbolized). While an apple, a peanut, a hamburger, and ice cream can be symbolized by the word "food," a pipe, a hammer, and a chair cannot. Strategies for discriminating among various classes of environmental stimuli that call for different symbol responses are included in the Non-SLIP Program (Carrier & Peak, 1975).

A third competency the client must have if his or her communication is to be more complex than the presentation of single symbols is the ability to discriminate among various sequential arrangements of symbols. The client has to be able to discriminate among the various types of permutations and combinations (orderings) of the symbols in the set that are usable for encoding messages. Tasks for providing such training are included in the Non-SLIP Program (Carrier & Peak, 1975).

Once the client can discriminate among the environmental stimuli (objects and events) that he or she will be taught to symbolize and the symbols used to represent them, he or she can be taught how symbols and environmental stimuli are associated. That is, the client can be taught that symbols can represent environmental stimuli even when they are not present. A person has to understand this relationship between symbol and referent intuitively before he or she can learn to use any symbol system. Several strategies have been reported for developing this awareness (see Brady & Saunders, 1991; Brown, 1988; Carrier & Peak, 1975; Sigafoos & Reichle, 1992).

After the client understands how individual symbols and environmental stimuli are related, he or she can be taught how combinations of symbols are related to environmental stimuli. Both the symbols with which a particular symbol is combined and its location in a series (or symbols) can influence its meaning. Ordered combinations of symbols, of course, can encode messages that it would not be possible to encode using single symbols. The Non-SLIP Program (Carrier & Peak, 1975) also includes tasks that are usable for developing an understanding of this concept.

A source of strategies for developing these competencies is the research of Premack (1970, 1971), Premack and Premack (1972, 1974), Rumbaugh and associates (Rumbaugh, 1977), and Gardner and Gardner (1969) on teaching symbols to subhuman primates. The approaches used by these investigators to teach the concept of symbol to such premates can be adapted for teaching this concept to mentally retarded children. Indeed, the Non-SLIP Program (Carrier & Peak, 1975), which was developed for teaching this general concept to mentally retarded children, is based on primate research by the Premacks.

Developing Awareness of the Pragmatics of Communication

Once the client understands that gestures, sounds, and printed configurations singly and in combination can represent (or symbolize) objects and events and is able to produce (or point to) at least one such symbol, he or she is ready to learn that transmission of an appropriate symbol (or combination of symbols) at an appropriate time can cause a desired event to occur (i.e., can manipulate the environment). It is desirable that the first symbols a client is taught allow him or her to ask for things that he or she needs or wants often; hunger, thirst, more, and wanting to go to the bathroom are primary examples.

To help the client become aware of how symbols can be used to manipulate his or her environment, it is desirable that you use tasks in which the client receives immediate reinforcement for producing or indicating a symbol, the reinforcement being successful manipulation of the environment. If, for example, the client knows a symbol for *more*, he or she can be given a small amount of food that he or she likes. The client can then be shown that producing (or indicating) the symbol for *more* results in him or her receiving more of it. It is desirable, incidentally, when teaching this symbol to use a number of different foods, liquids, and other objects as reinforcers. Otherwise, the client might interpret it as meaning more of a specific thing.

Some of the strategies used in the subhuman primate research of the Premacks, the Gardners, and Rumbaugh and his associates for teaching pragmatics of communication can be adapted for teaching this concept to severely communicatively impaired children and adults. The language program developed by Kent (1974) also has some tasks that can be used for this purpose. For additional strategies, see Kouri (1988), Kozleski (1991), Mount and Shea (1982), Shea and Mount (1982), and Woolman (1980).

NEED FOR A DIAGNOSTIC TRIAL

If an electronic communication aid is being recommended, its purchase should follow a diagnostic trial with it (Bruno & Romich, 1989). A device that seems to be helpful in the therapy room may not be so in the real world. Consequently, devices recommended solely by the results of an evaluation may end up being poorly utilized. Companies that manufacture and/or distribute communication aids are usually agreeable to such a trial (Bruno & Romich, 1989). Also, some state- and federal-funded AAC resource centers (e.g., ones in New Jersey and the United Kingdom) maintain a short-term communication aid loan program for this purpose (Enstrom, 1990, 1992; Enstrom & Littman, 1992; Fuller, Donegan, & Jolleff, 1993).

WHEELCHAIR POSITIONING

The position of a client in a wheelchair can influence his or her use of a communication board or an electronic device. Adjustment of positioning by an occupational or physical therapist can align a person in space appropriately for communication (e.g., enabling him or her to have adequate head control to direct gaze straight ahead rather than at the ceiling); provide support for an upper or lower extremity, thereby enabling the person to activate a switching mechanism or point to items on a communication board; and reduce involuntary movements and abnormal reflex activity that can interfere with these (Bay, 1991; MacNeela, 1987; McCormack, 1990; McEwen, 1992; McEwen & Karlan, 1988, 1989; McEwen & Lloyd, 1990; Nelson et al., 1989; Stowers, Altheide, & Shea, 1987; Trefler, 1984; Vanderheiden, 1987b). All clients in wheelchairs should be evaluated to determine whether their positioning in them is optimal for the particular communication strategy, or strategies, being considered or used.

FACILITATED COMMUNICATION

There have been a number of reports of autistic children and adults being taught to communicate by typing or otherwise generating message components while someone holds their hand, wrist, or arm (Anderson & Harrison, 1992; Batt, Remington-

Gurney, & Crossley, 1990; Beukelman, 1993; Biklen, 1988, 1990a, 1990b, 1992a, 1992b; Biklen & Crossley, 1990; Biklen et al., 1991; Bilkin & Schubert, 1991; Calculator, 1992a, 1992b; Crossley, 1988a, 1988b, 1990, 1991, 1992; Crossley & McDonald, 1984; Crossley, Remington-Gurney, & Batt, 1990; Cummins & Prior, 1992; Friedrich, 1992; Grandin, 1989; Hudson, Melita, & Arnold, 1993; McClennen & Gabel, 1992; McLean, 1992; Prior & Cummins, 1992; Prizant & Schuler, 1987; Remington-Gurney, Crossley, & Batt, 1990; Rimland, 1992; Smith & Belcher, 1993). This method has been referred to as facilitated communication. The reason why they are able to communicate while being held has not been established empirically. However, it has been hypothesized that their failure to do so when not being held is because of neuromotor difficulties (possibly an apraxia) and/or a lack confidence in their ability to communicate (Bilken, 1992a).

The basic elements of the method can be described as follows (Bilken, 1992a, p. 16):

1. *Physical support.* The facilitator does not assist the communication user in making a selection of letters or other targets but may help the student to isolate the index finger and stabilize the student at the hand, wrist, or arm during typing, while generally pulling the student's arm back after each selection.
2. *Initial training/introduction.* Students are given activities with fairly predictable answers initially, for example, spelling their names, matching exercises, and cloze exercises. They are then encouraged to progress to open-ended typed conversation.
3. *Maintaining focus.* Where necessary, the facilitator reminds the communication user to keep his or her eyes on the keyboard or other communication aid, to maintain isolation of the index finger used for pointing, to reduce extraneous actions such as screeches, slapping of objects, or biting, and, if the student exhibits echoed or stereotyped spoken language, to type what he or she intends to communicate.
4. *Avoid testing for competence.* A key element of the method is emotional support or encouragement; it is important to treat the person as competent with the knowledge that the person's thinking and literacy abilities will reveal themselves over time.
5. *Generalizing.* Communication users will often develop a high level of communication ability with one or two facilitators and will need encouragement and repeated attempts to generalize to more facilitators.
6. *Fading.* Students become more independent over time; thus, it is important to work on fading physical support.

The following comments by Crossley (1992, pp. 16–17) clarify the nature of the facilitator's role:

> *The facilitator does not point for the user or move the user's hand toward a selection. If the user has low muscle tone, the facilitator provides support,*

such as a hand under the user's forearm; if the user tends to perseverate, the facilitator withdraws the user's hand from the display after every selection; if the user moves impulsively without looking as the display, the facilitator inhibits the user from pointing until the facilitator has observed the user scanning the display; and so on.

Facilitated communication may be helpful to persons who are severely communicatively impaired for reasons other than autism (e.g., Down syndrome; see Crossley, 1990) and for learning communication strategies other than those involving typing. Merely being held, for example, could give some potential AAC users the confidence they need to learn a direct-selection communication strategy.

SELECTING A LEXICON

One aspect of intervention with all augmentative communication strategies except those that rely solely on the alphabet is deciding what messages the client will be able to transmit. The number of messages in such a lexicon ordinarily has to be relatively small.

Several factors you should be considered when selecting a lexicon—particularly an initial lexicon—to augment a client's communication ability:

1. The messages the client needs to be able to communicate immediately for informing caregivers about basic needs (Bryen, Goldman, & Quinlisk-Gill, 1988)
2. The messages the client needs to be able to communicate to facilitate his or her vocational, educational, and recreational objectives
3. The messages the client needs to be able to communicate to express positive feelings (e.g., love) and negative feelings (e.g., anger) (Beukelman, 1989)
4. The client's level of awareness of the ability of communication to enable him or her to manipulate the activity of caregivers (Bryen, Goldman, & Quinlisk-Gill, 1988)
5. The numbers of messages that the symbols in the lexicon—singly or in combination—would allow the client to communicate that he or she needs to be able to communicate.
6. The client's preference for and competency to utilize the two language styles—referential and expressive (Iacono, 1992)

What concepts/messages would it be useful for a person to be able to communicate? Obviously these would vary from person to person, but there are some that would facilitate communication for all persons. Social-regulative ones—no, yes, be quiet, help, stop, wait, I want, I'm finished, goodbye, hello, excuse me, I'm sorry, please, thank you, more, and good—tend to be used as soon as they are introduced (Adamson et al., 1992). In addition to facilitating conversation, their use may cause severely communicatively impaired persons to be viewed more positively than they would be otherwise.

Karlan and Lloyd (1983) had a group of judges rate a number of lexical items on whether or not they would be essential for elementary school–age children and adolescents or adults. The items for elementary school children rank ordered according to the proportion of judges who rated them as essential were the following: bathroom/ toilet/potty, eat/food, name sign (i, me, my), drink, no, help, mother/mommy, more, father/daddy, water, stop, bed/sleep, look/watch, milk, go, happy, hot, good, coat. I would add to this list sad and angry/mad. Those for adolescents and adults rank ordered according to the same criterion were the following: bathroom/toilet/potty, eat/food, no, drink, stop, name sign (I, me, my) help, water, go, bed/sleep, cold, hot, you, coat, good, more, work, come, wash, clean, in, sad, shoes, walk, angry/mad, open, shirt, milk. I would add yes to this list. Considerable caution should be exercised when using these lists because vocabulary that intuitively would seem to be very useful is not included.

There have also been a number of attempts to define an initial vocabulary for preschoolchildren who are severely communicatively impaired. Fried-Oken and More (1992) present a comprehensive review of this literature through 1991 and a single-word composite vocabulary list for preliterate, preschoolchildren based on word lists generated by parents and clinicians of 15 severely communicatively impaired preschoolchildren and language samples elicited from 30 matched normally developing ones along with word lists generated by their parents.

Walker and her associates in the United Kingdom have developed an open-ended lexicon based around a common core of 350 functional concepts, known as the Makaton Vocabulary (Byler, 1985; Carpenter, 1987; Cooney & Knox, 1981; Grove, 1990; Grove & McDougall, 1990, 1991; Grove & Walker, 1990; Le Prevost, 1983; Mountain, 1984, 1987; Park, 1986; Walker, 1986, 1987; Walker & Grove, 1986; Walker et al., 1985). It is taught with manual signs (in the United States, Signing Exact English ones) and/or graphic symbols, accompanied by speech. This lexicon is intended for providing basic communication while facilitating more comprehensive language use. It is not intended to be an end in itself. The 350 core concepts are taught in a series of nine stages. Those concepts that are needed earlier and used most frequently are taught first. For a list of these concepts, arranged by stages, see Table 1 in Grove and Walker (1990).

One group that tends to have special vocabulary needs are persons who are at the end stage of a progressive disease, such as multiple sclerosis. Because they are likely to want to communicate about religious/spiritual matters (e.g., God, eucharist, confession, death, prayer, heaven, hell), it is important that they be provided with the vocabulary needed to do so (see Porter, 1989).

Whenever possible, users should be involved extensively in the selection and retention of vocabulary, and they should be given the consultative support that will make this task a pleasant one for them (Beukelman, McGinnis, & Morrow, 1991). They obviously know better than anyone else what they want to be able to communicate efficiently that they cannot at present.

Also whenever possible, the word usage of users' nondisabled peers should be taken into consideration when developing a lexicon, particularly when they are going to be in an integrated classroom. Beukelman, Jones, and Rowan (1989) and Fried-Oken and More (1992) report data that may be helpful when developing lexicons for preschoolers.

For further information about factors to consider when selecting a lexicon, see the following: Adamson et al. (1992); Beukelman, McGinnis, and Morrow (1991), Blackstone (1988f), Blau (1983b), Bryen, Goldman, and Quinlisk-Gill (1988), Carlson (1981), Dennis et al. (1982), Francis (1990), Gerber and Kraat (1992), Karlan and Lloyd (1983), McGinnis, 1991; McGinnis and Beukelman, 1989, Morrow, Beukelman, and Mirenda (1989), Morrow et al. (in press), Schlosser & Lloyd, 1991; Yorkston et al. (1987, 1988, 1989, 1990), Yorkston, Fried-Oken, and Beukelman (1988), Yorkston and Karlan (1986), and Yorkston, Smith, and Beukelman (1990).

MAXIMIZING SPEED OF MESSAGE TRANSMISSION

Normal conversation proceeds at 120 to 200 words per minute, whereas that of motor-impaired communication aid users who compose messages on a letter-by-letter or word-by-word basis typically proceeds at a rate of 2 to 10 words per minute (Alm et al., 1993). This slow rate may not be particularly handicapping for basic needs communication with family and caregivers, but it can limit other types of communication. It may partly explain, for example, why severely communicatively impaired children spend more time interacting with people when there is an unequal relationship—such as parents, therapists, and teachers—and less time interacting with peers (Light, Collier, & Parnes, 1985a). It may also partly explain why communication aid users tend to initiate conversations less frequently than do their peers (Alm et al., 1993). Slow rates of message transmission are particularly frustrating to those communication aid users who are not cognitively impaired in any way, such as the well-known cosmologist Dr. Stephen Hawking (Alm, Arnott, & Murray, 1992).

Fortunately, conversations do not consist entirely of novel material. Words, phrases, and entire messages are used again and again. Consequently, many utterances and parts of utterances can be prefabricated. The use of prefabricated message components can increase communication rate for both communication board and electronic aid users. For the former, this can be done by including frequently used words and phrases on their boards. For the latter, particularly for those using a microcomputer-based system, it can be done in a number of ways (see Alm, Arnott, & Murray, 1992; Alm, Arnott, & Newell, 1992a, 1992b; Alm et al., 1993).

Another type of strategy that can be used with microcomputer-based electronic aids to speed up message transmission is letter and word prediction (see Newell et al., 1992). With it, the computer completes words after the first few letters have been keyboarded and/or fills in words after the first few are entered. One such strategy, Minspeak, is described in chapter 5.

CLUES FOR MAKING "20 QUESTIONS" MORE EFFICIENT

Unaided communication with clients whose expressive ability is limited to signaling yes and no tends to be a game of 20 questions. Those communicating with them attempt to guess the message by asking "Is it . . . ?", "Do you want . . . ?", or other questions until they are successful. The number of questions needed to be asked is likely to be fewer if they are aware of (have a clue about) the general nature of the message before attempting to guess it (Garrett, Beukelman, & Low-Morrow, 1989). Persons communicating with such clients should be encouraged to establish, by questioning them, whether a message is about a person, place, event, thing, or time before attempting to guess it.

PERIODICALLY REASSESSING COMMUNICATION NEEDS

After a person has been taught the use of an augmentative communication strategy, it is necessary periodically to reevaluate its ability to meet his or her communication needs. (See Light, Beesley, & Collier, 1988, for a case study that illustrates why it is essential to do so.)

Both the symbol set and the manner in which it is used for encoding and transmitting messages may have to be modified from time to time. The symbol set with which a person is initially provided probably will have to be added to periodically because the things he or she will need to communicate about are likely to change. It also may be necessary to delete some symbols from this set when new ones are added if he or she uses a communication board or an electronic communication aid that only can display or generate a finite number of symbols.

Further, the person may improve in the ability to use symbols or regress in this ability to the point that he or she needs a different symbol set. A young child who uses a communication board may begin with a symbol set that consists of pictures and then improve to the point that he or she can handle one consisting of Blissymbols and words. An adult who has a degenerative central nervous system disease may begin with one consisting of printed words and then regress to the point where he or she is severely dyslexic and can only utilize one consisting of pictures.

The response mode that a person uses for encoding and transmitting messages also may have to be changed. It may be necessary to make such a change because either the person has become capable of using a more efficient strategy for encoding and transmitting message components or the person can no longer use a strategy he or she used previously because of additional central nervous system damage. The person may be able to go from a scanning to a direct-selection response mode, or he or she may regress from a direct-selection response mode to a scanning one.

Another reason why the approach a person uses for encoding and transmitting messages may have to be changed periodically is either that he or she has become capable of using a display containing a larger number of message components or is no longer able to utilize as large a one as previously because of additional central nervous system damage. A third reason is the person's changing communication needs. When a child who lacks normal use of his or her upper extremities reaches the point in school that he or she is expected to do written assignments, the child may have to be interfaced with a microcomputer system with a printer. It is desirable when selecting a communication aid to anticipate the user's future communication needs and make certain that necessary components (peripherals) are likely to be available for the aid for meeting them.

FUNDING COMMUNICATION AID COMPONENTS

The components of an electronic communication aid may cost more than a potential user can afford. There are sources from which it may be possible to obtain funding in such cases, including the following:

1. The school system in which a child is enrolled (see Haney, 1992). Public Law 94-142 mandates that school systems must provide access to augmentative communication aids to children who need them to meet their educational objectives.
2. The vocational rehabilitation commission in the person's state (if it can be argued that providing him with such an aid will make him more employable).
3. A community organization such as the Kiwanis Club, Sertoma International, the Telephone Pioneers of America, or a computer-user group. With regard to the latter, one based in Connecticut, Voice for Joanie, has loaned computer-based communication aids to more than 50 persons who have ALS.
4. Litigation (particularly if the cause of the person becoming severely communicatively impaired was negligence, e.g., malpractice).
5. Private, state, or federal health insurance programs.
6. The State Bureau for Crippled Children (or other state agency that performs this function).
7. United Cerebral Palsy, the National Easter Society for Crippled Children and Adults, or some other voluntary organization that assists persons who have the condition that caused the client's communicative disorder.
8. "Title funds" available from the state.
9. Trust funds administered by local banks or foundations that are intended for helping crippled children or adults.
10. Bake sales, rummage sales, and similar community-based fund-raising activities.

Unfortunately, funding is often a problem. As Blackstone (1989, p. 62) has stated:

The lack of funding for devices is a concern heard everywhere. Third party agencies, both private and public, are "considering the problem" and "study-

ing solutions." In the interim, each case must be fought and won. As professionals, we can do our part for the "funding cause" by demonstrating through our research and case studies the efficacy of using assistive technologies, materials, and strategies to improve communication. If we do not, our piece of the technology funding pie will be . . . gobbled up by some other group.

The use of the term *communication prosthesis* to label such aids may be helpful when seeking funding from private, state, and federal insurance programs. For further information about funding communication aids, see Beukelman, Yorkston, and Smith (1985).

TELECOMMUNICATION

There are a number of devices and services that severely speech impaired persons can use to communicate by telephone. Those discussed in this section include devices for generating speech, devices for generating noise, telecommunication devices for the deaf (TDDs), videotelephones, and telecommunication relay services.

Devices for Generating Speech

Both microcomputers and some dedicated augmentative communicative devices can be used for generating speech. If the loudspeaker on the device is placed close to the telephone or if the volume is turned up (if the speaker cannot be moved), the resulting speech should be intelligible to the person at the other end of the line. Although a regular telephone can be used, a speaker phone would be more efficient.

An inexpensive audiocassette tape recorder can be used for limited telephone communication, particularly for emergencies. If a client is going to be spending time at home alone and has no other means of communicating by telephone, a message can be recorded that indicates he needs help and gives his name and address. The client would dial 911 or a friend or family member and play the tape. The words yes, no, and I don't know could also be recorded on the tape. The client could be trained to locate them quickly using the fast-forward and rewind controls and the tape counter.

Devices for Generating Noise

Inexpensive noise-generating devices are available at Radio Shack and similar stores that are used by persons learning international Morse code. These can be operated with any type of single-switch switching mechanism. If the device is placed by a telephone, a client can communicate to the person at the other end of the line by generating sequences of dots and dashes. An advantage of this approach is that the necessary equipment is inexpensive. A disadvantage is that it can only be used for communicating with persons who are willing to learn the code.

Telecommunication Devices for the Deaf (TDDs)

These devices, also known as text telephones (TTs), can be used for communicating with anyone who has one. They are actually limited microcomputers with built-in software, keyboards, monitor screens, modems, and sometimes printers. They are attached to a telephone line the same way as a telephone. A message that is typed by a client is displayed on the screen of the TDD at the other end of the line and vice versa. Some TDDs are relatively inexpensive (less than $300). In most states they can be leased from telephone companies and in some states they are distributed free to severely communicatively impaired persons, particularly those with low incomes.

Videotelephones

Videotelephones have been used by persons who communicate with graphic symbols (e.g., Blissymbols) to enable them to communicate by telephone (Brodin, 1992b; Brodin & Björck-Åkesson, 1993a, 1993b; Brodin, Fahlén, & Nilsson, 1993; Brodin & Magnusson, 1992a, 1992b, 1993). The symbols are transmitted to the screen of the videotelephone at the other end of the line and vice versa.

Telecommunication Relay Services

Telecommunication relay services (TRSs) are available in all 50 states. Their establishment was mandated by Title IV of the Americans with Disabilities Act, which was passed by the Congress in 1990. They enable persons who are severely speech impaired and have either a microcomputer and modem or a TTD to initiate and receive telephone calls. They also enable those who have dedicated augmentative communication devices that contain a microcomputer and modem to do this.

Relay services operate 24 hours a day, 365 days a year. Telephone calls made through them cost no more than regular ones. Most can be used for both long-distance and local calls. Full confidentiality is maintained, and no records of the contents of calls are retained by the TRS.

A user usually contacts a TRS by dialing an 800 number. When the operator (referred to as a communication assistant, or CA) answers, the user types the telephone number that he or she wants to call. The CA dials this number and when the party answers, the user types the first thing that he or she wants to say. The CA "voices" this to the party and when the party responds, the CA types what was said. This interaction can go on for as long as the people want to "talk." If the person initiating the call can talk, he or she would dial the same 800 number and when the CA answers, "voice" the telephone number of the speech- (and/or hearing-) impaired person whom he or she wants to contact.

The user can hear the contacted person's response rather than having it typed by the CA if the caller has a TDD (TT) and the TRS offers "hearing passthrough." Unfortunately, this was not possible when this chapter was written if the user had a microcomputer.

Information about accessing the TRS in your state can be obtained from your local telephone company. TRSs also exist in Canada and other countries. In some they are run by private rather than government organizations. Information about their availability can be obtained from local organizations for the deaf. For further information about TRSs, see Strauss (1992).

GAINING ADMINISTRATIVE SUPPORT

Your supervisor and other administrators of the institution where you are employed initially may not be enthusiastic about the use of augmentative intervention programs with clients. This lack of enthusiasm is likely to be due to their not understanding the positive impacts that such intervention programs can have on severely communicatively impaired persons and that intervention with such programs does not reduce motivation for learning speech. The outcome data summarized in chapter 2 should be useful when attempting to convince such persons that these programs are of value.

TRAINING PERSONS TO SERVE AS FACILITATORS

Facilitators can enhance the communication abilities of augmentative communication users in several ways. First, they can make certain that the equipment the user needs is in operating condition and available. If the equipment is electronic, they can do what is necessary to maintain it, including preventive maintenance and recharging (or changing) batteries. They also make certain that the person can access the system whenever he or she wants to communicate.

Facilitators can make certain the message component (symbol) set is adequate for meeting the user's communication needs. If, for example, the client is using a communication board with a graphic symbol set (e.g., Blissymbols), facilitators can periodically update the board so that needed symbols become available. Or if a speech-generating device with Minspeak is being used, facilitators can assist the client in programming it.

Also, facilitators can be interpreters. They voice (speak) what the user communicates to them that he or she wants to say. While a message may be communicated to them by in a short-hand (telegraphic) form, they voice it in grammatical sentences. Consequently, they function in much the same way as interpreters do for the deaf. Interpreters for the deaf voice in grammatical English (or another language) what their clients sign. Because the syntax of American Sign Language (ASL) differs from that of spoken English, they do not directly translate messages. When they voice them, the syntax is that of spoken English rather than ASL.

Facilitators may also interpret (voice) for dysarthrics whose speech is likely to be unintelligible to persons who are not used to communicating with them. These would be dysarthrics who choose to speak rather than use augmentative communication. Facilitators while doing so are functioning like portable speech-generating communication devices.

An augmentative communication user may have more than one facilitator. Beukelman (1991) reported, for example, that one school-age child during a five-year period had 16.

Several programs have been described for training facilitators (see Calculator & Luchko, 1983a; Culp & Carlisle, 1988c; Light et al., 1992; McNaughton & Light, 1989; Light, McNaughton, & Parnes, 1986a, 1986b). However, few data have been reported on their relative effectiveness (Beukelman, 1991).

INTRODUCTION CARDS AND OTHER METHODS FOR TRAINING PERSONS IN A USER'S ENVIRONMENT TO INTERPRET MESSAGES TRANSMITTED BY AUGMENTATIVE COMMUNICATION

If the person is using a symbol set that is unfamiliar to those with whom he or she has to communicate, it is necessary to train them to interpret messages encoded using the symbols. It also may be necessary to train them how to communicate with a person if he or she is using a communication aid. For example, it may be necessary to teach them how to facilitate communication for a communication board user by utilizing a scanning strategy.

One approach is to have users give persons with whom they communicate an explicit, printed introduction card that states they cannot speak and directs them to the relevant features of their communication systems (Doss et al., 1991). For example, an introduction card for a person who uses a portable communication board in a wallet could have the following message printed on it (Doss et al., 1991, p. 261):

> *Hi! My name is Susan. I cannot speak. I talk by showing you pictures and words in my wallet. Thank you!*

And one for a person who uses an electronic speech-generating communication aid could contain a message such as the following (Doss et al., 1991, p. 261):

> *Hi! My name is Susan. I cannot speak. I talk by using this machine. Please follow these steps in order to understand my message. 1) Wait for me to push buttons. 2) Listen to my message. Thank you!*

An introduction card, of course, would only be practical for persons who have the physical ability to show it (Hanagan, 1991).

It is important that the training be as brief and as readily available as possible. The less time and energy necessary to learn to use a communication strategy and to interpret messages transmitted by it, the more likely those in the person's environment are to take the time to learn to use and interpret it. This is particularly likely to be true if the person lives in an institution such as a residential facility for the mentally retarded or a nursing home. Also, the more readily available such training, the more likely those interacting with the person are to take it (Craven & Cotter, 1985; Faw et al., 1981; Fitzgerald et al., 1984). If the person is in a hospital or nursing home and training in using the communication strategy is available on the ward, nurses and others who interact with the user probably are more likely to take the time to learn to use it than they would be if they had to go elsewhere to receive the training.

How can persons in a user's environment be trained to assist him or her in transmitting and interpreting messages? There are several general approaches that can be used singly or in combination.

1. *Written instructions*, possibly with drawings or photographs, can be prepared on how to assist the person in transmitting messages, on how to interpret the symbols he or she uses, or both. A photocopy of the instructions should be kept near the user (attached to the bed, wheelchair, or communication aid). Other copies should be given to persons who will be communicating with him or her often. The writing should be as clear as possible, no technical jargon should be used, and the level of vocabulary and syntax should be no higher than sixth grade (because it is important that the instructions be understandable to members of the user's family, including older children).
2. *Videotaped or audiotaped instructions* can be prepared on how to assist the person in transmitting messages and/or how to interpret the symbols he or she uses. This approach using videotape can be quite effective for teaching interpretation of manual gestural signs (Bady & Silverman, 1978). For such an approach to be practical, it would, of course, be necessary to have an appropriate audiotape or videotape player readily available to those who would be communicating with the person.
3. *Training sessions* can be conducted by the user's clinician (or someone trained by him or her) on how to assist the user in transmitting messages and/or on how to interpret the symbols. This approach is the least desirable of the three because of the demands it tends to place on the clinician's time and because this training only can be available at certain times. These times would not necessarily coincide with occasions during which an untrained person would have to communicate with the user.

ENHANCING INTERACTION BETWEEN AUGMENTATIVE COMMUNICATION USERS AND OTHERS

A person who has and/or knows how to use an augmentative communication strategy or aid will not necessarily use it effectively to initiate and participate in conversations (Angelo & Goldstein, 1990; Basil, 1992; Beukelman, 1988; Beukelman & Yorkston,

1982; Calculator & Delaney, 1986; Green & Scherer, 1985; Harris & Vanderheiden, 1980; Higginbotham, 1986, 1989; Higginbotham, Mathy-Laikko, & Yoder, 1988; Higginbotham & Yoder, 1982; Jolleff et al., 1992; Kraat, 1985a; Light, 1988; Light, Collier, & Parnes, 1985a, 1985b; Newell, 1992). According to Angelo and Goldstein (1990, p. 231), when augmented communicators engage in conversations

> *the augmented speaker typically assumes the role of responder and seldom initiates conversations with others. When initiations do occur, they are often limited to object or action requests . . . . Far less common are requests for information that could enable the augmented speaker to actively initiate and participate in conversations.*

There can be several reasons why an augmentative user's interactions with speaking partners during conversations could be highly asymmetrical. First, the user may not have available all of the symbols needed for encoding the types of messages needed to initiate and participate in everyday conversations. This is particularly apt to be a problem when he or she is using a symbol set other than the alphabet (possibly combined with commonly used words and phrases) or American Sign Language.

Second, persons with whom he or she could communicate may not understand the symbols in which messages are being encoded. For example, a preschoolchild probably would be unable to understand messages encoded using letters printed on a communication board. Third, the user may be embarrassed about being unable to speak and having to rely on augmentative communication. Consequently, he or she may avoid using it.

Fourth, the user may not know how to utilize the system to initiate conversations (Light, McNaughton, & Parnes, 1986) and/or to keep them going (Buzolich, King, & Baroody, 1991). The user must have a way to signal that he or she wants to communicate—for example, a noise-making device such as a bell attached to a toe (Schreiber, 1979) or a modified portable transistor radio (King, 1991) or an easily seen arm gesture (DeRuyter & Donoghue, 1989). And to keep conversations going the "listener" must know how to promote turn taking (Hunt, Alwell, & Goetz, 1991b)—for example, by encouraging the user to comment on what is being said by communicating messages such as That's great!, Wow!, Oh no!, Sounds good!, and Yuck! (Buzolich, King, & Baroody, 1991). The listener must have what Lindblom (1990) has referred to as communicative empathy for the user; that is, he or she must be sensitive to the user's feelings about communicating and adapt to them in accordance with his or her communicative goals.

And fifth, the user's pattern of passivity could be the result of learned helplessness and learned dependency. This refers to a decrease in motivation on the part of the user to produce goal-directed responses because of a combination of having experienced "failure" in the past when attempting to produce them and caregivers not expecting them to be produced and consequently providing few opportunities for their production (Basil, 1992). The consequence is diminished social independence

(Reichle, Feeley, & Johnston, 1993). This learning of passivity in communication may begin in infancy. Babies affected with cerebral palsy give fewer cues than their peers, and, consequently, their parents often become more controlling and directive in order to have successful communication (Jolleff & McConachie, 1992). Encouraging caregivers to provide more opportunities for symmetrical communication—for example, asking more open-ended questions—can reduce user passivity (Basil, 1992).

An important aspect of any augmentative communication intervention program is encouraging and facilitating the use of the strategy, technique, or aid for initiating and participating in conversations (Basil, 1992). It isn't safe to assume that once a person has learned it, he or she will do so. There are several pragmatically oriented teaching strategies that could be helpful for achieving this goal (Angelo & Goldstein, 1990; Basil, 1992; Glennen, 1992; Glennen & Calculator, 1985).

EMOTIONAL ASPECTS OF INTERVENTION

All augmentative communication intervention programs should take into consideration the emotional needs of the client and his or her significant others. Meeting these would include for the client development of the ability to communicate feelings, both positive and negative, and for the client and his or her significant others the development of an "objective attitude" toward the pathological condition and the limitations imposed on it.

Development of the ability to communicate feelings involves providing clients with appropriate symbols and a means for indicating them. It is particularly important that symbols be provided for expressing messages about trust and closeness as well as negative feelings (Beukelman, 1989). Those for expressing the latter should include symbols for swearing (e.g., $@%[SHHH!!!]?) and for encoding the message "Please don't patronize me!" (Creech & Viggiano, 1981).

If a client is using a communication aid that generates synthesized speech, it may be possible to program it to provide information about current emotional state (e.g., tension or anger). This information would be conveyed, as it is for normal speakers, through changes in voice parameters (Alm et al., 1993).

Both clients and their significant others are likely to react emotionally to the conditions that caused the clients to be severely communicatively impaired. It is normal for a person to grieve after experiencing a loss. The stages that people go through while grieving are predictable: denial, anger, bargaining, depression, and finally acceptance (Clark, 1990; Tanner, 1980). If the client and his or her significant others are not progressing through these stages in the expected manner (or appear unlikely to do so), they may require psychotherapy (Broder & Hinton, 1982, 1984). A client who has fixated at the denial stage may believe that the loss of speech is only temporary and would, therefore, be unwilling to use augmentative communication. Or a client who has fixated at the depression stage may not be interested in communicating. There may be difficulty in locating a psychiatric social worker, clinical psychologist, or psychiatrist who can work effectively with a patient who cannot speak.

ASSESSING THE IMPACT OF AUGMENTATIVE INTERVENTION PROGRAMS

One aspect of every augmentative communication intervention program should be a periodic systematic assessment of its impact on the user. This information is needed for at least two reasons. One reason is to inform the clinician periodically whether the program is having the desired effect. If it does not appear to be achieving the clinician's goals, it may have to be modified.

Another reason why such information is needed is to add to our knowledge concerning the impacts of particular augmentative strategies on children and adults who are severely communicatively impaired for various reasons. Some information about them has been reported (e.g., Beukelman, 1986; Beukelman & Yorkston, 1980; Beukelman et al., 1981; Cook et al., 1983; Culp et al., 1985; Enderby & Hamilton, 1981; and Roper & Kalbe, 1984). The more information that is available, the better able we will be as clinicians to select the optimal strategy for each of our clients.

When evaluating the effectiveness of augmentative intervention programs, the focus should be on their utilization beyond the clinical setting—that is, on functional communication in daily interactions. Among the factors that should be considered in such evaluations are the ability of the client to utilize augmentative communication in interactions (situations) in which he or she was not specifically instructed to utilize it and the extent to which the client continues to utilize augmentative communication in the natural environment following intervention (Calculator, 1988b, 1988c). Some clients experience difficulty (or reticence) using augmentative communication for purposes other than those directly taught (Calculator, 1988b, 1988c; Glennen & Calculator, 1985; Reichle & Yoder, 1985). And if the client reverted after a period of time to his or her preintervention communication mode, the effectiveness of the intervention would be questionable.

Several kinds of information are needed to assess systematically the impacts of intervention with augmentative communication on clients. This information can be abstracted from observations that are made to answer questions such as the following (Silverman, 1993):

1. What are the effects of the therapy on specific behaviors that contribute to a client's communicative disorder?
2. What are the effects of the therapy on other attributes of a client's communicative behavior?
3. What are the effects of the therapy on the client other than those directly related to communicative behavior?

4. What are the client's attitudes toward the therapy and its effects on his or her communicative and other behaviors?
5. What are the attitudes of the client's clinician, family, friends, and others toward the therapy and toward its effects on the client's communicative behavior and other attributes of behavior?
6. What investment is required of client and clinician?
7. What is the probability of relapse following termination of the therapy?

These questions can be used to assess the impacts of any therapy on persons who have a communicative disorder. Their application to the assessment of the impacts of augmentative intervention programs is illustrated in chapter 2. Methodology that can be used for generating the observations needed to answer each question and respond to each Inventory item is described in Silverman (1993, Chapter 13).

PREVENTIVE MAINTENANCE FOR COMMUNICATION AIDS

If a person will be using a gestural-assisted or neuro-assisted communication aid, it is necessary to make some provision for the maintenance of that aid. Such a maintenance program may include the following:

1. Arranging to have the batteries checked periodically and recharged or replaced before they fail
2. Periodically checking electric cables used to interconnect system components and switching mechanisms for signs of wear and replacing them when necessary
3. Cleaning the surfaces of communication boards and other displays

Someone in a user's environment should be trained to perform as many of these functions as possible. The person should be taught how to test batteries and replace or recharge them. It may also be possible to train the person to troubleshoot problems with connecting cables, switching mechanisms, and a microcomputer. He or she should also be provided with information about where batteries and other materials needed for maintaining the aid can be purchased and where the aid can be repaired.

UTILIZING MICROCOMPUTER-BASED AIDS FOR RECREATION AND EDUCATION

One advantage of a microcomputer-based augmentative communication aid over a dedicated one is that it can be used for purposes other than communication. There is software available for all microcomputers that enable them to be used for both recreation and education. Some software can be used by persons who can control only a single switch. There is even a single-switch scanning program that enables a severely motor-handicapped child to draw (*PIC-MAN*, 1984). For further information, see Goldenberg, Russell, and Carter (1984).

UTILIZING MICROCOMPUTER-BASED AIDS FOR ENVIRONMENTAL CONTROL

A switching mechanism used for activating a microcomputer-based communication aid may also be used to control other devices. Such devices could include a nurse call system, a television set, a book-page turner, a thermostat (to make the room warmer or colder), and an automatic telephone dialer. Configuring a microcomputer for controlling electrical devices usually requires the addition of both hardware—including an digital-to-analog converter (see Silverman, 1987b)—and software. For further information about the use of microcomputer-based augmentative communication aids for environmental control, see Copeland (1974a), Dymond et al., (1988), Parish (1979–1980), Peizer, Lorenze, and Dixon (1982), Pollak and Gallagher (1989), and Thornett, Langer, and Brown (1990).

LITERACY LEARNING

Children who are severely speech impaired may have difficulty learning to read, write, and spell (Koppenhaver, Evans, & Yoder, 1991; Koppenhaver et al., 1992; Koppenhaver & Yoder, 1988, 1990a, 1990b, 1990c, 1992; Light & Smith, 1993; Pierce & McWilliams, 1993; Smith, 1989, 1990, 1992a, 1992b, 1992c, 1992d; Steelman, 1992; Steelman, Coleman, & Koppenhaver, 1992; Steelman et al., 1993; Steelman, Pierce, & Koppenhaver, 1993). In addition to the educational consequences of these types of impairments, there are also communicative ones. Persons who are severely speech impaired who can read and spell can use a communication board with a national language symbol system. And those who can read, write, and spell can communicate with a microcomputer and word processing software (Scull & Hill, 1988; Smith et al., 1989). Their ability to do these is likely to be enhanced by providing them with abundant reading and writing materials and immersing them in varied and regular experiences with print materials (Koppenhaver, Evans, & Yoder, 1991).

VOCATIONAL REHABILITATION AND EMPLOYMENT RIGHTS

Title I of the Americans with Disabilities Act of 1990 (ADA, PL 101-336) prohibits discrimination against people with disabilities in all employment, including application procedures, hiring, firing, advancement, compensation, and training. In particular, the ADA requires that employers make reasonable accommodation. Reasonable accommodation could include use of a communication device and the services of a sign language interpreter (Employment rights of people . . . , 1992). This law does not, however, require that employers give special attention or consideration to the applications of persons with disabilities.

The ADA should be a boon to many severely communicatively impaired adults, particularly those who have normal (or above normal) intelligence and have attended a college or university (Huer, 1990, 1991). Most of the latter are capable of gainful employment regardless of the degree of impairment in their upper and lower extremities. Although they may perform tasks more slowly than able-bodied workers, they are likely to be more accurate and reliable because they tend to be more highly motivated (Pierce & Kublin, 1993). Some have (or are capable of acquiring) the skills needed to be computer programmers. A slogan that has been used for promoting the educational and vocational interests of another minority group is also appropriate for promoting these for this one: "A mind is a terrible thing to waste."

One type of reasonable accommodation a severely communicatively impaired person may request is to work at home, as do millions of able-bodied persons in the United States.

LEKOTEKS AND TOY LIBRARIES

Toys can be used as tools for stimulating augmentative communication between severely communicatively impaired children and their parents, siblings, and others in the home environment (Brodin, 1991a, 1991b). Libraries from which appropriate toys can be borrowed exist in the United States and at least 36 other countries (Björck-Åkesson and Brodin, 1992; Brodin & Björck-Åkesson, 1992). Toy libraries that specialize in servicing children with disabilities sometimes are referred to as lekoteks. Lekoteks are often affiliated with rehabilitation centers as a part of their assessment and educational services. The age group on which they focus usually is preschool. The lekotek staff can be helpful when selecting toys for accomplishing specific goals, such as encouraging augmentative communication.

SWITCH TRAINING

Before a person can learn to use an electronic gestural-assisted communication device, he or she must be taught to operate its switching mechanism. Sometimes, particularly with young children, the use of a switching mechanism is taught with a device other than a communication aid (e.g., a toy). Almost any battery-operated toy can easily be modified so that it can be turned on and off with any single-switch switching mechanism (Backiel, 1985; Burkhart, 1985a, 1985b). A cable is attached to the toy (see Figure 8–2) into which the switching mechanism can be plugged.

With very young children, an attempt may be made to teach the function of a

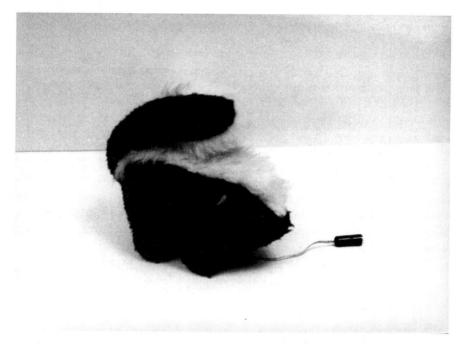

FIGURE 8–2   **A toy with a cable attached for a switching mechanism.**

switch rather than the use of a particular switching mechanism. The devices in Figure 8–3 are intended for this purpose. The child learns that by pushing the clown he or she can cause something to happen (e.g., the cars to move on the track).

ADVOCACY

We have a responsibility to persons who are severely communicatively impaired that goes beyond augmenting their ability to communicate. It is to be their advocate, to promote their overall welfare. As Pat Mirenda of the University of Nebraska-Lincoln has stated (1993, p. 8):

> *Whenever I talk about communication contexts and opportunities and how important it is to get people out of their burning buildings and into truly inclusive contexts, people invariably say to me "Yeah, you're right, but I don't have time for that," or "Yeah, but that's not my job." Well, I suggest, with all due respect, that that is just not true. It is our job. For we are not just in the business of communication, or mobility, or literacy, or behavior management, or whatever our specialty area happens to be. We are in the busi-*

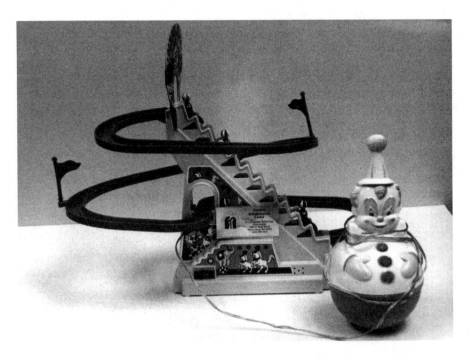

FIGURE 8–3   **A toy for teaching the function of a switching mechanism. Pushing the clown causes the cars to move on the track.**

ness of liberating the human spirit—*we are in the business, in many cases, of* giving people lives—*and, in many situations, that requires ongoing and persistent advocacy efforts that go far beyond what we might conceive of as our traditional roles and job descriptions.*

For further information about advocacy, see Zangari, Kangas, and Lloyd (1988).

References and Bibliography

This bibliography and reference list, which was updated at the beginning of 1993, includes almost all papers that to my knowledge contain information about augmentative and alternative communication (AAC). It is an updated version of the one I began compiling in 1976 that appeared in the first two editions of this text. The list is international in scope and includes both published and unpublished material. A number of sources were consulted in compiling this bibliography, including *Asha* (convention paper abstracts), *Dissertation Abstracts, Index Medicus,* the MEDLINE data base, bibliographies published by the Trace Center and the International Society for Augmentative and Alternative Communication, and the references lists of the papers located. A few of the references obtained from secondary sources are incomplete but are included to make this bibliography as comprehensive as possible.

The bibliography items are from my book *Comprehensive Bibliography on Augmentative and Alternative Communication: A Key to the AAC Literature for Clinicians and Researchers.* This book, which is updated periodically and contains both author and subject indices, can be ordered from CODI Publications, Box 261, Greendale, WI 53129.

Abelson, C., & Pfeiffer, D. (1975). Communication aids for the non-verbal severely handicapped child—A multidimensional challenge. *Canadian Journal of Occupational Therapy*, 42, 141–144.

Abkarian, G. G. (1981). A nonverbal child in a regular classroom. *Journal of Learning Disabilities*, 14(3), 138–139.

Abkarian, G. G., Dworkin, J., & Brown, S. (1978). An adventitiously non-verbal child: Signed English as a transitional step in Reye's syndrome. Paper presented at the annual meeting of the American Speech-Language-Hearing Association, San Francisco.

Abrahamsen, A. A., Romski, M. A., & Sevcik, R. A. (1989). Concomitants of success in acquiring an augmentative communication system: Changes in attention, communication, and sociability. *American Journal on Mental Retardation*, 93(5), 475–496.

Abrams, P. (1975). *Simultaneous Language Program for Non-verbal Preschool Children.* Chicago: Dysfunctioning Child Center, Michael Reese Medical Center.

Adams, M. R. (1966). Communication aids for patients with amyotrophic lateral sclerosis. *Journal of Speech and Hearing Disorders,* 31, 274–275.

Adamson, L. B., & Dunbar, B. (1991). Communication development of young children with tracheostomies. *Augmentative and Alternative Communication,* 7, 275–283.

Adamson, L. B., Romski, M. A., Deffebach, K., & Sevcik, R. A. (1992). Symbol vocabulary and the focus of conversations: Augmenting language development for youth with mental retardation. *Journal of Speech and Hearing Research,* 35, 1333–1343.

Ahlers, J., Bortnem, P., Brady, H., & Leite, J. (1987). Weekly communication group: Adult mediated, same-age and cross-age discourse activities. Intervention strategy developed under Contract No. 300-85-0139 (*Implementation Strategies for Improving the Use of Communication Aids in Schools Serving Handicapped Children*) from the U.S. Department of Education distributed by the American Speech-Language-Hearing Association.

Aiello, S. (1980). Non-oral communication survey: A summary report. Paper presented at the annual meeting of the American Speech-Language-Hearing Association, Detroit.

Alant, E. (1992). AAC: Accessibility and implementation in South Africa. *Augmentative and Alternative Communication,* 8, 112.

Albanese, M. K., Jerrell, N. F., Follansbee, R., & Carpenter, T. (1990). A computer-based communication system and tutorial for adults with ALS. *Augmentative and Alternative Communication,* 6, 100.

Albanese, M. K., Sauer, M., & Jarrell, N. F. (1990). A communication system for a cognitively intact, physically disabled, deaf-blind user. *Augmentative and Alternative Communication,* 6, 110.

Albert, M., Pare, L., & Goodenough-Trepagnier, C. (1992). ECRIRE from the perspective of ten years of experience. *Augmentative and Alternative Communication,* 8, 112.

Allaire, J. H., & Gressard, R. P. (1989). Nonspeaking children: Characteristics and parent perceptions. Paper presented at the annual meeting of the American Speech-Language-Hearing Association, St. Louis.

Allaire, J. H., Gressard, R. P., Blackman, J. A., & Hostler, S. L. (1991). Children with severe speech impairments: Caregiver survey of AAC use. *Augmentative and Alternative Communication,* 7, 248–255.

Allaire, J. H., Gressard, R. R., & Van Dyck, M. C. (1990). Parent perceptions of augmentative and alternative communication. *Augmentative and Alternative Communication,* 6, 119.

Allen, D., Moore, E., Dunn, N., & Anderson, V. (1986). Transition from an urban residential setting to a rural public school setting: Do augmentative communication systems work in the real world? *Augmentative and Alternative Communication,* 2, 69.

Allen, J. B. (April 30, 1974). Nu-Life for amputees and paralyzed patients. *Congressional Record-Extensions of Remarks.*

Allen, J. M. (1988). Teaching interaction skills to caregivers of aided communicators. *Augmentative and Alternative Communication,* 4, 167–168.

Alm, N. (1986). Applying lessons from conversation analysis to the design of communication aids. *Augmentative and Alternative Communication,* 2, 69–70.

Alm, N., Arnott, J. L., & Murray, I. R. (1992). Bypassing communication difficulties to allow satisfying conversational participation by a non-speaking person. *Proceedings of the Institute of Acoustics,* 14 (Part 6), 637–644.

Alm, N., Arnott, J. L., & Newell, A. F. (1992a). Evaluation of a text-based communication system for increasing conversational participation and control. Paper presented at RESNA International '92.

Alm, N., Arnott, J. L., & Newell, A.F. (1992b). Prediction and conversational momentum in an augmentative communication system. *Communications of the ACM* [Association for Computing Machinery], 35(5), 46–57.

Alm, N., Brophy, B., Arnott, J. L., & Newell, A. F. (1988). Preliminary evaluation of a conversation aid based on speech acts. *Augmentative and Alternative Communication*, 4, 153.

Alm, N., McGregor, A., Arnott, J. L., & Newell, A. F. (1992). Using prestored text in conversation by an AAC user. *Augmentative and Alternative Communication*, 8, 112.

Alm, N., Murray, I. R., Arnott, J. L., & Newell, A. F. (March 1993). Pragmatics and affect in a communication system for non-speakers. *Journal of the American Voice I/O Society,* 13, 1–15.

Alpert, C. (1980). Procedures for determining the optimal nonspeech mode with the autistic child. In Richard Schiefelbusch (Ed.), *Nonspeech Language and Communication: Analysis and Intervention.* Baltimore: University Park Press, 389–420.

Altheide, M. R., & Hough, S. D. (1986). Introducing augmentative communication: A model for parent education. *Augmentative and Alternative Communication*, 2, 70.

Alwell, M., Hunt, P., Goetz, L., & Sailor, W. (1989). Teaching generalized communicative behaviors within interrupted behavior chain contexts. *Journal of the Association for Persons with Severe Handicaps*, 14, 91–100.

American Indian Sign: Gestural Communication for the Speechless (1974). A series of four videotapes (VC 1 PT. 1–PT. 4) distributed by the Learning Resources Center, Veterans Administration Hospital, St. Louis.

American Speech-Language-Hearing Association (1991a). Augmentative and alternative communication. *Asha*, 33 (Suppl. 5), 8.

American Speech-Language-Hearing Association (1991b). Report: Augmentative and alternative communication. *Asha*, 33 (Suppl. 5), 9–12.

American Speech-Language-Hearing Association (1993). Preferred practice patterns for the professions of speech-language pathology and audiology. *Asha*, 35 (Suppl. 11), 61–62, 87–88.

Amer-Ind Video Dictionary (1975). A series of four videotapes (VC 76 PT. 1–PT. 4) distributed by the Learning Resources Center, Veterans Administration Hospital, St. Louis.

Anderson, J. D. (1980). Spatial arrangement of stimuli and the construction of communication boards for the physically handicapped. *Mental Retardation*, 18(1), 41–42.

Anderson, K. (1978). An eye position controlled typewriter. In P. Nelson (Ed.), *Proceedings of Workshop on Communication Aids*. Ottawa: Canadian Medical and Biological Engineering Society, National Research Council.

Anderson, K., & Neuman, S. (1977). *Total communication for mentally retarded children.* Videotape presented at the annual meeting of the American Speech-Language-Hearing Association, Chicago.

Anderson, P. M., & Kiernan, S. C. (1988), Cost effectiveness issues in augmentative and alternative communication—In the black. *Augmentative and Alternative Communication*, 4, 142,

Anderson, P. M., Kiernan, S. C., & Ashida, K. (1988). More for your money: An arena assessment for AAC. *Augmentative and Alternative Communication*, 4, 170.

Anderson, P. M., Wood, J., & Kiernan, S. C. (1988). A clinical comparison of six commercially available speech synthesizers. *Augmentative and Alternative Communication*, 4, 163.

Anderson, S. S., & Harrison, J. S. (1992). Comparison of augmentative devices used in "facilitated communication." Paper presented at the annual meeting of the American Speech-Language-Hearing Association, San Antonio.

Andrews, I. M. (1986). Improvements in communication and capability through the use of the Queenwood special computer system. *Augmentative and Alternative Communication*, 2, 70.

Angelo, D. H. (1988). Effects of pragmatic teaching on information-requesting behaviors of augmented speakers. Paper presented at the annual meeting of the American Speech-Language-Hearing Association, Boston.

Angelo, D. H., & Goldstein, H. (1990). Effects of a pragmatic teaching strategy for requesting information by communication board users. *Journal of Speech and Hearing Disorders*, 55, 231–243.

Angelo, D. H., & Jones, S. D. (1992). Family stressors, needs, and resources of children using assistive devices. *Augmentative and Alternative Communication*, 8, 112–113.

Angelo, J. (1987). A comparison of three coding methods for abbreviation expansion in acceleration vocabularies. Unpublished doctoral dissertation, University of Wisconsin-Madison.

Angelo, J. (1992). Comparison of three computer scanning modes as an interface method for persons with cerebral palsy. *American Journal of Occupational Therapy*, 46(3), 217–222.

Archer, L. (1977). Blissymbolics—A non-verbal communication system. *Journal of Speech and Hearing Disorders*, 42, 568–579.

Armfield, A. (1986a). Demonstration of Makaton to begin learning Chinese. *Augmentative and Alternative Communication*, 2, 70–71.

Armfield, A. (1986b). Makaton in USA. *Augmentative and Alternative Communication*, 2, 71.

Armstrong, B. L. (1990). Integrating environmental control, computer access, communication with developmentally disabled persons. *Augmentative and Alternative Communication*, 6, 138.

Armstrong, B. L., Brown III, F. R. (1988). Management of augmentative communication: Selecting a system and intervention course. Paper presented at the annual meeting of the American Speech-Language-Hearing Association, Boston.

Arnott, J. L. (1986). Speech synthesizer control by stenotype keyboard. *Augmentative and Alternative Communication*, 2, 71.

Arnott, J. L., & Javed, M. Y. (1992). Probabilistic character disambiguation for reduced keyboards using small text samples. *Augmentative and Alternative Communication*, 8, 215–223.

Arruabarrena, A., Buldain, G., Gardeazabal, L., Gomez, E., & Gonzalez, J. (1989). JAL2: An integrated tool to enhance communication and autonomy of disabled people. *Journal of Medical Engineering and Technology*, 13(1–2), 28–33.

Arthur, G. (1952). *The Arthur Adaptation of the Leiter International Performance Scale.* Washington, DC: Psychological Service Center Press.

Ashida, K., Kiernan, S. C., & Anderson, P. M. (1988). Follow-up: If you don't call us, we'll call you. *Augmentative and Alternative Communication*, 4, 142.

Assal, G., & Buttet, J. (1976). Non-verbal vocal expression in aphasics. *Review of Otoneuroophthalmology*, 48, 373–379.

Assistive Devices for Handicapped Students: A Model and Guide for a State Wide Delivery System (1980). Washington, DC: National Association of State Directors of Special Education.

Astros aid quadriplegic (March 21, 1974). *Atlantic City Press* (Atlantic City, NJ).

Attermeir, S. (Ed.) (1987). *Augmentative Communication: Clinical Issues.* New York: Haworth. [Also published in *Physical and Occupational Therapy in Pediatrics,* 7, 1987.]

Augmentative and alternative communication (June–July 1992). *Asha,* 34, 86.

Augmentative and alternative communication devices: 1991 buyers' guide (December 1990). *Asha,* 32, 12–13, 16.

Augmentative and alternative communicative devices: 1993 buyers' guide (December 1992). *Asha,* 34, 50, 52.

Australian News and Information Bureau. Blissymbolics (1973). *Hearing and Speech News,* 41(5), 6–7.

Backiel, T. C. (1985). Additional resources—Supplement to information on battery-operated toys. *Language, Speech, and Hearing Services in Schools,* 16, 79.

Bady, J. A., & Silverman, F. H. (1978). A videotape approach to teaching interpretation of Amer-Ind signs. *Perceptual and Motor Skills,* 47, 530.

Bailey, S. (1983). Blissymbolics and aphasia therapy: A case study. In C. Code & D. Muller (Eds.), *Aphasia Therapy.* London: Edward Arnold, pp. 178–186.

Baker, B. R. (September 1982). Minspeak: A semantic compaction system that makes self-expression easier for communicatively disabled individuals. *Byte,* 7, 186–202.

Baker, B. R. (1983). Chopsticks and Beethoven. *Communication Outlook,* 5, 8–11.

Baker, B. R. (1985). The use of words and phrases on a Minspeak communication system. *Communication Outlook,* 7(1), 8–10.

Baker, B. R. (1986a). *How to Establish a Core Vocabulary Through the Dialogue Method and How to Write Dialogue.* Pittsburgh: Author.

Baker, B. R. (1986b). Using images to generate speech. *Byte,* 11, 160–168.

Baker, B. R., & Higgins, J. M. (1988). Syntactical issues in augmentative and alternative communication. *Augmentative and Alternative Communication,* 4, 136.

Baker, L. A. (1992). Plan for success: Curriculum design for the AAC student. *Augmentative and Alternative Communication,* 8, 113.

Baker, M. (1984). Who knows what the future holds? In *Conversations with Nonspeaking People.* Toronto: Rehabilitation Council for the Disabled.

Balandin, S., Wallbrink, A., & Beedham, J. (1992). Focus on dinner. *Augmentative and Alternative Communication,* 8, 113.

Balick, S., Spiegel, D., & Greene, G. (1976). Mime in language therapy and clinician training. *Archives of Physical Medicine and Rehabilitation,* 57, 35–38.

Balkon, J. J. M., Blom, C. L., & Soede, M. (1987). *Efficient Input Systems for Augmentative Communication.* Hoensbroek, Norway: Institute for Rehabilitation Research.

Barker, M. R. (1992). Input systems for integrated AAC and power mobility devices. *Augmentative and Alternative Communication,* 8, 113.

Barnes, N., Aguirre, N., & Schulte, L. (1988). Computer adaptations—From device training to functional classroom use. *Augmentative and Alternative Communication,* 4, 165.

Barnes, S. (1973). The use of sign language as a technique for language acquisition in autistic children: An applied model for bridging verbal and nonverbal theoretical systems. Unpublished doctoral dissertation, California School of Professional Psychology, San Francisco.

Barnhart, K. S., & Keenan, J. E. (1988). Early communication systems for the severely brain-injured patient. *Augmentative and Alternative Communication*, 4, 146–147.

Baron, N., Isensee, L., and Davis, A. (1977). Iconicity and learnability: Teaching sign language to autistic children. Paper presented at the Second Boston University Conference on Language Development, Boston.

Barrera, R. D., Lobato-Barrera, D., & Sulzer-Azaroff, B. (1980). A simultaneous treatment comparison of three expressive language training programs with a mute autistic child. *Journal of Autism and Developmental Disorders*, 10, 21–37.

Barrera, R. D., & Sulzer-Azaroff, B. (1983). An alternating treatment comparison of oral and total communication training programs with echolalic autistic children. *Journal of Applied Behavior Analysis*, 16, 379–394.

Barron-Jadd, E., & Weitzner-Lin, B. (1992). Using EZ Keys: A case study with a dysgraphic adolescent. *Augmentative and Alternative Communication*, 8, 113–114.

Bartak, L., Rutter, M., & Cox, A. (1975). A comparative study of infantile autism and specific developmental receptive language disorders: 1. The children. *British Journal of Psychiatry*, 126, 127–145.

Basil, C. (1986). Social interaction and learned helplessness in nonvocal severely handicapped children. *Augmentative and Alternative Communication*, 2, 71–72.

Basil, C. (1992). Social interaction and learned helplessness in severely disabled children. *Augmentative and Alternative Communication*, 8, 188–199.

Basil, C., & Ruiz, R. (1985). *Sistemas de Communication No Vocal para Ninos con Disminuciones Fisicas* [Nonvocal Communication Systems for Children with Physical Handicapps]. Madrid: Los Libros de Fundesco.

Batstone, S., & Bailey, S. (1990). Baileywick: VOCA for the multiply disabled low vision user. *Augmentative and Alternative Communication*, 6, 110.

Batt, M., Remington-Gurney, J., & Crossley, R. (1990). Facilitated communication—Parent perspectives. *Augmentative and Alternative Communication*, 6, 92.

Battison, R., & Markowicz, H. (1976). *Sign Aphasia and Neurolinguistic Theory*. Washington, DC: Linguistics Research Laboratory, Gallaudet College.

Battison, R., & Padden, C. (1974). Sign language aphasia: A case study. Paper presented at the annual meeting of the Linguistic Society of America, New York.

Baumgarner, J. R., & Karadin, K. A. (1987). Differing outcomes in assessment for augmentative communication. Paper presented at the annual meeting of the American Speech-Language-Hearing Association, New Orleans.

Baumgarner, J. R., Manning, A., & Caswell, S. (1989). The effects of structured vision training on communication board use. Paper presented at the annual meeting of the American Speech-Language-Hearing Association, St. Louis.

Baumgart, D., Johnson, J., & Helmstetter, E. (1990). *Augmentative and Alternative Communication Systems for Persons with Moderate and Severe Disabilities*. Baltimore: Paul H. Brookes.

Bay, J. L. (1991). Positioning for head control to access an augmentative communication machine. *American Journal of Occupational Therapy*, 45(6), 544–549.

Beasley, M. (1977). The role of the occupational therapist in interfacing communication aids. *Proceedings of the Workshop on Communication Aids for the Handicapped*. Ottawa: University of Ottawa, pp. 55–67.

Beasley, M. (1978). The importance of positioning and seating for the cerebral palsied child. In

P. Nelson (Ed.), *Proceedings of the Workshop on Communication Aids*. Ottawa: Canadian Medical and Biological Engineering Society, National Research Council.

Beattie, W., Booth, L., Newell, A. F., & Arnott, J. L. (1990). The role of predictive computer programs in special education. *Augmentative and Alternative Communication*, 6, 89–90.

Beattie, W., Booth, L., Newell, A. F., & Ricketts, I. W. (1992). Predictive systems for reluctant writers and hesitant spellers. *Augmentative and Alternative Communication*, 8, 114.

Bebko, J. M. (1990). Echolalia, mitigation, and autism: Indicators from child characteristics for the use of sign language and other augmentative language systems. *Sign Language Studies*, 66, 61–78.

Bedrosian, J. L., & Hoag, L. A. (1992). Effects of variables on perceptions of communicative competence. Paper presented at the annual meeting of the American Speech-Language-Hearing Association, San Antonio.

Bedrosian, J. L., Hoag, L. A., Calculator, S. N., & Molineux, B. (1992). Variables influencing perceptions of the communicative competence of an adult augmentative and alternative communication system user. *Journal of Speech and Hearing Research*, 35, 1105–1113.

Bedwinek, A. P. (1983). The use of PACE to facilitate gestural and verbal communication in a language-impaired child. *Language, Speech, and Hearing Services in Schools*, 14, 2–6.

Beliveau, C., & Pendergast, L. G. (1988). Critical issues in service delivery. *Augmentative and Alternative Communication*, 4, 150.

Bell, D. J., et al. (1976). *Let Your Fingers Do the Talking: A Teaching Manual for Use with Non-verbal Retardates*. Sonyea, NY: Craig Development Center. Copies can be obtained from the ERIC Document Reproduction Service, Box 190, Arlington, VA.

Benaroya, S., Wesley, S., Ogilvie, H., Klein, L. S., & Clarke, E. (1979). Sign language and multisensory input training of children with communication and related developmental disorders; Phase II. *Journal of Autism and Developmental Disorders*, 9(2), 219–220.

Benaroya, S., Wesley, S., Ogilvie, H., Klein, L. S., & Meaney, M. (1977). Sign language and multisensory input training of children with communication and related developmental disorders. *Journal of Autism and Childhood Schizophrenia*, 7, 23–31.

Bender, M., Valletutti, P., & Bender, P. (1985). *Teaching the Moderately and Severely Handicapped. Volume II: Communication, Socialization, Safety, and Leisure Skills*. Austin, TX: Pro-Ed.

Bennett, D. L., Gast, D. L., Wolery, M., & Schuster, J. (1986).The use of PACE to facilitate gestural and verbal communication in a language-impaired child. *Education and Training of the Mentally Retarded*, 21, 117–129.

Bergen, A., & Colangelo, C. (1982). *Positioning the Client with Central Nervous System Deficits. The Wheelchair and Other Adapted Equipment*. Valhalla, NY: Valhalla Rehabilitation Publications.

Berliss, J., Borden, P., & Vanderheiden, G. (1989). *Trace Resourcebook: Assistive Technologies for Communication, Control, and Computer Access, 1989–90 Edition*. Madison, WI: Trace Research and Development Center.

Berlowitz, C. (January 13, 1991). Ana begins to speak. *This World*, p. 16.

Berninger, V. (1989). Comparison of two microcomputer-assisted methods of teaching word decoding and encoding to non-vocal, non-writing and learning disabled students. *Learning and Educational Technology*, 23, 124–129.

Berninger, V. W., & Gans, B. M. (1986a). Assessing word processing capability of the nonvocal, nonwriting. *Augmentative and Alternative Communication*, 2(2), 56–63.

Berninger, V. W., & Gans, B. M. (1986b). Language profiles in nonspeaking individuals with normal intelligence with severe cerebral palsy. *Augmentative and Alternative Communication*, 2(2), 45–50.

Bernstein, L. (Ed.) (1988). *The Vocally Impaired: Clinical Practice and Research*. Needham Heights, MA: Allyn & Bacon.

Berry, J. O. (1986). Augmentative and alternative communication: Impact on the family. *Augmentative and Alternative Communication*, 2, 72.

Berry, J. O. (1987). Strategies for involving parents in programs for young children using augmentative and alternative communication. *Augmentative and Alternative Communication*, 3(2), 90–93.

Berry, J. O. (1988). AAC (Attitudes, Advocacy and Community) for people using AAC. *Augmentative and Alternative Communication*, 4, 138.

Berry, J. O., Ashbaugh, J. A., Thompson, A. S., & Losoncy, M. A. (1984). Training in nonvocal communication implementation. *Communication Outlook*, 6(2), 14, 16–17.

Beukelman, D. R. (1985). The weakest link is better than the strongest memory. *Augmentative and Alternative Communication*, 1(2), 55–57.

Beukelman, D. R. (1986). Evaluating the effectiveness of intervention programs. In Sarah W. Blackstone (Ed.), *Augmentative Communication: An Introduction*. Rockville, MD: American Speech-Language-Hearing Association, pp. 423–445.

Beukelman, D. R. (1987). When you have a hammer, everything looks like a nail. *Augmentative and Alternative Communication*, 3(2), 94–96.

Beukelman, D. R. (1988). She was setting a world's record, and we thought she was drowning, right dad? *Augmentative and Alternative Communication*, 4, 122–123.

Beukelman, D. R. (1989). There are some things you just can't say with your right hand. *Augmentative and Alternative Communication*, 5, 257–258.

Beukelman, D. R. (1990). AAC in the 1990s: A clinical perspective. In *Proceedings of the Visions Conference: Augmentative and Alternative Communication in the Next Decade*. Wilmington, DE: Alfred I. duPont Institute, pp. 109–113.

Beukelman, D. R. (1991). Magic and cost of communicative competence. *Augmentative and Alternative Communication*, 7, 2–10.

Beukelman, D. R., & Garrett, K. L. (1986). Personnel preparation in augmentative communication. *Nebraska Speech, Language, and Hearing Journal*, 24, 5–8.

Beukelman, D. R., & Garrett, K. L. (1988). Augmentative and alternative communication for adults with acquired severe communication disorders. *Augmentative and Alternative Communication*, 4, 104–121.

Beukelman, D. R., Garrett, K. L., Lange, U., & Tice, R. (1988). *Cue-Write: Word Processing with Spelling Assistance and Practice Manual*. Tucson, AZ: Communication Skill Builders.

Beukelman, D. R., Jones, R. S., & Rowan, M. (1989). Frequency of word usage by nondisabled peers in integrated preschool classrooms. *Augmentative and Alternative Communication*, 5, 243–248.

Beukelman, D. R., Kraft, G., & Freal, J. (1985). Expressive communication disorders in persons with multiple sclerosis: A survey. *Archives of Physical Medicine and Rehabilitation*, 66, 675–677.

Beukelman, D. R., McGinnis, J., & Morrow, D. (1991). Vocabulary selection in augmentative and alternative communication. *Augmentative and Alternative Communication*, 7, 171–185.

Beukelman, D. R., & Mirenda, P. (1988). Communication options for persons who cannot speak: Assessment and evaluation. In C. A. Coston (Ed.), *Proceedings of the National Planners Conference on Assistive Device Service Delivery.* Washington, DC: RESNA, Association for the Advancement of Rehabilitation Technology.

Beukelman, D. R., & Mirenda, P. (1992). *Augmentative and Alternative Communication: Management of Severe Communication Disorders in Children and Adults.* Baltimore: Paul H. Brooks.

Beukelman, D. R., Traynor, C., Poblete, M., & Warren, C. G. (1984). Microcomputer-based communication augmentation systems for two nonspeaking, physically handicapped persons with severe visual impairment. *Archives of Physical Medicine and Rehabilitation,* 65(2), 89–91.

Beukelman, D. R., Wolverton, R., & Hiatt, E. (1988). Augmented literacy for nonspeaking/nonwriting persons. *Augmentative and Alternative Communication,* 4, 170.

Beukelman, D. R., & Yorkston, K. M. (1977). A communication system for the severely dysarthric speaker with an intact language system. *Journal of Speech and Hearing Disorders,* 42, 265–270.

Beukelman, D. R., & Yorkston, K. M. (1978). A series of communication options for individuals with brain stem lesions. *Archives of Physical Medicine and Rehabilitation,* 59, 337–342.

Beukelman, D. R., & Yorkston, K. M. (1980). Nonvocal communication: Performance evaluation. *Archives of Physical Medicine and Rehabilitation,* 61, 272–275.

Beukelman, D. R., & Yorkston, K. M. (1982). Communication interaction of adult communication augmentation system users. *Topics in Language,* 2, 39–54.

Beukelman, D. R., & Yorkston, K. M. (1984). Computer enhancement of message formulation and presentation for communication augmentation system users. *Seminars in Speech and Language,* 5, 1–10.

Beukelman, D. R., & Yorkston, K. M. (1985). Frequency of letter occurrence in the communication samples of augmented communicators. Unpublished manuscript, University of Washington, Seattle.

Beukelman, D. R., & Yorkston, K. M. (1989). Augmentative and alternative communication for persons with severe acquired communication disorders: An introduction. *Augmentative and Alternative Communication,* 5, 42–48.

Beukelman, D. R., Yorkston, K. M., & Dowen, P. (1985). *Augmentative Communication: A Casebook of Clinical Management.* San Diego: College Hill.

Beukelman, D. R., Yorkston, K. M., Gorhoff, S. C., Mitsuda, P. M., & Kenyon, V. T. (1981). Canon Communicator use by adults: A retrospective study. *Journal of Speech and Hearing Disorders,* 46, 374–378.

Beukelman, D. R., Yorkston, K. M., & Lossing, C. A. (1984). Functional communication assessment of adults with neurogenic disorders. In A. S. Halpren & M. J. Fuhrer (Eds.), *Functional Assessment in Rehabilitation.* Baltimore: Paul H. Brookes.

Beukelman, D. R., Yorkston, K. M., Poblete, M., & Naranjo, C. (1984). Frequency of word occurrence in communication samples produced by adult communication aid users. *Journal of Speech and Hearing Disorders,* 49, 360–367.

Beukelman, D. R., Yorkston, K. M., & Smith, K. (1985). Third-party payer response to requests for purchase of communication augmentation systems: A study of Washington State. *Augmentative and Alternative Communication,* 1(1), 5–9.

Beukelman, D. R., Yorkston, K. M., & Waugh, P. F. (1980). Communication in severe aphasia:

Effectiveness of three instruction modalities. *Archives of Physical Medicine and Rehabilitation*, 61, 248–252.

Bialik, P., & Lebel, T. (1992). We couldn't see the forest for the trees. *Augmentative and Alternative Communication*, 8, 114.

Bicker, D. D. (1972). Imitative sign training as a facilitator of word-object association with low-functioning children. *American Journal of Mental Deficiency*, 76, 509–516.

Bigge, J. L. (1977). Severe communication problems. In J. L. Bigge and P. A. O'Donnell (Eds.), *Teaching Individuals with Physical and Multiple Disabilities*. Columbus, OH: Charles C. Merrill, pp. 108–136.

Bigge, J. L. (1991). *Teaching Individuals with Physical and Multiple Disabilities*. 3rd ed. Westerville, OH: Charles E. Merrill.

Biklen, D. (Producer) (1988). *Regular Lives* [Videotape]. Washington, DC: State of the Art.

Biklen, D. (1990a). Are the words theirs? An observational study of facilitated communication. *Augmentative and Alternative Communication*, 6, 91.

Biklen, D. (1990b). Communication unbound: Autism and praxis. *Harvard Educational Review*, 60, 291–314.

Biklen, D. (1992a). Typing to talk: Facilitated communication. *American Journal of Speech-Language Pathology*, 1(2), 15–17.

Biklen, D. (1992b). Facilitated communication: Biklen responds. *American Journal of Speech-Language Pathology*, 1(2), 21–22.

Biklen, D., & Crossley, R. (1990). Facilitated communication: The Syracuse and Melbourne experiences. Paper presented at the seventeenth annual conference of the Association for Persons with Severe Handicaps, Chicago.

Biklen, D., Morton, M., Saha, S., Duncan, J., Gold, D., Hardardottir, M., Karna, E., O'Connor, S., & Rao, S. (1991). "I AMN NOT A UTISTIVC OH THJE TYP" (I am not autistic on the typewriter). *Disability, Handicap, and Society*, 6(3), 161–180.

Biklen, D., & Schubert, A. (1991). New words: The communication of students with autism. *Remedial and Special Education*, 12(6), 46–57.

Binion, M. O., & Todd, J. H. (1988). Augmentative and alternative communication: One state's initiative. *Augmentative and Alternative Communication*, 4, 139.

Bioengineering Research Team of the Association for Retarded Citizens of the United States (1992). Eye on the Horizon. *Augmentative and Alternative Communication*, 8, 114.

Bioengineering Research Team of the Association for Retarded Citizens of the United States (1992). Voices of the future. *Augmentative and Alternative Communication*, 8, 114–115.

Bird, F., Dores, P. A., Moniz, D., & Robinson, J. (1989). Reducing severe aggressive and self-injurious behaviors with functional communication training. *American Journal on Mental Retardation*, 94(1), 37–48.

Björck-Åkesson, E. (1990). Communicative interaction of young nonspeaking children and their parents. *Augmentative and Alternative Communication*, 6, 87–88.

Björck-Åkesson, E., & Brodin, J. (1992a). Evaluation of a visual telecommunication system for persons with moderate mental retardation. *Augmentative and Alternative Communication*, 8, 115.

Björck-Åkesson, E. & Brodin, J. M. (1992b). International diversity of toy libraries. *TECSE*, 12(4), 528–543.

Björck-Åkesson, E., Brodin, J., Granlund, M., & Olsson, C. (1992). Communicative competence in profoundly disabled persons: A Scandinavian perspective. *Augmentative and Alternative Communication*, 8, 115.

Blacher, J. (Ed.) (1984). *Severely Handicapped Young Children and Their Families: Research in Review.* Orlando, FL: Academic Press.

Blackoe, V., Potter, R., Dymond, E., & McClemont, E. (1990). Provision of AAC in Huntington's Chorea—A case study. *Augmentative and Alternative Communication,* 6, 106.

Blackstien-Adler, S., Ryan, S., Parnes, P., & Naumann, S. (1990). Development of an integrated wheelchair tray system for augmentative and alternative communication. *Augmentative and Alternative Communication,* 6, 111.

Blackstone, S. W. (Ed.) (1986a). *Augmentative Communication: An Introduction.* Rockville, MD: American Speech-Language-Hearing Association.

Blackstone, S. W. (1986b). Augmentative communication: Preservice education in speech-language pathology and audiology. *Augmentative and Alternative Communication,* 2, 72.

Blackstone, S. W. (1986c). Training strategies. In Sarah W. Blackstone (Ed.), *Augmentative Communication: An Introduction.* Rockville, MD: American Speech-Language-Hearing Association, pp. 267–421.

Blackstone, S. W. (1988a). Amyotrophic lateral sclerosis. *Augmentative Communication News,* 1(3).

Blackstone, S. W. (1988b). Augmentative communication: A clinical management process model. In L. Bernstein (Ed.), *The Vocally Impaired: Clinical Practice and Research.* Needham Heights, MA: Allyn & Bacon.

Blackstone, S. W. (1988c). Auditory scanning (AS) techniques. *Augmentative Communication News,* 1(5), 4–5, 8.

Blackstone, S. W. (1988d). Dual sensory impairments. *Augmentative Communication News,* 1(4).

Blackstone, S. W. (1988e). Light pointing technologies and training. *Augmentative Communication News,* 1(2).

Blackstone, S. W. (1988f). Vocabulary selection issues and practices. *Augmentative Communication News,* 1(5).

Blackstone, S. W. (1989a). AAC after TBI: Silenced by the epidemic. *Augmentative Communication News,* 2(6), 1–5.

Blackstone, S. W. (1989b). Augmentative communication services in the schools. *Asha,* 31(1), 61–64.

Blackstone, S. W. (1989c). For consumers: Societal rehabilitation. *Augmentative Communication News,* 2(3), 1–3.

Blackstone, S. W. (1989d). Individuals with developmental apraxia of speech (DAS). *Augmentative Communication News,* 2(2), 1–4, 6.

Blackstone, S. W. (1989e). Integration of school, work, and community. *Augmentative Communication News,* 2(5).

Blackstone, S. W. (1989f). M & Ms: Meaningful, manageable measurement. *Augmentative Communication News,* 2(3), 3–5.

Blackstone, S. W. (1989g). The 3 R's: Reading, writing, and reasoning. *Augmentative Communication News,* 2(1) 1–6, 8.

Blackstone, S. W. (1989h). Traumatic brain injury and AAC. *Augmentative Communication News,* 2(6).

Blackstone, S. W. (1989i). Visual scanning: What is it all about? Visual scanning: Training approaches. *Augmentative Communication News,* 2(4), 1–5.

Blackstone, S. W. (1990a). AAC service delivery issues. *Augmentative Communication News,* 3(4).

Blackstone, S. W. (1990b). Adults with severe-profound mental challenges. *Augmentative Communication News*, 3(3).

Blackstone, S. W. (1990c). Assistive technology in the classroom. *Augmentative Communication News*, 3(6).

Blackstone, S. W. (1990d). Early communication training approaches. *Augmentative Communication News*, 3(1), 3–5.

Blackstone, S. W. (1990e). Early prevention of severe communication disorders. *Augmentative Communication News*, 3(1), 1–3.

Blackstone, S. W. (1990f). Examining issues of rate and rate enhancement in AAC. *Augmentative Communication News*, 3(5), 1–3.

Blackstone, S. W. (1990g). Graphic symbols: Issues and practices. *Augmentative Communication News*, 3(2).

Blackstone, S. W. (1990h). Infant, toddler, & preschool applications. *Augmentative Communication News*, 3(1).

Blackstone, S. W. (1990i). Rate enhancement in AAC. *Augmentative Communication News*, 3(5).

Blackstone, S. W. (1991a). AAC and autism. *Augmentative Communication News*, 4(5).

Blackstone, S. W. (1991b). Effects of world-wide recession on assistive technology programs. *Augmentative Communication News*, 4(6).

Blackstone, S. W. (1991c). Issues and practices in aphasia. *Augmentative Communication News*, 4(1).

Blackstone, S. W. (1991d). Telecommunications: Options for people with severe speech impairments. *Augmentative Communication News*, 4(4).

Blackstone, S. W. (1991e). Training partners to facilitate interaction. *Augmentative Communication News*, 4(2).

Blackstone, S. W. (1991f). Training partners to facilitate the use of technology. *Augmentative Communication News*, 4(3).

Blackstone, S. W. (1992a). Communication options with tracheostomies and mechanical ventilators. *Augmentative Communication News*, 5(6).

Blackstone, S. W. (1992b). Down syndrome: AAC intervention. *Augmentative Communication News*, 5(2).

Blackstone, S. W. (1992c). Equipment abandonment: The need for consumer participation. *Augmentative Communication News*, 5(3).

Blackstone, S. W. (1992d). Hearing and listening: Considerations for people who use AAC. *Augmentative Communication News*, 5(5).

Blackstone, S. W. (1992e). Language issues and AAC: What master clinicians think and do. *Augmentative Communication News*, 5(4).

Blackstone, S. W. (1992f). Speech recognition: Applications in AAC. *Augmentative Communication News*, 5(1).

Blackstone, S. W., Berg, M. H., Stokes, L. , Boltz, I., & Kaiser, H. (1992). Instructional strategies for helping children learn symbols on communication displays. *Augmentative and Alternative Communication*, 8, 115–116.

Blackstone, S. W., Bristow, D., & LaBran, J. (1992). Strategies for interfacing assistive technologies: A case example. *Augmentative and Alternative Communication*, 8, 116.

Blackstone, S. W., Carter, G., Berg, M. H., & Biondi, J. (1992). Quality in the schools: An AAC consumer satisfaction questionnaire. *Augmentative and Alternative Communication*, 8, 116.

Blackstone, S. W., & Cassatt-James, E. (1984). Communicative competence in communication aid users and their partners. Paper presented at the Third International Conference on Augmentative and Alternative Communication, Boston.

Blackstone, S. W., & Cassatt-James, E. L. (1986). Exemplary communication aid programs serving school-age children in the United States. *Augmentative and Alternative Communication*, 2, 72–73.

Blackstone, S. W., Cassatt-James, E. L., & Bruskin, D. (Eds.) (1988). *Augmentative Communication: Implementation Strategies.* Rockville, MD: American Speech-Language-Hearing Association.

Blackstone, S. W., Dawson, K., Baker, L. W., Glicksman, M., & Yoder, D. (1992). Dispelling the myths of segregation: A panel discussion. *Augmentative and Alternative Communication*, 8, 116–117.

Blackstone, S. W., & Isaacson, R. (1888). Service delivery in augmentative communication. In L. Bernstein (Ed.), *The Vocally Impaired: Clinical Practice and Research.* Needham Heights, MA: Allyn & Bacon.

Blackstone, S. W., & Painter, M. (1985). Speech problems in multihandicapped children. In J. Darby (Ed.), *Speech and Language Evaluation in Neurology: Childhood Disorders.* Orlando, FL: Grune & Stratton, pp. 219–242.

Blau, A. F. (1983a). On interaction. *Communicating Together*, 1, 10–12.

Blau, A. F. (1983b). Vocabulary selection in augmentative communication: Where do we begin? In H. Winitz (Ed.), *Treating Language Disorders: For Clinicians by Clinicians.* Baltimore: University Park Press, pp. 205–233.

Blau, A. F. (1984). *Dial Scan Manual: Suggestions for Training and Use.* Lake Zurich, IL: Don Johnston Developmental Equipment.

Blau, A. F. (1986a). Back–channel communication: Message reformation in nonspeech/speech interaction and intervention. *Augmentative and Alternative Communication*, 2, 73.

Blau, A. F. (1986b). The development of literacy skills for severely speech- and writing-impaired children. In Sarah W. Blackstone (Ed.), *Augmentative Communication: An Introduction.* Rockville, MD: American Speech-Language-Hearing Association, pp. 293–299.

Blau, A. F. (1987). Resolution strategies and revision behaviors: Evidence from augmentative communicators. Paper presented at the annual meeting of the American Speech-Language-Hearing Association, New Orleans.

Blischak, D. M. (1992). Vocabulary selection in multi-modal communication. *Augmentative and Alternative Communication*, 8, 117.

Bliss, C. K. (1965). *Semantography (Blissymbolics).* 2nd ed. Sydney, Australia: Semantography (Blissymbolics) Publications.

Bliss, C. K. (1975). *Syntax Supplement No. 1.* Toronto: Blissymbolics Communication Institute.

Bliss, C. K., & McNaughton, S. (1975). *The Book to the Film "Mr. Symbol Man."* Sydney, Australia: Semantography Publications.

Blissymbolics Communication International (1984). *Picture Your Blissymbols Instructional Manual.* Toronto, Ontario: Author.

Blissymbolics Communication International (1985a). *Blissymbol Applications Readings from B.C.I. Newsletters 1974–1982.* Monograph No. 2. Toronto: Author.

Blissymbolics Communication International (1985b). *Blissymbolics Independent Study Guide.* Toronto: Author.

Blissymbolics Communication International (1985c). *Teaching Aids and Ideas.* Monograph No. 9. Toronto: Author.

Blockberger, S., Armstrong, R. W., O'Connor, A., & Freeman, R. (1990). Children's attitudes toward a nonspeaking child using various augmentative and alternative communication techniques. Paper presented at the fifth biennial conference of the International Society for Augmentative and Alternative Communication, Stockholm.

Blockberger, S., Armstrong, R. W., Freeman, R., & O'Connor, A. (1990). Augmentative and alternative communication (AAC) techniques and children's attitudes toward a nonspeaking child. *Augmentative and Alternative Communication, 6,* 139.

Blockberger, S., Field, D., & Cooper, D. (1992). Issues when mounting augmentative communicative devices. *Augmentative and Alternative Communication, 8,* 117.

Blockberger, S., & Kamp, L. (1990). The use of voice output communication aids (VOCAs) by ambulatory children. *Augmentative and Alternative Communication, 6,* 127–128.

Bloomberg, K. P. (1984). The comparative translucency of initial lexical items represented by five graphic symbol systems. Unpublished master's thesis, Purdue University.

Bloomberg, K. P. (1986). Compic—Computer Pictographs for Communication. *Augmentative and Alternative Communication, 2,* 73–74.

Bloomberg, K. P. (1990). Computer pictographs for communication. *Communication Outlook,* 12(1), 17–18.

Bloomberg, K. P., Dunne, L., & Snelleman, J. (1988). COMPIC—Stage 2. *Augmentative and Alternative Communication, 4,* 153.

Bloomberg, K. P., & Johnson, H. (1990a). Practical augmentative strategies. *Augmentative and Alternative Communication, 6,* 92–93.

Bloomberg, K. P., & Johnson, H. (1990b). Servicing a state. The scoop on S.C.I.O.P. *Augmentative and Alternative Communication, 6,* 119.

Bloomberg, K. P., & Johnson, H. (1990c). A statewide demographic survey of people with severe communication impairments. *Augmentative and Alternative Communication, 6,* 50–60.

Bloomberg, K. P., Karlan, G. R., & Lloyd, L. L. (1990). The comparative translucency of initial lexical items represented in five graphic symbol systems and sets. *Journal of Speech and Hearing Research, 33,* 717–725.

Bloomberg, K. P., & Lloyd, L. L. (1986). Graphic/aided symbols and systems: Resource information. *Communication Outlook, 7,* 24–30.

Blyden, A. E. (1989). Survival word acquisition in mentally retarded adolescents with multi-handicaps: Effects of color—revised stimulus materials. *Journal of Special Education,* 22(4), 493–501.

Bobby, B. (1976). *Say It with Symbols* (filmstrip). Toronto: Blissymbolics Communication Institute.

Bodine, C., & Beukelman, D. R. (1991). Prediction of future speech performance among potential users of AAC systems: A survey. *Augmentative and Alternative Communication, 7,* 100–111.

Bolling, J. F. (1985). A decision-making matrix for determining non-oral communication alternatives. Paper presented at the annual meeting of the American Speech-Language-Hearing Association, Washington, DC.

Bolton, M. P., & Taylor, A. C. (1981). A universal computer and interface system for the disabled (UNICAID). *Journal of Biomedical Engineering,* 3(4), 281–284.

Bolton, S., & Dashiell, S. (1984). *INteraction CHecklist for Augmentative Communication.* Huntington Beach, CA: INCH Associates.

Bonvillian, J. D., & Friedman, R. (1978). Language development in another mode: The acquisition of sign by a brain-damaged adult. *Sign Language Studies*, 19, 111–120.

Bonvillian, J. D., & Nelson, K. E. (1976). Sign language acquisition in a mute autistic boy. *Journal of Speech and Hearing Disorders*, 41, 339–347.

Bonvillian, J. D., & Nelson, K. E. (1978). Development of sign language in autistic children and other language handicapped individuals. In P. Siple (Ed.), *Understanding Language Through Sign Language Research*. New York: Academic Press, pp. 187–209.

Bonvillian, J. D., Nelson, K. E., & Rhyme, J. (1981). Sign language and autism. *Journal of Autism and Developmental Disorders*, 11(1), 125–137.

Boonzaier, D. A., & Shalit, A. (1990). Intercultural problems in "transplanting" western AAC technologies in developing countries. *Augmentative and Alternative Communication*, 6, 105.

Booth, T. (1978). Early receptive language training for the severely and profoundly retarded. *Language, Speech, and Hearing Services in Schools*, 9, 142–150.

Borkowski-Rice, G., & Larkin, C. (1992). IEP development to facilitate inclusion of augmentative communication device users. *Augmentative and Alternative Communication*, 8, 117.

Bornstein, H. A. (1974). Signed English: A manual approach to English language development. *Journal of Speech and Hearing Disorders*, 39, 330–343.

Bornstein, H. A., & Jordan, I. D. (1984).*Functional Signs: A New Approach from Simple to Complex*. Austin, TX: Pro-Ed.

Bornstein, H. A., Saulnier, K. L., & Hamilton, L. B. (1983). *Comprehensive Signed English Dictionary*. Washington, DC: Gallaudet University Press.

Bottorf, L., & DePape, D. (1982). Initiating communication systems for severely speech-impaired persons. *Topics in Language Disorders*, 2(2), 55–71.

Boubekker, M., Foulds, R., & Norman, C. (1986). Human quality synthetic speech based on concatenated diphones. *Proceedings of the RESNA Ninth Annual Conference*. Washington, DC: RESNA, Association for the Advancement of Rehabilitation Technology, pp. 405–407.

Boumans, T., & Bristow, D. (1992). Consumers' perspective. *Augmentative and Alternative Communication*, 8, 117–118.

Bourgeois, M. S. (1990). Enhancing communication skills in patients with Alzheimer's disease using a prosthetic memory aid. *Journal of Applied Behavioral Analysis*, 23, 29–42.

Bourgeois, M. S. (1991). Communication treatment for adults with dementia. *Journal of Speech and Hearing Research*, 34, 831–844.

Bourgeois, M. S. (1992). Evaluating memory wallets in conversations with patients with dementia. *Journal of Speech and Hearing Research*, 35, 1344–1357.

Bourgeois, M. S. (1993). Effects of memory aids on the dyadic conversations of individuals with dementia. *Journal of Applied Behavioral Analysis*, 26, 77–87.

Bowler, D. M. (1991). Need for theory in studies of augmentative and alternative communication. *Augmentative and Alternative Communication*, 7, 127–132.

Bowles-Bridwell, L. (1987). Writing with computers: Implications from research for the language impaired. *Topics in Language Disorders*, 7(4), 78–85.

Brady, D. O., & Smouse, A. D. (1978). A simultaneous comparison of three methods for language training with an autistic child: An experimental single case analysis. *Journal of Autism and Childhood Schizophrenia*, 8(3), 271–279.

Brady-Dobson, G. (1982). *Brady-Dobson Alternative Communication (B-DAC)*. Elmira, OR: Author.

Brady, N. C., & Saunders, K. J. (1991). Considerations in the effective teaching of object-to-symbol matching. *Augmentative and Alternative Communication, 7,* 112–116.

Braille (1990). *The New Encyclopaedia Britannica.* 15th ed.

Bralley, R. C., & Ormond, T. F. (1970). *Communication for the Laryngectomized.* Danville, IL: Interstate Printers and Publishers.

Brandenberg, S., & Vanderheiden, G. (1987a). *Rehabilitation Resource Book Series—Book1: Communication Aids.* San Diego: College-Hill.

Brandenberg, S., & Vanderheiden, G. (1987b). *Rehabilitation Resource Book Series—Book2: Switches, Training, and Environmental Control.* San Diego: College-Hill.

Brandenberg, S., & Vanderheiden, G. (1987c). *Rehabilitation Resource Book Series—Book3: Software and Hardware for Individuals with Sensory and Physical Disabilities.* San Diego: College-Hill.

Braun, U., & Stuckenschneider-Braun, M. (1990). Adapting [Minspeak] "word strategy" to the German language and culture. *Augmentative and Alternative Communication, 6,* 115.

Bray, N. W., & Goossens', C. (1991). Salient letter, letter category, and multimeaning iconic encoding with AAC systems: A comment on Light et al. (September 1990). *Augmentative and Alternative Communication, 7,* 290–293.

Brenner, A. C. (1986). The effect of total communication on vocabulary comprehension: A study using the PPVT-R on trainable mentally handicapped students. *Augmentative and Alternative Communication, 2,* 74.

Brewin, G., & Farrar, P. (1992). Augmenting communication on sexual assault. *Augmentative and Alternative Communication, 8,* 118.

Bricker, D. (1983). Early communication: Development and training. In M. Snell (Ed.), *Systematic Instruction for the Moderately and Severely Handicapped.* 2nd ed. Columbus, OH: Charles E. Merrill, pp. 269–288.

Bricker, D., & Dennison, L. (1978). Training prerequisites to verbal behavior. In M. Snell (Ed.), *Systematic Instruction for the Moderately and Severely Handicapped.* Columbus, OH: Charles E. Merrill, pp. 157–178.

Bridges-Freeman, S. (1990). Children's attitudes toward synthesized speech varying in quality. Unpublished doctoral dissertation, Michigan State University.

Bridgman, P. W. (1927). *The Logic of Modern Physics.* New York: Macmillian.

Brightman, A. (Ed.) (1985). *Ordinary Moments: The Disabled Experience.* Syracuse, NY: Human Policy Press.

Brindle, B. R. (1989). Incidental teaching techniques modified for manual communication with multihandicapped adults. Paper presented at the annual meeting of the American Speech-Language-Hearing Association, St. Louis.

Bristow, D. C., Byers, V.W., & DeLaCruz, A. F. (1988). Adapting speech audiometry testing for the nonspeaking physically impaired population. *Augmentative and Alternative Communication, 4,* 147–148.

Bristow, D. C., & Caldwell, T. (1984). Utilization of the communication system to achieve the curriculum goals. Paper presented at the annual meeting of the American Speech-Language-Hearing Association, San Francisco.

Bristow, D. C., & Damico, J. S. (1988). Comparison of acquired or congenital nonspeaking adults communications interactions. Paper presented at the annual meeting of the American Speech-Language-Hearing Association, Boston.

Bristow, D. C., & Fristoe, M. W. (1982). Design and construction of individualized nonspeech communication systems. Paper presented at the annual meeting of the American Speech-Language-Hearing Association, Toronto.

Bristow, D. C., & Fristoe, M. W. (1984a). Learning of Blissymbols and manual signs. *Journal of Speech and Hearing Disorders*, 49, 145–151.

Bristow, D. C., & Fristoe, M. (1984b). Systematic evaluation of the nonspeaking child. Miniseminar presented at the annual meeting of the American Speech-Language-Hearing Association, San Francisco.

Bristow, D. C., & Fristoe, M. W. (1987a). Effects of test adaptations on test performance. Paper presented at the annual meeting of the American Speech-Language-Hearing Association, New Orleans.

Bristow, D. C., & Fristoe, M. W. (1987b). Learnability of signs and symbols with the mentally retarded. Paper presented at the annual meeting of the American Speech-Language-Hearing Association, New Orleans.

Bristow, D. C., & Fristoe, M. W. (1988). Effects of test adaptations on test performance. *Augmentative and Alternative Communication*, 4, 171.

Bristow, D. C., Fristoe, M. W., & Juneau, M. L. (1986). The effects of test adaptations on test performance. Paper presented at the annual meeting of the American Speech-Language-Hearing Association, Detroit.

Bristow, D. C., & Pickering, G. L. (1988). "I want to participate too." *Augmentative and Alternative Communication*, 4, 143.

Bristow, D. C., & Pickering, G. L. (1990). Integrating visual aids with augmentative communication devices. Paper presented at the annual meeting of the American Speech-Language-Hearing Association, Seattle.

Bristow, D. C., Pickering, G. L., & Ballinger, B. (1992). Impact of vision in operating assistive technology: A case study. *Augmentative and Alternative Communication*, 8, 118.

Broder, H., & Hinton, G. (1982). Preventive psychotherapeutic measures for use with nonvocal clients: A case study. *Journal of Rehabilitation*, 48(4), 24–27, 80.

Broder, H., & Hinton, G. (1984). Preventive psychotherapeutic measures for use with nonvocal clients. *Communication Outlook*, 5(3), 10–11.

Brodin, J. (1990). Communication with children with profound mental retardation and multiple disabilities. *Augmentative and Alternative Communication*, 6, 140.

Brodin, J. (1991a). To interpret children's signals: Play and communication in profoundly mentally retarded and multiply handicapped children. Unpublished doctoral dissertation, University of Stockholm.

Brodin, J. M. (1991b). To interpret non-verbal communication in profoundly mentally retarded and multiply handicapped children. Paper presented at the Third Nordic Child Language Symposium, Oulo, Finland.

Broden, J. M. (1992a). Qualitative research and ethical aspects in AAC. Paper presented at the Second ISAAC Research Symposium in Augmentative and Alternative Communication, Philadelphia.

Brodin, J. M. (1992b). *Telecommunication for People with Mental Retardation. Requirements and Services*. Report No. 3 in the series *Technology, Communication, and Disability*. Department of Education, Stockholm University, Sweden.

Brodin, J. M., & Björck-Åkesson, E. (1992). Toy libraries/Lekoteks in an international perspective. *EuroRehab*, 2, 97–102.

Brodin, J. M., & Björck-Åkesson, E. (1993a). *Evaluation of Still Picture Telephone for Mentally Retarded Persons*. Vällingby, Sweden: Swedish Telecom Group, Box 510, S-162 15.

Brodin, J. M., & Björck-Åkesson, E. (1993b). *Still Picture Telephones for Persons with Profound Mental Retardation*. Vällingby, Sweden: Swedish Telecom Group, Box 510, S-162 15.

Brodin, J. M., Fahlén, M., & Nilsson, S. (1993). *MINITRIAL. A Limited Study of the Use of Videotelephony for People with Moderate Mental Retardation.* Report No. 7 in the series *Technology, Communication, and Disability.* Department of Education, Stockholm University, Sweden.

Brodin, J. M., & Magnússon, M. (1992a). *Still Picture Telephones for People with Aphasia and Mental Retardation.* Report No. 4 in the series *Technology, Communication, and Disability.* Department of Education, Stockholm University, Sweden.

Brodin, J. M., & Magnússon, M. (1992b). *Technology and People with Disability.* Report No. 2 in the series *Technology, Communication, and Disability.* Department of Education, Stockholm University, Sweden.

Brodin, J. M., & Magnússon, M. (1993). *Videotelephony and Disability: A Bibliography.* Report No. 5 in the series *Technology, Communication, and Disability.* Department of Education, Stockholm University, Sweden.

Broehl, D. (1990). Hear our voices—An empowerment initiative. *Communication Outlook,* 12(2), 12–13.

Broehl, M. E. (1992). Legal issues in AAC in law and in practice. *Augmentative and Alternative Communication,* 8, 118.

Brookner, S. P., & Harris, C. A. (1977). Interactive techniques to facilitate communication in non-vocal children. Poster presentation at the annual meeting of the American Speech-Language-Hearing Association, Chicago.

Brookner, S. P., & Murphy, N. O. (1975). The use of a total communication approach with a nondeaf child: A case study. *Language, Speech, and Hearing Services in Schools,* 6, 131–137.

Brooks, J., Musselwhite, C., & Norris, L. (1988). Advocacy in AAC: Resources and experiences. *Augmentative and Alternative Communication,* 4, 169.

Brophy, B., Fuller, D., Newell, A. F., & Arnott, J. L. (1988). A survey of the communication disordered population in Tayside. *Augmentative and Alternative Communication,* 4, 137–138.

Brophy, B., & Sutherland, C. (1990). A conversation aid's contribution to communication by nonvocal speakers. *Augmentative and Alternative Communication,* 6, 98.

Broumley, L., Cairns, A. Y., & Arnott, J. L. (1992). Using artificial intelligence techniques in a personal communication aid. *Augmentative and Alternative Communication,* 6, 95–96

Broumley, L., Cairns, A. Y., & Arnott, J. L. (1992). Evaluation of a personalized communication system developed with aphasic adults. *Augmentative and Alternative Communication,* 8, 118–119.

Browder, D., Morris, W., & Snell, M. (1981). Using time delay to teach manual signs to a severely retarded student. *Education and Training of the Mentally Retarded,* 16, 252–258.

Brown, C. (1954). *My Left Foot.* London: Secker and Warburg.

Brown, C. C., Cavalier, A. R., & Mineo, B. A. (1988). A new horizon: Independence for persons with severe handicaps. *Augmentative and Alternative Communication,* 4, 164–165.

Brown, C. C., Cavalier, A. R., Mineo, B. A., & Buckley, R. (1988). Sound-to-sound translation and environmental control for people with mental retardation. *Augmentative and Alternative Communication,* 4, 172.

Brown, C. C., Cavalier, A. R., Wyatt, C., & Kostraba, J. (1992). Eyegaze/headpointing technology research with persons having mental retardation. *Augmentative and Alternative Communication,* 8, 119.

Brown, C. C., Mineo, B. A., & Cavalier, A. R. (1986). Freedom of choice and expression through voice recognition and eyegaze for persons with profound mental retardation. *Augmentative and Alternative Communication, 2,* 74–75.

Brown, C. C., Sauer, M., Cavalier, A. R., & Wyatt, C. (1992). Speech recognition and graphics research for persons having mental retardation. *Augmentative and Alternative Communication, 8,* 119–120.

Brown, V. (1988). Integrating drama and sign language. *Teaching Exceptional Children,* 21(1), 4–8.

Brown, W. P., Vanderheiden, G. C., & Harris, D. (1977). 1977 Bibliography on Non-vocal Communication Techniques and Aids. Madison: Trace Research and Development Center for the Severely Communicatively Handicapped, University of Wisconsin.

Brown-Herman, C., Calculator, S. N., Connelly, J. A., & Reinhardt, D. (1989). Caregiver accuracy in identifying nonverbal communication. Paper presented at the annual meeting of the American Speech-Language-Hearing Association, St. Louis.

Browning-Gill, N. (1992). Introducing augmentative communication in a Brazilian center. *Augmentative and Alternative Communication, 8,* 120.

Brunn, G., Jarkler, B., & Speldt, B. (1974). Communication display/printout aid with a memory. In Keith Copeland (Ed.), *Aids for the Severely Handicapped.* New York: Grune & Stratton, pp.116–118.

Bruno, J. (1986). Modeling procedures for increased use of communicative functions in communication aid users. In Sarah W. Blackstone (Ed.), *Augmentative Communication: An Introduction.* Rockville, MD: American Speech-Language-Hearing Association, pp. 301–305.

Bruno, J. (1988). The Minspeak technique, association performance, and the preliterate child. *Augmentative and Alternative Communication, 4,* 148.

Bruno, J. (1989). Customizing a Minspeak system for a preliterate child: A case example. *Augmentative and Alternative Communication, 5,* 89–100.

Bruno, J. (1990). Maximizing classroom participation for nonspeaking children. *Augmentative and Alternative Communication, 6,* 91.

Bruno, J. (1991). How will I talk tomorrow?—Continuity and transition in AAC. Paper presented at the annual meeting of the American Speech-Language-Hearing Association, Atlanta.

Bruno, J., & Baker, B. (1986). Minspeak and children: A two year clinical prospective. *Augmentative and Alternative Communication, 2,* 75.

Bruno, J., & Bryen, D. (1986). The impact of modeling procedures on physically disabled nonspeaking children. *Augmentative and Alternative Communication, 2,* 75.

Bruno, J., & Goehl, H. (1991). Comparison of picture and word association performance in adults and preliterate children. *Augmentative and Alternative Communication, 7,* 70–79.

Bruno, J., & Hunnicutt, S. (1990). Voice output communication systems: Considerations in designing systems for international use. *Augmentative and Alternative Communication, 6,* 126.

Bruno, J., & Romich, B. (1989). Beyond device characteristics: A response to Woltosz. *Augmentative and Alternative Communication, 5,* 203–205.

Bruno, J., & Sauer, M. (1992). AAC services: Impact of the service delivery model. *Augmentative and Alternative Communication, 8,* 120.

Bruno, J., & Stoughton, A. M. (1984). Computer-aided communication device for a child with cerebral palsy. *Archives of Physical Medicine and Rehabilitation,* 65(10), 603–605.

Bruno, J., Young, J. A., Thomas, B., & Gough, M. (1989). Developing a short-term intensive treatment program for AAC users. Paper presented at the annual meeting of the American Speech-Language-Hearing Association, St. Louis.

Bryen, D. N., & Baker, D. B. (1992). Successful models of AAC intervention for adults in the community. *Augmentative and Alternative Communication*, 8, 120.

Bryen, D. N., Goldman, A. S., & Quinlisk, G. S. (1988). Sign language with students with severe/profound mental retardation: How effective is it? *Education and Training of the Mentally Retarded*, 23(2), 129–137.

Bryen, D. N., & Joyce, D. (1985). Language intervention with the severely handicapped: A decade of research. *Journal of Special Education*, 19, 7–39.

Bryen, D. N., & Joyce, D. (1986). Sign language and the severely handicapped. *Journal of Special Education*, 20, 183–194.

Bryen, D. N., & Laurent, D. (1990). Finding a voice: Summer campus institute on augmentative communication. *Augmentative and Alternative Communication*, 6, 140–141.

Bryen, D. N., & McGinley, V. (1991). Sign language input to community residents with mental retardation. *Education and Training in Mental Retardation*, 26(2), 207–213.

Buck, M. (1968). *Dysphasia: Professional Guidance for Family and Patient.* Englewood Cliffs, NJ: Prentice Hall.

Buhr, P. A., & Holte, R. C. (1981). Some considerations in the design of communication aids for the severely physically handicapped. *Medical and Biological Engineering and Computing*, 19, 725–733.

Bullock, A., Dalrymple, G. F., & Danca, J. M. (1975). The Auto-Com at Kennedy Memorial Hospital: Rapid and accurate communication by a multihandicapped student. *American Journal of Occupational Therapy*, 29, 150–152.

Bunnell, H. T., Polikoff, J., Peters, S., Kadambe, S., & Mineo, B. (1992). Progress in computer enhancement of dysarthric speech. *Augmentative and Alternative Communication*, 8, 121.

Burd, L., Hammes, K., Bornhoeft, D., & Fisher, W. (1988). A North Dakota prevalence study of nonverbal school-age children. *Language, Speech, and Hearing Services in Schools*, 19, 371–383.

Burke, E. H. (1986). Maintaining the use of communication aids—Problems encountered among a clinic population. *Augmentative and Alternative Communication*, 2, 75.

Burkhart, L. J. (1985a). *Homemade Battery Powered Toys and Educational Devices for Severely Handicapped Children.* College Park, MD: Linda J. Burkhart, Box 793.

Burkhart, L. J. (1985b). *More Homemade Battery Devices for Severely Handicapped Children with Suggested Activities.* College Park, MD: Linda J. Burkhart, 8503 Rhode Island Avenue.

Burkhart, L. J. (1987). *Using Computers and Speech Synthesis to Facilitate Communicative Interaction with Young and/or Severely Handicapped Children.* Wauconda, IL: Don Johnston Developmental Equipment.

Burkhart, L. J. (1990). Self-selection of communication systems by preschool children: Suggested strategies. *Augmentative and Alternative Communication*, 6, 146.

Burkhart, L. J., West, S., & Garber, S. (1992). Empowering local teams: Training augmentative and alternative communication strategies through direct service. *Augmentative and Alternative Communication*, 8, 121.

Burnside, S. (March 21, 1974). All he could do was breathe—It's enough to run computer. *Miami Herald.*

Burroughs, J. A., Albritton, E. G., Eaton, B. B., & Montague, J. C. (1990). A comparative study of language delayed preschool children's ability to recall symbols from two symbol systems. *Augmentative and Alternative Communication*, 6, 202–206.

Burroughs, J. A., Albritton, E. G., Montague, J. C., & Eaton, B. B. (1989). The acquisition of contrasting symbol systems by language delayed children. Paper presented at the annual meeting of the American Speech-Language-Hearing Association, St. Louis.

Burstein, D., Gough, M., Thomas, B., Patton-Thompas, S., Young, J., Howell, D., & Profeta, H. (1992). Widener Memorial Public School: Teaching with technology. *Augmentative and Alternative Communication*, 8, 122.

Butler, O., & Fouldes, J. (1974). Typing aid remote controlled (TARC). In Keith Copeland (Ed.), *Aids for the Severely Handicapped*, New York: Grune & Stratton, pp. 83–88.

Butt, D. S. (1992). Let's begin at the beginning: Easy visual scanning techniques. Paper presented at the annual meeting of the American Speech-Language-Hearing Association, San Antonio.

Butt, D. S., & de Zaldo, G. F. (1992). The birth of augmentative communication in Mexico. Paper presented at the annual meeting of the American Speech-Language-Hearing Association, San Antonio.

Buzolich, M. J. (1984). Interaction analysis of augmented and normal adult communicators. Unpublished doctoral dissertation, University of California, San Francisco.

Buzolich, M. J. (1986). Cognitive and communicative development in severely physically handicapped nonspeaking children. *Augmentative and Alternative Communication*, 2, 75–76.

Buzolich, M. J. (1987a). Children in transition: Implementing augmentative communication systems with severely speech-handicapped children. *Seminars in Speech and Language*, 8, 199–213.

Buzolich, M. J. (1987b). Creative funding for services. Intervention strategy developed under Contract No. 300-85-0139 (*Implementation Strategies for Improving the Use of Communication Aids in Schools Serving Handicapped Children*) from the U.S. Department of Education distributed by the American Speech-Language-Hearing Association.

Buzolich, M. J. (1987c). Facilitating early motor, perceptual-motor, and communicative development using computers. Intervention strategy developed under Contract No. 300-85-0139 (*Implementation Strategies for Improving the Use of Communication Aids in Schools Serving Handicapped Children*) from the U.S. Department of Education distributed by the American Speech-Language-Hearing Association.

Buzolich, M. J. (1987d). Facilitating interaction in communication groups involving individuals who use augmentative communication aids and techniques and their speaking peers. Intervention strategy developed under Contract No. 300-85-0139 (*Implementation Strategies for Improving the Use of Communication Aids in Schools Serving Handicapped Children*) from the U.S. Department of Education distributed by the American Speech-Language-Hearing Association.

Buzolich, M. J. (1987e). Teaching students and their speaking peers to repair communication breakdowns caused by unintelligible speech. Intervention strategy developed under Contract No. 300-85-0139 (*Implementation Strategies for Improving the Use of Communication Aids in Schools Serving Handicapped Children*) from the U.S. Department of Education distributed by the American Speech-Language-Hearing Association.

Buzolich, M. J., & King, J. S. (1988). Bridge School: A program for severely physically disabled nonspeaking students. *Augmentative and Alternative Communication*, 4, 139.

Buzolich, M. J., & King, J. S. (1992). Auditory scanning: Communication systems for the visually impaired AAC system user. *Augmentative and Alternative Communication*, 8, 122.

Buzolich, M. J., King, J. S., & Baroody, S. M. (1990). The acquisition of the commenting function among AAC users. *Augmentative and Alternative Communication*, 6, 136.

Buzolich, M. J., King, J. S., & Baroody, S. M. (1991). Acquisition of the commenting function among system users. *Augmentative and Alternative Communication*, 7, 88–99.

Buzolich, M. J., & Lunger, J. G. (1992). Empowering system users in peer training. *Augmentative and Alternative Communication*, 8, 122–123.

Buzolich, M. J., & Weimann, J. (1988). Turn taking in atypical conversations: The case of the speaker/augmented communicator dyad. *Journal of Speech and Hearing Research*, 31, 3–18.

Byler, J. K. (1985). The Makaton vocabulary: An analysis based on recent research. *British Journal of Special Education*, 12, 113–120.

Calculator, S. N. (n.d.). *Design and Revision of Non-Oral Systems of Communication for the Mentally Retarded Physically Handicapped: A Discussion of the Unicolor Binary Visual Encoding Board with General Implications for Communication.* Working Paper 101. Madison: Department of Communicative Disorders, University of Wisconsin.

Calculator, S. N. (1984). Communication board: Prop or tool? *Communicating Together*, 2(2), 15–16.

Calculator, S. N. (1988a). Designing functional and integrated communication programs for severely handicapped children. *Augmentative and Alternative Communication*, 4, 172.

Calculator, S. N. (1988b). Evaluating the effectiveness of AAC programs for persons with severe handicaps. *Augmentative and Alternative Communication*, 4, 177–179.

Calculator, S. N. (1988c). Promoting the acquisition and generalization of conversational skills by individuals with severe disabilities. *Augmentative and Alternative Communication*, 4, 94–103.

Calculator, S. N. (1991). Best practices in providing AAC services to students with severe disabilities. Paper presented at the annual meeting of the American Speech-Language-Hearing Association, Atlanta.

Calculator, S. N. (1992a). Perhaps the emperor has clothes after all: A response to Biklen. *American Journal of Speech-Language Pathology*, 1(2), 18–20.

Calculator, S. N. (1992b). Facilitated communication: Calculator responds. *American Journal of Speech-Language Pathology*, 1(2), 23–24.

Calculator, S. N., & Bedrosian, J. (Eds.) (1988). *Communication Assessment and Intervention for Adults with Mental Retardation.* San Diego: College-Hill.

Calculator, S. N., & Delaney, D. (1986). Comparison of nonspeaking and speaking mentally retarded adults' clarification strategies. *Journal of Speech and Hearing Disorders*, 51, 252–259.

Calculator, S. N., & Dollaghan, C. (1982). The use of communication boards in a residential setting: An evaluation. *Journal of Speech and Hearing Disorders*, 47, 281–287.

Calculator, S. N., & Hicks, P. (1987). Augmentative communication instruction in the classroom: An integrated approach. Paper presented at the annual meeting of the American Speech-Language-Hearing Association, New Orleans.

Calculator, S. N., & Jorgensen, C. M. (1990). Incorporating AAC instruction in the classroom. *Augmentative and Alternative Communication*, 6, 134–135.

Calculator, S. N., & Jorgensen, C. M. (1991). Integrating AAC instruction into regular education settings: Expounding on best practices. *Augmentative and Alternative Communication*, 7, 204–214.

Calculator, S., & Luchko, C. (1983a). Evaluating the effectiveness of a communication board training program. *Journal of Speech and Hearing Disorders*, 48, 185–191.

Calculator, S., & Luchko, C. (1983b). The use of communication boards in a residential setting: An evaluation. *Journal of Speech and Hearing Disorders*, 48, 281–287.

Calculator, S., Nadeau, G., Brown-Herman, C., & Reinhardt, D. (1988a). Evaluating the AAC interaction competencies of adults with severe/profound disabilities. *Augmentative and Alternative Communication*, 4, 148.

Calculator, S., Nadeau, G., Brown-Herman, C., & Reinhardt, D. (1988b). Recognizing and responding to communicative attempts by severely handicapped adults. Paper presented at the annual meeting of the American Speech-Language-Hearing Association, Boston.

California Research Institute (1990). *The Way to Go* [videotape]. Available from TASH, 11201 Greenwood Ave. North, Seattle, WA 98113.

Camarata, S. M., & Dattilo, J. (1988). Facilitating conversational initiations in augmentative users. Paper presented at the annual meeting of the American Speech-Language-Hearing Association, Boston.

Campbell, A., & Lloyd, L. (1986). Graphic symbols and symbol systems: What research and clinical practice tell us. Paper presented at the Conference of the American Association on Mental Deficiency, Denver.

Campbell, P. H., & Wilcox, M. J. (1986). Communication effectiveness of movement patterns used by nonvocal children with severe handicaps. *Augmentative and Alternative Communication*, 2, 76.

Canadian Rehabilitation Council for the Disabled (1984). *Conversations with Nonspeaking People*. Toronto: Author for the International Project on Communication Aids for the Speech Impaired (IPCAS). [Also published as *Samtal Med Personer Som Inte Talar* by Handikappinstitutet, the Swedish Institute for the Handicapped.]

Capelovitch, S., & Seela, S. (1992). Motor changes in children with cerebral palsy. *Augmentative and Alternative Communication*, 8, 123.

Cappa, S. F., Pirovano, C., & Vignolo, L. A. (1985). Chronic "locked-in" syndrome: Psychological study of a case. *Eur-Neurol*, 24(2), 107–111.

Carin, S. (1988). Development and integration of a system for a severely impaired brain injured adult. *Augmentative and Alternative Communication*, 4, 156.

Carlisle, M., & Culp, D. (1988). Evolutionary stages in intervention for brain-injured patients: Clinical framework. *Augmentative and Alternative Communication*, 4, 144.

Carlson, C. E., & Cameron, D. J. (1988). Analysis of conversational dyads between adult speakers. *Augmentative and Alternative Communication*, 4, 162.

Carlson, C. E., & Kowalski, K. R. (1986). Long-term communication training: Selected case studies of nonspeaking adults with acquired neurogenic disorders. *Augmentative and Alternative Communication*, 2, 76–77.

Carlson, C. E., & Kowalski, K. R. (1990). The use of multiple AAC systems in progressive disease. *Augmentative and Alternative Communication*, 6, 100.

Carlson, C. E., & Kowalski, K. R. (1992). The challenge of keep AAC users interactive: Lay inservice training. *Augmentative and Alternative Communication*, 8, 123.

Carlson, F. L. (1976). An adapted communication project for a nonspeaking child. Paper presented at the annual meeting of the American Speech-Language-Hearing Association, Houston.

Carlson, F. L. (1981). A format for selecting vocabulary for the nonspeaking child. *Language, Speech, and Hearing Services in Schools*, 12, 240–245.

Carlson, F. L. (1982a). *Alternate Methods of Communication*. Danville, IL: Interstate Printers and Publishers.

Carlson, F. L. (1982b). *Prattle and Play*. Omaha, NE: Media Resource Center, MCRI, 444 S. 4th Street.

Carlson, F. L. (1984). *Picsyms Categorical Dictionary*. Lawrence, KS: Baggeboda Press.

Carlson, F. L. (1987). Communication strategies for infants. In E. McDonald (Ed.), *Treating Cerebral Palsy: For Clinicians by Clinicians*. Austin, TX: Pro-Ed.

Carlson, F. L., Hough, S., Lippert, E., & Young, C. (1987). Developing augmentative communication signaling behaviors in severely/profoundly developmentally delayed children. Intervention strategy developed under Contract No. 300-85-0139 (*Implementation Strategies for Improving the Use of Communication Aids in Schools Serving Handicapped Children*) from the U.S. Department of Education distributed by the American Speech-Language-Hearing Association.

Carlson, F. L., Hough, S., Lippert, E., & Young, C. (1988). Facilitating interaction during mealtime. In S. Blackstone, E. Cassatt-James, & D. Bruskin (Eds.), *Augmentative Communication: Implementation Strategies*. Rockville, MD: American Speech-Language-Hearing Association, pp. 5.8-10–5.8-20.

Carlson, F. L., & James, C. (1980). Picsyms systems and symbol systems. Unpublished paper. Omaha: Meyer Children's Rehabilitation Institute, University of Nebraska Medical Center.

Carlson, F. L., & Kovarik, A. M. (1985). Developmental comprehension of PICSYMS, an augmentative communication symbol system. Paper presented at the annual meeting of the American Speech-Language-Hearing Association, Washington, DC.

Carlson, R., Galyas, K., Granstron, B., Hunnicutt, S., Larsson, B., & Neovius, L. (1981). A multi-language portable text-to-speech system for the disabled. *Journal of Biomedical Engineering*, 3(4), 285–288.

Carmel, S. (1982). *International Hand Alphabet Charts*. Rockville, MD: Author.

Carmeli, S., Loeb, N., Yaniv, K., & Seligman-Wine, J. (1990). Factors in introducing VOCA's to a young, competent AAC user. *Augmentative and Alternative Communication*, 6, 116–117.

Carpenter, B. (1987). A formative evaluation of a Makaton-based reading scheme. Unpublished master's thesis, Nottingham University, England.

Carr, E. G. (1979). Teaching autistic children to use sign language: Some research issues. *Journal of Autism and Developmental Disorders*, 9(4), 345–359.

Carr, E. G. (1981). *How to Teach Sign Language to Developmentally Disabled Children*. Austin, TX: Pro-Ed.

Carr, E. G. (1982). Sign language. In R. Koegel, A. Rincover, & A. Egel (Eds.), *Educating and Understanding Autistic Children*. San Diego: College-Hill, pp. 142–157.

Carr, E. G., Binkoff, J. A., Kologinsky, E., & Eddy, M. (1978). Acquisition of sign language by autistic children. Part 1: Expressive labelling. *Journal of Applied Behavior Analysis*, 11, 489–501.

Carr, E. G., & Dores, P. (1981). Patterns of language acquisition following simultaneous communication with autistic children. *Analysis and Intervention in Developmental Disabilities*, 1, 1–15.

Carr, E. G., & Durand, V. M. (1985). Reducing behavior problems through functional intervention training. *Journal of Applied Behavior Analysis*, 18, 111–126.

Carr, E. G., & Durand, V. M. (November 1987). See me, help me. *Psychology Today*, 21(11), 62–64.

Carr, E. G., & Kemp, D. C. (1989). Functional equivalence of autistic leading and communicative pointing: Analysis and treatment. *Journal of Autism and Developmental Disorders*, 19(4), 561–578.

Carr, E. G., & Kologinsky, E. (1983). Acquisition of sign language by autistic children: II. Spontaneity and generalization. *Journal of Applied Behavior Analysis*, 16, 297–314.

Carr, E. G., Kologinsky, E., & Leff, S. S. (1987). Acquisition of sign language by autistic children: III. Generalized descriptive phases. *Journal of Autism and Developmental Disorders*, 17(2), 217–229.

Carr, E. G., Pridal, C., & Dores, P. A. (1984). Speech versus sign comprehension in autistic children: Analysis and prediction. *Journal of Experimental Child Psychology*, 37(3), 587–597.

Carrier, Jr., J. K. (1974a). Application of functional analysis and a non-speech response mode to teaching language. In L. V. McReynolds (Ed.), *Developing Systematic Procedures for Training Children's Language*, ASHA Monograph No. 18.

Carrier, Jr., J. K. (1974b). Nonspeech noun usage training with severely and profoundly retarded children. *Journal of Speech and Hearing Research*, 17, 510–517.

Carrier, Jr., J. K. (1976). Application of a nonspeech language system with the severely language handicapped. In Lyle L. Lloyd (Ed.), *Communication Assessment and Intervention Strategies*. Baltimore: University Park Press, pp. 523–547.

Carrier, Jr., J. K., & Peak, T. (1975). *Program Manual for Non-SLIP (Non-Speech Language Initiation Program)*. Lawrence, KS: H & H Enterprises.

Carroll-Thomas, S. (1986a). Adult aphasia: Assessment and training for communication board use. *Augmentative and Alternative Communication*, 2, 77.

Carroll-Thomas, S. (1986b). A triage approach to communication augmentation in intensive care units. *Augmentative and Alternative Communication*, 2, 77.

Carroll-Thomas, S. (1988). Predictive planning in progressive neurological disease. *Augmentative and Alternative Communication*, 4, 159.

Carter, G., Atkinson, P., Barton, M., & Stephens, R. (1988). Toys and playing for pleasure. *Augmentative and Alternative Communication*, 4, 137.

Cartmell, D. J. (1986). Speech technology—A tutorial. *Augmentative and Alternative Communication*, 2, 77–78.

Casali, S. P., & Williges, R. C. (1990). Data bases of accommodative aids for computer users with disabilities. *Human Factors*, 32(4), 407–422.

Casby, M. W. (1984). Simple switch modifications for use in augmentative communication. *Language, Speech, and Hearing Services in Schools*, 15, 216–220.

Cascella, P. W., & Laurent, D. L. (1989). Computer applications with adult mentally retarded individuals. Paper presented at the annual meeting of the American Speech-Language-Hearing Association, St. Louis.

Casey, L. O. (1978). Development of communicative behavior in autistic children: A parent program using manual signs. *Journal of Autism and Childhood Schizophrenia*, 8(1), 45–59.

Cassatt-James, E. L. (1986). Establishing the use of multimodalities using the communicative interaction assessment procedure. In Sarah W. Blackstone (Ed.), *Augmentative Communication: An Introduction*. Rockville, MD: American Speech-Language-Hearing Association, pp. 307–319.

Cerreti, S., Emiliani, P. L., & Troncini, A. (1986). Computerized communication aid for Italian motor-disabled people. *Augmentative and Alternative Communication*, 2, 78.

Chan, E., & Charbonneau, E. J. (1986). An experimental test battery in French evaluating various morpho-phonemic analysis skills in users of alphabetical (phonological) communication systems versus users of nonalphabetical communication systems. *Augmentative and Alternative Communication*, 2, 78–79.

Chapman, R. S., & Miller, J. F. (1980). Analyzing language and communication in the child. In R. L. Schiefelbusch (Ed.), *Nonspeech Language and Communication*. Baltimore, MD: University Park Press, pp. 159–196.

Charbonneau, J. R., Cote, C., & Roy, O. Z. (1974). NRC's "Comhandi" communication system technical description and application at the Ottawa Crippled Children's Treatment Center. Paper presented at the seminar on Electronic Controls for the Severely Physically Handicapped, Vancouver, British Columbia.

Charlebois-Marois, C. (1985). *Everybody's Technology: A Sharing of Ideas in Augmentative Communication*. Montreal: Charlecoms Enr., Box 419, Jean-Talon Station.

Charlebois-Marois, C. (1986). Communication: It takes two people . . . and a few other things: Developing preliminary skills. *Augmentative and Alternative Communication*, 2, 79.

Chase, J. B., Tallman, T. M., & Herbly, H. (1990). Mental health professionals: AAC training and clinical services. *Augmentative and Alternative Communication*, 6, 114–115.

Chavis, M. C., Cooper-Glenn, J., Perkins-Faulk, J., & Caragher, A. (1989). Conversing with augmentative communication systems: An "after school club" approach. Paper presented at the annual meeting of the American Speech-Language-Hearing Association, St. Louis.

Chen, L. Y. (1968). "Talking hands" for aphasic patients. *Geriatrics*, 23, 145–148.

Chen, L. Y. (1971). Manual communication by combined alphabet and gestures. *Archives of Physical Medicine and Rehabilitation*, 52, 381–384.

Chester, S. L., & Egolf, D. B. (1972). Nonverbal communication and aphasia therapy. Paper presented at the annual meeting of the American Speech-Language-Hearing Association, San Francisco.

Christensen, J., & Brandt, Å. (1990). Service delivery in Denmark: Support must go on. *Augmentative and Alternative Communication*, 6, 141.

Christopher, F., Salciccia, C., Parathyras, A., Zaretsky, H., & Kerman-Lerner, P. (1986). Innovative group psychotherapeutic techniques with quadriplegic nonspeaking adults. *Augmentative and Alternative Communication*, 2, 79–80.

Christopoulou, C., & Bonvillian, J. D. (1985). Sign language, pantomine, and gestural processing in aphasic persons: A review. *Journal of Communication Disorders*, 18(1), 1–20.

Chubon, R. A., & Hester, M. R. (1988). An enhanced standard computer keyboard system for single-finger and typing-stick typing. *Journal of Rehabilitation Research and Development*, 25(4), 17–24.

Chusid, J. G., & McDonald, J. J. (1960). *Correlative Neuroanatomy and Functional Neurology*. Los Altos, CA: Lange Medical Publications.

Clagett, S. M., & Haberbosch, S. (1992). It happened on the way to communication. *Augmentative and Alternative Communication*, 8, 123.

Clappe, C., Grant, M., Hazard, G., Lang, J., & Tomlinson, R. (1973). The Morse code visual translator—A means of communication for the anarthric patient. Paper presented at the annual meeting of the American Speech-Language-Hearing Association, Detroit.

Clark, C. R. (1981). Learning words using traditional orthography and the symbols of Rebus, Bliss, and Carrier. *Journal of Speech and Hearing Disorders*, 46, 191–196.

Clark, C. R. (1984). A close look at the standard Rebus system and Blissymbolics. *Journal of the Association for Persons with Severe Handicaps*, 9, 37–48.

Clark, C. R., Davies, C. O., & Woodcock, R. W. (1974). *Standard Rebus Glossary*. Minneapolis: American Guidance Service.

Clark, C. R., & Greco, J. A. (1973). *MELDS Glossary of Rebuses and Signs*. Minneapolis: Research, Development, and Demonstration Center in Education of Handicapped Children, University of Minnesota.

Clark, C. R., Moores, D. F., & Woodcock, R. W. (1973). *Minnesota Early Language Development Sequence*. Minneapolis: Research, Development, and Demonstration Center in Education of Handicapped Children, University of Minnesota.

Clark, C. R., & Woodcock, R. W. (1976). Graphic systems of communication. In Lyle L. Lloyd (Ed.), *Communication Assessment and Intervention Strategies*. Baltimore: University Park Press.

Clark, J. G. (June/July 1990). Emotional response transformations: Redirections and projections. *Asha*, 32, 67–68.

Clark, M., Kearns, T., Meldon, D., Malocca, A., O'Connell, A., & Rafferty, M. (1984). *Language Alternatives for Mentally Handicapped (LAMH) Manual*. Dublin, Ireland: St. Michael's House, Ballymun Road.

Clark, P., & Evans, A. L. (1986). A single switch operated portable word processor. *Augmentative and Alternative Communication*, 2, 80.

Clark, T. A. (1976). American sign language and the recently devised sign systems. Paper presented at the annual meeting of the American Speech-Language-Hearing Association, Houston.

Clarke, S., Remington, B., & Light, P. (1986). An evaluation of the relationship between receptive speech skills and expressive signing. *Journal of Applied Behavior Analysis*, 19, 231–239.

Clarke, S., Remington, B., & Light, P. (1988). The role of referential speech in sign learning by mentally retarded children: A comparison of total communication and sign-alone training. *Journal of Applied Behavior Analysis*, 21(4), 419–426.

Clayton, C. J. (1990). A tongue sensing [switching] system. *Augmentative and Alternative Communication*, 6, 136.

Clayton, C. J. (1992). Software tailored access. *Augmentative and Alternative Communication*, 8, 123–124.

Clement, M. (September-October, 1961). Morse code method of communication for the severely handicapped cerebral palsied child. *Cerebral Palsy Review*, 15–16.

Clements, N., & Taylor, J. (1992). Successful AAC system use: A model and process. *Augmentative and Alternative Communication*, 8, 124.

Cockerill, H. (1992). "Shut up and let me talk"—Child-directed therapy. *Augmentative and Alternative Communication*, 8, 124.

Coelho, C. A., Purdy, M. H., & Clarkson, J. V. (1992). Clinical utility of an AAC device with a severely aphasic adult. Paper presented at the annual meeting of the American Speech-Language-Hearing Association, San Antonio.

Cohen, C., & Palin, M. (1986). Speech synthesis and speech recognition devices. In M. Grossfeld & C. Grossfeld (Eds.), *Microcomputer Applications in Rehabilitation of Communication Disorders*. Rockville, MD: Aspen Systems, pp. 183–211.

Cohen, C. G. (1985). Augmentative communication: A perspective for pediatricians. *Pediatric Annals*, 14(3), 232–234, 236–237, 240.

Cohen, C. G. (1986). Total habilitation and lifelong management. In Sarah W. Blackstone (Ed.), *Augmentative Communication: An Introduction*. Rockville, MD: American Speech-Language-Hearing Association, pp. 447–469.

Cohen, C. G. (1987). Establishing equipment requirements for an evaluation facility: A generic guide. Intervention strategy developed under Contract No. 300-85-0139 (*Implementation Strategies for Improving the Use of Communication Aids in Schools Serving Handicapped Children*) from the U.S. Department of Education distributed by the American Speech-Language-Hearing Association.

Cohen, C. G., Frumkin, J., & Geiger, C. (1988). Interactive language instruction using video and computer technology. *Augmentative and Alternative Communication*, 4, 164.

Cohen, C. G., & Shane, H. C.(1988). Successful employment resulting from AAC intervention strategies. *Augmentative and Alternative Communication*, 4, 149.

Cohen, L. K. (1976). *Communication Aids for the Brain Damaged Adult*. Minneapolis: Sister Kenny Institute.

Colby, K. M., Christinoz, D., & Grahm, S. (n.d.). A personal, portable, and intelligent speech prosthesis (working paper). Los Angeles: Department of Psychiatry, University of California School of Medicine.

Colby, K. M., Christinaz, D., Parkinson, R. C., Graham, S., & Karpf, C. (1981). A word-finding computer program with a dynamic lexical-semantic memory for patients with anomia using an intelligent speech prosthesis. *Language and Speech*, 14, 272–281.

Coleman, C. L. (1988). Computer recognition of the speech of adults with cerebral palsy. *Augmentative and Alternative Communication*, 4, 143.

Coleman, C. L., Cook, A. M., & Meyers, L. S. (1980). Assessing non-oral clients for assistive communication devices. *Journal of Speech and Hearing Disorders*, 45, 515–526.

Coleman, C. L., & Meyers, L. S. (1991). Computer recognition of the speech of adults with cerebral palsy and dysarthria. *Augmentative and Alternative Communication*, 7, 34–42.

Coleman, P. P., & Steelman, J. D. (1992a). Emergent Literacy and AAC users: Research and practice. *Augmentative and Alternative Communication*, 8, 124.

Coleman, P. P., & Steelman, J. D. (1992b). Project A*C*S*E*S: Adaptive Computer Solutions for Employment Skills. *Augmentative and Alternative Communication*, 8, 125.

Coleman, R. F., & Gutnick, H. N. (1988). Intelligibility of three ACDs varying in synthesis strategy. Paper presented at the annual meeting of the American Speech-Language-Hearing Association, Boston.

Collier, B. (1991). Report of ISAAC developing countries seminar. *Augmentative and Alternative Communication*, 7, 138–146.

Collier, B., Blackstein-Adler, S., & Thomas, D. (1988). Visual functional issues in AAC—Clinical observations and implications. *Augmentative and Alternative Communication*, 4, 158.

Collier, B., Norris, L., & Rothschild, N. (1990). Technology—What's working, what's not and why? *Augmentative and Alternative Communication*, 6, 119–120.

Collins, D. W. (1974). Patient initiated light operated telecontrol (PILOT). In Keith Copeland (Ed.), *Aids for the Severely Handicapped*. New York: Grune & Stratton, pp. 31–41.

Colven, D., & Poon, P. (1990). A proposed standard for switch operated systems. *Augmentative and Alternative Communication*, 6, 141.

Combs, R. G. (1969). Myocom: Communication for non-verbal handicapped. *Transactions of the Missouri Academy of Science*, 3, 102.

Competencies for speech-language pathologists providing services in augmentative communication (1988). *Asha*, 30(1), 55–58.

Computerized device speaks for handicapped youngsters (1976). *Journal of the Acoustical Society of America*, 59, 1520–1521.

Conrad, S. L. (1982). An investigation of the performance rate of non-verbal, hospitalized children using an electronic communication system. Unpublished Ph.D. dissertation, University of Texas, Dallas.

Constable, C. (1983). Creating communicative context. In H. Winitz (Ed.), *Treating Language Disorders: For Clinicians by Clinicians*. Austin, TX: Pro-Ed.

Cook, A. M., & Coleman, C. L. (1987). Selecting augmentative communication systems by matching client skills and needs to system characteristics. *Seminars in Speech and Language*, 8, 153–167.

Cook, A. M., Coleman, C. L., Preszler, A. M., & Dahlquist, D. L. (1983). A hierarchy of augmentative communication system characteristics useful for matching devices to clients' needs and skills. *Proceedings of the Sixth Annual Conference on Rehabilitation Engineering*. Bethesda, MD: Rehabilitation Engineering Society of North America, pp. 185–186.

Cook, A. M., Coleman, C. L., Preszler, A. M., Dahlquist, D. L., & Meyers, L. S. (1983). Matching non-oral subjects needs and skills to augmentative communication systems: Results of a three year study. Paper presented at the Sixth Annual Conference on Rehabilitation Engineering, San Diego.

Cook, A. M., Hussey, S. M., & Murphy, J. W. (1988). Using technology in a diagnostic-therapeutic paradigm for severely disabled clients. *Augmentative and Alternative Communication*, 4, 172–173.

Cook, A. M., Woodall, H. E., & LeGare, M. C. (1988). Contributions of neuroscience to the use of communication devices. *Augmentative and Alternative Communication*, 4, 166.

Cook, S. (1987a). Referral mechanisms for a communication aids program within an urban school district. Intervention strategy developed under Contract No. 300-85-0139 (*Implementation Strategies for Improving the Use of Communication Aids in Schools Serving Handicapped Children*) from the U.S. Department of Education distributed by the American Speech-Language-Hearing Association.

Cook, S. (1987b). Using "topic specific" miniboards to allow individuals who use augmentative communication aids to initiate communication with school staff members. Intervention strategy developed under Contract No. 300-85-0139 (*Implementation Strategies for Improving the Use of Communication Aids in Schools Serving Handicapped Children*) from the U.S. Department of Education distributed by the American Speech-Language-Hearing Association.

Cook, S. (1988). Using topic specific miniboards to allow individuals who use augmentative communication aids to initiate communication with school staff menbers. In S. Blackstone, E. Cassatt-James, & D. Bruskin (Eds.), *Augmentative Communication: Implementation Strategies*. Rockville, MD: American Speech-Language-Hearing Association, pp. 5.3-24–5.3-30.

Coon, R., Kremer, G., & Hilderbrand-Nilshon, M. (1992). Demographic analysis of people with speech impairments in Berlin, Germany. *Augmentative and Alternative Communication*, 8, 125.

Cooney, A., & Knox, G. (1981). An evaluation of a sign language programme taught to a group of severely/profoundly retarded children. In G. McIntyre & T. R. Parmenter (Eds.), *Preparation for Life: Programmes for Mentally Handicapped People in Australia in the 80's*. Sydney, Australia: Prentice Hall, pp. 350–364.

Copeland, K. (Ed.) (1974a). *Aids for the Severely Handicapped*. New York: Grune & Stratton.

Copeland, K. (1974b). Simplified communication system for the aged infirm. In Keith Copeland (Ed.), *Aids for the Severely Handicapped*. New York: Grune & Stratton, pp. 99–103.

Corley, P., & Follansbee, R. (1990). Teaching early literacy skills to nonspeaking physically challenged adults. *Augmentative and Alternative Communication*, 6, 131–132.

Costa, G., Giannoni, P., Schiaffino, A., & Veruggio, G. (1986). Written communication: An experience of system for severe motor handicapped. *Augmentative and Alternative Communication*, 2, 80–81.

Costello, J. M., & Sauer, M. (1988). Computer technology as a tool for developing communicative competence. *Augmentative and Alternative Communication*, 4, 166–167.

Costello, J. M., & Sauer, M. (1990a). Augmentative communication system options for the "eight hour nonspeaker." *Augmentative and Alternative Communication*, 6, 117.

Costello, J. M., & Sauer, M. (1990b). Teaching single switch visual scanning: An instruction model. *Augmentative and Alternative Communication*, 6, 147.

Coston, C. (Ed.) (1988). *Proceedings of the National Planners Conference on Assistive Device Service Delivery*. Washington, DC: RESNA, Association for the Advancement of Rehabilitation Technology.

Cottier, C. A. (1989). Providing options for augmentative communication users. Paper presented at the annual meeting of the American Speech-Language-Hearing Association, St. Louis.

Cottier, C. A. (1992a). Most common obstacles when mainstreaming AAC-using students. Paper presented at the annual meeting of the American Speech-Language-Hearing Association, San Antonio.

Cottier, C. A. (1992b). Sofia—"Your opinion of me when I use AAC." *Augmentative and Alternative Communication*, 8, 126.

Crabtree, M., Mirenda, P., & Beukelman, D. R. (1989). Attitudes of listeners in two age groups toward natural and synthetic speech. Paper presented at the annual meeting of the American Speech-Language-Hearing Association, St. Louis.

Crabtree, M., Mirenda, P., & Beukelman, D. R. (1990). Age and gender preferences for synthetic and natural speech. *Augmentative and Alternative Communication*, 6, 256–261.

Craven, C. G., & Cotter, P. T. (1985). A comprehensive total communication training package for staff. Paper presented at the annual meeting of the American Speech-Language-Hearing Association, Washington, DC.

Creech, R. (1980). Do you like your larynx? *Communication Outlook*, 2(4), 1–10.

Creech, R. (1984). The key that releases the soul of a man. In *Conversations with Non-speaking Persons.* Toronto: Canadian Rehabilitation Council for the Disabled.

Creech, R. (1988a). Paravocal communicators speak out. *Aug-Communique: North Carolina Augmentative Communication Newsletter,* 6(3), 12.

Creech, R. (1988b). Technology without training: A boat without oars. *Augmentative and Alternative Communication,* 4, 141–142.

Creech, R. (1990a). Facilitating education, work, and social interaction with AAC. *Augmentative and Alternative Communication,* 6, 136.

Creech, R. (1990b). Practical augmentative and alternative communication: The ultimate goal. *Augmentative and Alternative Communication,* 6, 150.

Creech, R. (1990c). Working toward a master's in speech pathology using AAC. *Augmentative and Alternative Communication,* 6, 137.

Creech, R., Kissick, L., Koski, M., & Musselwhite, C. (1988). Paravocal communicators speak out: Strategies for encouraging communication aid use. *Augmentative and Alternative Communication,* 4, 168.

Creech, R., & Viggiano, J. (1981). Consumers speak out on the life of the nonspeaker. *Asha,* 23(8), 550–552.

Creedon, M. P. (1973). Language development in nonverbal autistic children using a simultaneous communication system. Paper presented at the annual meeting of the Society for Research in Child Development, Philadelphia.

Creedon, M. P. (Ed.) (1975). *Appropriate Behavior Through Communication: A New Program in Simultaneous Language.* Chicago: Dysfunctioning Child Center. [Available from Developmental Institute, Humana Hospital, 31st at Lake Shore Drive, Chicago, IL 60616.]

Cregan, A. (1980). *Sigsymbols: A Nonvocal Aid to Communication and Language Development.* Cambridge, England: Cambridge Institute of Education.

Cregan, A. (1982). *Sigsymbol Dictionary.* Hatfield, Herts AL10 8TX, England: A. Cregan, 76 Wood Close.

Cregan, A. (1984). Sigsymbols: A graphic aid to communication and language development. Paper presented at the Curriculum Conference, Cambridge Institute of Education, Cambridge, England.

Cregan, A. (1986). Group work and play: Interactive communication via graphic symbols. *Augmentative and Alternative Communication,* 2, 81.

Cregan, A. (1990). Meaningful abstracts: Symbol assistance with "real" reading. *Augmentative and Alternative Communication,* 6, 130–131.

Cregan, A., & Lloyd, L. (1984a). *Sigsymbol Dictionary: American Edition.* West Lafayette, IN: Lyle Lloyd, Speech Clinic, Purdue University.

Cregan, A., & Lloyd, L. (1984b). Sigsymbols: Graphic symbols conceptually linked with manual signs. Paper presented at the Third International Conference on Augmentative and Alternative Communication (sponsored by the International Society for Augmentative and Alternative Communication), Cambridge, MA.

Cregan, A., & Lloyd, L. L. (1988). *Sigsymbols: American Edition.* Wauconda, IL: Don Johnston Development Equipment.

Cregan, A., & Lonnquist, B. (1990). Sigsymbols and manual signs: Keeping open options for expression. *Augmentative and Alternative Communication,* 6, 125.

Cress, C. J. (1986). *Bibliography of Vocabulary Frequency and Wordset Analysis Studies.* Madison: Trace Research and Development Center, University of Wisconsin.

Cress, C. J., & French, G. J. (1992). Computer interface training for children with and without cognitive disabilities. *Augmentative and Alternative Communication, 8,* 126.

Cress, C. J., Vanderheiden, G. C., & Kelso, D. P. (1987). Word frequency implications for exact communication in augmentative system users. Paper presented at the annual meeting of the American Speech-Language-Hearing Association, New Orleans.

Critcher, C. G., Carrier Jr., J. K., & LaCroix, Z. E. (1973). Speech and language training using a nonspeech response mode. Paper presented at the annual meeting of the American Speech-Language-Hearing Association, Detroit.

Crochetiere, J. W., Foulds, R. A., & Sterne, R. G. (1974). Computer-aided motor communication. Paper presented at the Conference on Engineering Devices in Rehabilitation, Boston. (Paper is published in the conference preceedings volume.)

Crossley, R. (1988a). Encouraging successes in nonvocal communication by people described as autistic. *Augmentative and Alternative Communication, 4,* 163.

Crossley, R. (1988b). Unexpected communication attachment by persons diagnosed as autistic and intellectually impaired. Paper presented at the fifth biennial conference of the International Society for Augmentative and Alternative Communication, Anaheim, CA.

Crossley, R. (1990). Literacy skills found in AAC users with Down syndrome. *Augmentative and Alternative Communication, 6,* 151.

Crossley, R. (1991). Communication training involving facilitated communication. *Communicating Together, 9*(2), 19–22.

Crossley, R. (May 1992). Lending a hand: A personal account of the development of facilitated communication training. *American Journal of Speech-Language Pathology, 1,* 15–18.

Crossley, R., & McDonald, A. (1984). *Annie's Coming Out.* New York: Viking Penguin.

Crossley, R., Remington-Gurney, J., & Batt, M. (1990). Communication training using facilitated communication. *Augmentative and Alternative Communication, 6,* 90–91.

Crystal, D. (1986). ISAAC in chains: The future of communication systems. *Augmentative and Alternative Communication, 2*(4), 140–145.

Culatta, B., & Blackstone, S. (1980). A program to teach non-oral communication symbols to multiple handicapped children. *Journal of Childhood Communication Disorders, 4,* 29–55.

Culatta, B., Colucci, S., Capozzi, M., & Schmidt, A. (1977). Spontaneous use of trained language symbols in multihandicapped children. Paper presented at the annual meeting of the American Speech-Language-Hearing Association, Chicago.

Culp, D. M. (1982). *Communication Interaction—Nonspeaking Children Using Augmentative Systems and Their Mothers.* Author.

Culp, D. M. (1987). Outcome measurement: The impact of augmentative communication. *Seminars in Speech and Language, 8,* 169–181.

Culp, D. M. (1989). Developmental apraxia and augmentative or alternative communication—A case example. *Augmentative and Alternative Communication, 5,* 27–34.

Culp, D. M., Ambrosi, D. M., Berniger, T. M., & Mitchell, J. E. (1985). A follow-up study of augmentative communication aid use. Paper presented at the annual meeting of the American Speech-Language-Hearing Association, Washington, DC.

Culp, D. M., Ambrosi, D. M., Berniger, T. M., & Mitchell, J. E. (1986). Augmentative communication aid use—A follow-up study. *Augmentative and Alternative Communication, 2*(1), 19–24.

Culp, D. M., & Carlisle, M. (1988a). Augmentative and alternative communication: "Locked-in" syndrome. *Augmentative and Alternative Communication, 4,* 149.

Culp, D. M., & Carlisle, M. (1988b). Evolutionary stages in augmentation for brain-injured patients: Clinical framework. Paper presented at the annual meeting of the American Speech-Language-Hearing Association, Boston.

Culp, D. M., & Carlisle, M. (1988c). *PACT: Partners in Augmentative Communication Training*. Tucson, AZ: Communication Skill Builders.

Culp, D. M., & Carlisle, M. (1990). Development of a center-based consumer newsletter. *Augmentative and Alternative Communication*, 6, 115.

Culp, D. M., & Stahlecker, J. (1986). Development and documentation of a communication facilitation program for nonspeaking children and their parents. *Augmentative and Alternative Communication*, 2, 81.

Cumley, G. D. (1991). AAC facilitator roles and responsibilities. Unpublished manuscript, University of Nebraska, Lincoln.

Cumley, G. D., & Beukelman, D. R. (1992). AAC facilitator model: Roles and responsibilities of AAC facilitators. *Augmentative and Alternative Communication*, 8, 126.

Cumley, G. D., & Swanson, S. (1992a). Developmental apraxia of speech (DAS): Communication options. *Augmentative and Alternative Communication*, 8, 126–127.

Cumley, G. D., & Swanson, S. (1992b). Facilitating communication skills in children with developmental apraxia of speech. Paper presented at the annual meeting of the American Speech-Language-Hearing Association, San Antonio.

Cummins, R., & Prior, M. (1992). Autism and assisted communication: A reply to Biklen. *Harvard Educational Review*, 62, 228–241.

Cumpata, J. E. F., & Donahue, E. (1985). Ventilator-dependent patients' use of speaking tracheostomy tubes: Nursing survey. Paper presented at the annual meeting of the American Speech-Language-Hearing Association, Washington, DC.

Cunningham, E., Gallagher, K., & Krawczyk, K. (1986). Assessment of communication aids with speech synthesis in acquired disability. *Augmentative and Alternative Communication*, 2, 81–82.

Cunningham, E., & Mackey, J. (1986). The use of synthetic speech in speech therapy. *Augmentative and Alternative Communication*, 2, 82.

Dabbagh, H. H., & Damper, R. I. (1985). Text composition by voice: Design issues and implementations. *Augmentative and Alternative Communication*, 1(2), 84–93.

Daharsh, P., & Mirenda, P. (1992). Communication and regular class inclusion for students who use AAC. *Augmentative and Alternative Communication*, 8, 127.

Dahl, I., & Galyas, K. (1990). Synthetic speech as an aid to communication and literacy. *Augmentative and Alternative Communication*, 6, 131.

Dahlberg, C., & Jaffe, J. (1977). *Stroke: A Doctor's Personal Story of His Recovery*. New York: W. W. Norton.

Dahle, A., & Goldman, R. (1990). Perception of synthetic speech by normal and developmentally disabled children. Paper presented at the annual meeting of the American Speech-Language-Hearing Association, Seattle.

Dalhoff, F. (1986). *Forstar Han Hvad Man Siger?* [Does He Understand What Is Said?]. Frederikshavn, Denmark: Dafalo Forlag.

Dalrymple, A. J., & Feldman, M. A. (1992). Effects of reinforced directed rehersal on expressive sign language learning by persons with mental retardation. *Journal of Behavioral Education*, 2(1), 1–16.

Damper, R. I. (1982). Speech technology—implications for biomedical engineering. *Journal of Medical Engineering and Technology*, 6(4), 135–149.

Damper, R. I. (1986a). Message composition by word abbreviation. *Augmentative and Alternative Communication*, 2, 82.

Damper, R. I. (1986b). Rapid message composition for large vocabulary speech output aids: A review of possibilities. *Augmentative and Alternative Communication*, 2(4), 152–159.

Damper, R. I., Burnett, J. W., Gray, P. W., Straus, L. P., & Symes, R.A. (1987). Hand-held text-to-speech device for the non-vocal disabled. *Journal of Biomedical Engineering*, 9(4), 332–340.

Daniels, L., & Worthingham, C. (1986). *Muscle Testing: Techniques of Manual Examination.* 5th ed. Philadephia: Saunders.

Daniloff, J. K. (1984). Comparison between the motoric constraints for Amer-Ind and ASL sign formation. *Journal of Speech and Hearing Research*, 27, 76–88.

Daniloff, J. K., Lloyd, L. L., & Fristoe, M. (1983). Amer-Ind transparency. *Journal of Speech and Hearing Disorders*, 48, 103–110.

Daniloff, J. K., Noll, J., Fristoe, M., & Lloyd, L. (1982). Gesture recognition in patients with aphasia. *Journal of Speech and Hearing Disorders*, 47, 43–47.

Daniloff, J. K., & Shafer, A. (1981). A gestural communication program for severely-profoundly handicapped children. *Language, Speech, and Hearing Services in Schools*, 12, 258–268.

Daniloff, J. K., & Vergara, D. (1984). Comparison between the motor constraints for Amer-Ind and ASL sign formation. *Journal of Speech and Hearing Research*, 27, 76–88.

Darley, F. L., Aronson, A. E., & Brown, J. R. (1975). *Motor Speech Disorders.* Philadelphia: Saunders.

Dashiell, S., Hanson, J., Hinchcliffe, M., & Hunt, J. (1987). Procedures for mainstreaming students who use communication aids. Intervention strategy developed under Contract No. 300-85-0139 (*Implementation Strategies for Improving the Use of Communication Aids in Schools Serving Handicapped Children*) from the U.S. Department of Education distributed by the American Speech-Language-Hearing Association.

Davis, G. A. (1973). Linguistics and language therapy: The sentence construction board. *Journal of Speech and Hearing Disorders*, 38, 205–214.

Davis, G. A. (1993). *A Survey of Adult Aphasia and Related Language Disorders.* Englewood Cliffs, NJ: Prentice Hall.

Dawson, K. (1982). *Standard Language Assessment Tests Capable of Modification and Use with Non-speaking Persons.* Boston: Communication Enhancement Clinic: Children's Hospital.

Day, R. M., Johnson, W. L., & Schussler, N. G. (1986). Determining the communicative properties of self-injury: Research, assessment, and treatment implications. In K. D. Gadow (Ed.), *Advances in Learning and Behavioral Disabilities.* Vol. 5. Greenwich, CT: JAI Press, pp. 117–139.

Dean, C. R., & Piccirilli, L. (1988). Communication partner preference for augmentative communication systems. Paper presented at the annual meeting of the American Speech-Language-Hearing Association, Boston.

Decker, M. Hoffmann, P., Schaffers, J., Wagener, T., Wagner, A., & Wehenkel, C. (1986). Development of a language-independent speech prosthesis. *Augmentative and Alternative Communication*, 2, 82–83.

Deegan, S. (1992). AAC training for professionals in Zimbabwe. *Augmentative and Alternative Communication*, 8, 127.

Deegan, S., & Robinson, C. (1988). "Speak out": A group for adolescents who use augmentative and alternative communication. *Augmentative and Alternative Communication*, 4, 136–137.

Deich, R. F., & Hodges, P. M. (1978). *Language Without Speech*. New York: Brunner/Mazel.

Deich, R. F., & Hodges, P. M. (1982). Teaching nonvocal communications to nonverbal retarded children. *Behavior Modification*, 6, 200–228.

Deliege, R. J., Speth-Lemmens, I. M., & Waterham, R. P. (1989). Development and primary evaluation of two speech communication aids. *Journal of Medical Engineering and Technology*, 13(1–2), 18–22.

Demasco, P. W. (1986). Progressive approaches to eye-tracking communication systems. *Augmentative and Alternative Communication*, 2, 83.

Demasco, P. W., Ball, J. E., Rookard, C., Quinlisk-Gill, S., & Kerly, P. (1990). The development of an AAC software architecture. *Augmentative and Alternative Communication*, 6, 116.

Demasco, P. W., Ball, J. E., Tyvand, S., Dunaway, J., Blodgett, D., & Bradley, W. (1992). A three level model for authoring in AAC systems. *Augmentative and Alternative Communication*, 8, 127.

Demasco, P. W., Jones, M., McCoy, K., & Pennington, C. (1992). Compansion: A rate enhancement technique for word-based AAC systems. *Augmentative and Alternative Communication*, 8, 127–128.

Demasco, P. W., & Mineo, B. A. (1992). Enhancing picture-based communication: Assessment and instruction. *Augmentative and Alternative Communication*, 8, 128.

Demasco, P. W., Mineo, B. A., & Foulds, R. A. (1990). Overview of Rehabilitation Engineering Center on Augmentative Communication. *Augmentative and Alternative Communication*, 6, 111.

Dennis, R., Reichle, J., Williams, W., & Vogelberg, R. T. (1982). Motoric factors influencing the selection of vocabulary for sign production programs. *Journal of the Association for the Severely Handicapped*, 7, 20–33.

DePape, D. J. (1979). *Guidelines for Seeking Funding for Communication Aids*. Madison: Trace Research and Development Center for the Severely Communicatively Handicapped, University of Wisconsin.

DePape, D. J., & Harris-Vanderheiden, D. (1977). *Selecting Initial Vocabulary Elements: Preliminary Notes*. Madison: Trace Research and Development Center for the Severely Communicatively Handicapped, University of Wisconsin.

DePape, D. J., & Vanderheiden, G. C. (1977). *Initial and Secondary Approaches for Developing a Means of Response and Expression for Non-vocal Severely Physically Handicapped Children and Adults:Preliminary Notes*. Madison: Trace Research and Development Center for the Severely Communicatively Handicapped, University of Wisconsin.

DePaul, R., & Yoder, D. E. (1986). Iconicity in manual sign systems for the augmentative communication user: Is that all there is? *Augmentative and Alternative Communication*, 2(1), 1–10.

DePaulo, B. M., & Coleman, L. M. (1987). Verbal and nonverbal communication of warmth to children, foreigners, and retarded adults. *Journal of Nonverbal Behavior*, 11(2), 75–88.

DeRuyter, F., & Beukelman, D. R. (1981). Efficiency of nonvocal switching patterns and effectiveness on alphabet arrangements. Paper presented at the annual meeting of the American Speech-Language-Hearing Association, Los Angeles.

DeRuyter, F., & Donoghue, K. A. (1989). Communication and traumatic brain injury: A case study. *Augmentative and Alternative Communication*, 5, 49–54.

DeRuyter, F., Doyle, M., & Kennedy, M. R. T. (1990a). ACS outcomes in traumatic brain injury: Are the data accurate? Paper presented at the annual meeting of the American Speech-Language-Hearing Association, Seattle.

DeRuyter, F., Doyle, M., & Kennedy, M. R. T. (1990b). ACS outcomes: Do the data tell the whole story? *Augmentative and Alternative Communication*, 6, 120.

DeRuyter, F., Doyle, M., & Kennedy, M. R. T. (1990c). Who is doing what for the nonspeaking person with traumatic brain injury? *Augmentative and Alternative Communication*, 6, 138–139.

DeRuyter, F., Doyle, M., & Kennedy, M. R. T. (1992). Interactive needs profile for nonspeaking brain injured adults. *Augmentative and Alternative Communication*, 8, 128.

DeRuyter, F., & Kennedy, M. R. T. (1991). Augmentative communication following traumatic brain injury. In D. Beukelman & K. Yorkston (Eds.), *Communication Disorders Following Traumatic Brain Injury: Management of Cognitive, Language, and Motor Impairments*. Austin, TX: Pro-Ed, pp. 317–365.

DeRuyter, F., Kennedy, M. R. T., & Doyle, M. (1990). Who is doing what for the nonspeaking traumatic brain injured? Paper presented at the annual meeting of the American Speech-Language-Hearing Association, Seattle.

DeRuyter, F., & Lafontaine, L. M. (1985). Relational data-base report of the nonspeaking population. Paper presented at the annual meeting of the American Speech-Language-Hearing Association, Washington, D. C.

DeRuyter, F., & Lafontaine, L. M. (1987). The nonspeaking brain-injured: A clinical and demographic database report. *Augmentative and Alternative Communication*, 3(1), 18–25.

DeTommaso, D., & Sterner, M. (1992). Learning/communicating: Can we do both at the same time? *Augmentative and Alternative Communication*, 8, 128–129.

Devereux, K., & van Oosterom, J. (1984). *Learning with Rebuses*. Stratford-upon-Avon, England: National Council for Special Education. Developing Horizons in Special Education Series Number 8. (Also available from EARD, Blackhill, Ely, Cambridgeshire, England)

Devices speak English for laryngectomy cases (1978). *Clinical Trends* (Opthalmology, Otolaryngology, & Allergy), 16(8), 6.

DeVilliers, J. G., & Naughton, J. M. (1976). Teaching a symbol language to autistic children. *Journal of Consulting and Clinical Psychology*, 42, 111–117.

Dewan, E. M. (1966). Communication for voluntary control of the electroencephalogram. *Proceedings of the Symposium on Biomedical Engineering*, 1, 349–351.

Diggs, C. C. (1990). Self-help for communication disorders. *Asha*, 32, 32–34.

DiSimoni, F. (1986). Alternative communication systems for the aphasic individual. In R. Chapey (Ed.), *Language Intervention in Adult Aphasia*. Baltimore: Williams & Wilkins, pp. 345–359,

Dixon, C. (August 1971). Electronic aids for the severely physically handicapped. *District Nursing*.

Dixon, C., & Curry, B. (1965). Some thoughts on the communication board. *Cerebral Palsy Journal*, 26, 12–13.

Dobres, R., White, L. C., & Haight, P. L. (1991). Introducing Minspeak™ to adults with neurological impairments: Assessing learning performance. Paper presented at the Sixth Annual Minspeak™ Conference, Minneapolis, MN.

Doherty, J. E. (1985a). The effects of sign characteristics on sign acquisition and retention: An integrative review of the literature. *Augmentative and Alternative Communication*, 1(3), 108–121.

Doherty, J. E. (1985b). The effects of translucency and handshape difficulty on sign acquisition and retention by preschool children. Unpublished doctoral dissertation, Purdue University.

Doherty, J. E. (1987). Handling, positioning, and adaptive equipment. In E. McDonald (Ed.), *Treating Cerebral Palsy: For Clinicians by Clinicians*. Austin, TX: Pro-Ed., pp. 153–170.

Doherty, J. E., Daniloff, J. K., & Lloyd, L. L. (1985). The effect of categorical presentation on Amer-Ind transparency. *Augmentative and Alternative Communication*, 1(1), 10–16.

Doherty, J. E., Karlan, G., & Lloyd, L. (1982). Establishing the transparency of two gestural systems by mentally retarded adults. Paper presented at the annual meeting of the American Speech-Language-Hearing Association, Toronto.

Dolz, J. L. (1990). Computer as an alternative evaluation system for disabled children. *Augmentative and Alternative Communication*, 6, 111.

Donker-Gimbrére, M. W., & van Balkom, H. (1988). A user's perspective on graphic systems. *Augmentative and Alternative Communication*, 4, 141,

Donnellan, A., Mirenda, P., Mesaros, R., & Fassbender, L. (1984). Analyzing the communicative functions of aberrant behavior. *Journal of the Association for Persons with Severe Handicaps*, 9, 201–212.

Donoghue, K. A. (1988). Speech-language pathologist's role in orthopedic management of nonoral brain injured individuals. *Augmentative and Alternative Communication*, 4, 156.

Donoghue, K. A., Doyle, M., & DeRuyter, F. (1990). Nonspeaking brain injured: Integrating augmentative and alternative systems with community college classrooms. *Augmentative and Alternative Communication*, 6, 139.

Doss, L. S., Locke, P. A., Johnston, S. S., Reichle, J., Sigafoos, J., Charpentier, P. J., & Foster, D. J. (1991). Initial comparison of the efficiency of a variety of AAC systems for ordering meals in fast food restaurants. *Augmentative and Alternative Communication*, 7, 256–265.

Doss, L. S., & Reichle, J. (1989). Establishing communicative alternatives to the emission of socially motivated excess behavior: A review. *Journal of the Association for Persons with Severe Handicaps*, 14, 101–112.

Doss, L. S., & Reichle, J. (1991a). Replacing excess behavior with initial communicative repertoire. In J. Reichle, J. Y. York, & J. Sigafoos, *Implementing Augmentative and Alternative Communication: Strategies for Learners with Severe Disabilities*. Baltimore: Paul H. Brookes, pp. 215–237.

Doss, L. S., & Reichle, J. (1991b). Using graphic organization aids to promote independent functioning. In J. Reichle, J. Y. York, & J. Sigafoos, *Implementing Augmentative and Alternative Communication: Strategies for Learners with Severe Disabilities*. Baltimore: Paul H. Brookes, pp. 275–288.

Dowden, P. A. (1986). Augmentative interventions in intensive care units. In Sarah W. Blackstone (Ed.), *Augmentative Communication: An Introduction*. Rockville, MD: American Speech-Language-Hearing Association, pp. 321–327.

Dowden, P. A., Beukelman, D. R., & Lossing, C. (1986). Serving nonspeaking patients in acute care settings: Intervention outcomes. *Augmentative and Alternative Communication*, 2(2), 38–44.

Dowden, P. A., Honsinger, M., & Beukelman, D. (1986). Serving non-speaking patients in acute care settings: An intervention approach. *Augmentative and Alternative Communication*, 2(1), 25–32.

Dowden, P. A., Yorkston, K. M., & Stoel-Gammon, C. (1987). Speech intelligibility of augmentative system users: Effect of context. Paper presented at the annual meeting of the American Speech-Language-Hearing Association, New Orleans.

Dowling, J., Harrington, K., Odell, S., & Running, A. (1988). Speaking for our selves. *Augmentative and Alternative Communication*, 4, 161.

Downing, O. J., & Tully, J. E. (1979). Telecad—A television communication aid for the disabled. *Medical and Biological Engineering and Computing*, 17, 476–480.

Doyle, M., Cottier, C., & Barua, C. (1992). Mainstreaming students with assistive technology. *Augmentative and Alternative Communication*, 8, 129.

Doyle, M., & DeRuyter, F. (1988). Chronic care rehabilitation team approach with a nonspeaking child. *Augmentative and Alternative Communication*, 4, 164.

Doyle, M., & DeRuyter, F. (1989). Vocabulary selection and expansion strategies for nonspeaking traumatic brain injured. Paper presented at the annual meeting of the American Speech-Language-Hearing Association, St. Louis.

Doyle, M., & DeRuyter, F. (1990). Unique issues in AAC intervention for different disability groups. Paper presented at the annual meeting of the American Speech-Language-Hearing Association, Seattle.

Doyle, M., DeRuyter, F., & Kennedy, M. (1990a). Influence of cognition on augmentative communication in nonspeaking persons with brain injury. *Augmentative and Alternative Communication*, 6, 141.

Doyle, M., DeRuyter, F., & Kennedy, M. (1990b). Selecting and expanding augmentative systems in nonspeaking persons with brain injury. *Augmentative and Alternative Communication*, 6, 90.

Doyle, M., & Palacios, K. (1992). Cognitive and language skills influencing AAC use in nonspeaking TBI. *Augmentative and Alternative Communication*, 8, 129.

Drazek, A. L., Lawrence-Dederich, S., Higginbotham, D. J., Scally, C. A., & Clark, L. (1992). Customizing a word prediction system: A case study. Paper presented at the annual meeting of the American Speech-Language-Hearing Association, San Antonio.

Drolet, C. (1982). *Unipex: Universal Language of Pictures*. Los Angeles: Imaginart Press.

Drommond, R. E., & Latson, L. F. (1989). Communication equipment selection protocol for clients with spinal cord injury. Paper presented at the annual meeting of the American Speech-Language-Hearing Association, St. Louis.

Drynan, D., & McGinnis, J. (1992). Clinical evaluation of rate enhancement techniques: A case study perspective. *Augmentative and Alternative Communication*, 8, 129.

Duffy, L. (1977). An innovative approach to the development of communication skills for severely speech handicapped cerebral palsied children. Unpublished master's thesis, University of Nevada, Las Vegas.

Duffy, R. J., & Duffy, J. R., (1984). *New England Pantomime Tests*. Austin, TX: Pro-Ed.

Duffy, R. J., Duffy, J. R., & Pearson, K. L. (1973). Impairment of gestural ability in aphasics. Paper presented at the annual meeting of the American Speech-Language-Hearing Association, Detroit.

Duffy, R. J., Duffy, J. R., & Pearson, K. L. (1975). Pantomime recognition in aphasics. *Journal of Speech and Hearing Research*, 18, 115–132.

Duganne, J. A., & Glicksman, M. A. (1993). Mac and me: Growing up with computers. *Augmentative and Alternative Communication*, 6, 93.

Duker, P. (1984). [Sign language: A gesture for and toward the mentally retarded.] *Tijdschr-Ziekenverpl*, 37(16), 512–515.

Duker, P. C., & Michielsen, H. M. (1983). Cross-setting generalization of manual signs to verbal instructions with severely retarded children. *Applied Research in Mental Retardation*, 4, 29–40.

Duker, P. C., & Moonen, X. M. (1985). A program to increase manual signs with severely/ profoundly mentally retarded children in natural environments. *Applied Research in Mental Retardation*, 6 (2), 147–158.

Duker, P. C., & Moonen, X. M. (1986). The effect of two procedures on spontaneous signing with Down's syndrome children. *Journal of Mental Deficiency Research*, 30, 335–364.

Duker, P. C., & Morsink, H. (1984). Acquisition and cross-setting generalization of manual signs with severely retarded individuals. *Journal of Applied Behavior Analysis*, 17(1), 93–103.

Duncan, J. L., & Silverman, F. H. (1977). Impacts of learning American Indian Sign Language on mentally retarded children. *Perceptual and Motor Skills*, 44, 1138.

Dunham, J. K. (1986). The transparency of manual signs in a linguistic and an environmental nonlinguistic context. Unpublished doctoral dissertation, Purdue University.

Dunham, J. K. (1989). The transparency of manual signs in a linguistic and an environmental nonlinguistic context. *Augmentative and Alternative Communication*, 5, 214–225.

Dunlop, E. (1986). A revised model of effective augmented communication: Some crude steps along the path of devising a useful clinical tool. *Augmentative and Alternative Communication*, 2, 83–84.

Dunn, L., & Dunn, L. (1981). *Peabody Picture Vocabulary Test*. Circle Pines, MN: American Guidance Service.

Dunn, M. (1982). *Pre-sign Language Motor Skills*. Tucson, AZ: Communication Skill Builders.

Dunn, N. (1987). Implementing a communication camp for individuals who use augmentative aids and techniques. Intervention strategy developed under Contract No. 300-85-0139 (*Implementation Strategies for Improving the Use of Communication Aids in Schools Serving Handicapped Children*) from the U.S. Department of Education distributed by the American Speech-Language-Hearing Association.

Dunn, N., Anderson, V., Allen, D., & Moore, E. (1986). Progression of augmentative communication systems in a severely handicapped child. *Augmentative and Alternative Communication*, 2, 84.

Dunn, N. S. (1990). Augmentative and alternative communication services in Arkansas. Paper presented at the annual meeting of the American Speech-Language-Hearing Association, Seattle.

Dunst, C. J., & Lowe, L. W. (1986). From reflex to symbol: Describing, explaining, and fostering communicative competence. *Augmentative and Alternative Communication*, 2(1), 11–18.

Durand, V. M. (1990). *Severe Behavior Problems: A Functional Communication Training Approach*. New York: Guilford Press.

Durand, V. M., & Berotti, D. (November 1991). Treating behavior problems with communication. *Asha*, 33, 37–39.

Durand, V. M., & Carr, E. (1991). Functional communication training to reduce challenging behavior: Maintenance and application in new settings. *Journal of Applied Behavior Analysis*, 24, 251–264.

Dutton, S. R., Davidheiser, C., & Tobias, S. (1929). Using a touch talker while having a severe hearing impairment. *Augmentative and Alternative Communication*, 8, 129–130.

Dyer, K., Dunlap, G., & Winterling, V. (1990). Effects of choice making on serious problem behaviors of students with severe handicaps. *Journal of Applied Behavior Analysis, 23,* 515–524.

Dymond, E. A., Potter, R., Griffiths, P. A., & McClemont, E. J. (1988). A week in the life of Mary: The impact of microtechnology on a severely handicapped person. *Journal of Biomedical Engineering,* 10(6), 483–490.

Dynes, D. T. (1992). Functional integration of multimodality AAC system. *Augmentative and Alternative Communication, 8,* 130.

Dyssegaard, B. (1990). Contact, communication, and computers—A continuum. *Augmentative and Alternative Communication, 6,* 149–150.

Eagleson, H. M., Vaughn, G. R., & Knudson, A. B. (1970). Hand signals for dysphasia. *Archives of Physical Medicine and Rehabilitation, 51,* 111–113.

Earl, C. (1972). *Don't Say a Word! The Picture Language Book.* London: Charles Knight & Co.

Easton, J. H. (1986). Group therapy for patients using speech synthesizers: Application. *Augmentative and Alternative Communication, 2,* 84–85.

Easton, J. H. (1988). Augmentative communication for patients in intensive care. *Intensive Care Nursing,* 4(2), 47–55.

Easton, J. H. (1989). Oh the frustration! *Communication Outlook,* 10(3), 16–17.

Easton, J. H., & Enderby, P. (1983). *The Acquisition Aids for the Speech Impaired.* Bristol, England: Assistive Communication Aids Centre, Frenchay Hospital.

Ecklund, S., & Reichle, J. (1987). A comparison of normal children's ability to recall symbols from two logographic systems. *Language, Speech, and Hearing Services in Schools, 18,* 34–40.

Edman, P. (1991). Relief Bliss: A low tech technique. *Communicating Together,* 9(1), 21–22.

Egan, J. J., Anthony, G. M., & Honke, L. E. (1976). Joan: A case study of manual communication with a severe cerebral palsied dysarthric. Paper presented at the annual meeting of the American Speech-Language-Hearing Association, Houston.

Egan, L. G. (1988). Cognitive development and use of switch-activated communication devices. *Augmentative and Alternative Communication, 4,* 166.

Egerton, S. W. (1976). Technical aids for the disabled. *The B. C. Professional Engineer,* 27(7), 25–27.

Egof, D. (1988). Coding communication devices: The effects of symbol set selection and code origin on the recall of utterances. Paper presented at the third annual CEC/TAM conference, Baltimore.

Ehrlich, M. D. (1974). The Votrax Voice Synthesizer as an aid for the blind. Paper presented at the 1974 Conference on Engineering Devices in Rehabilitation, Boston.

Eichler, J. H. (1973). *Instructions for the ETRAN Eye Signaling System.* Ridgefield, CT: Jack H. Eichler, 5 Beaver Brook Road.

Einis, L. P., & Báiley, D. M. (1990). The use of powered leisure and communication devices in a switch training program. *American Journal of Occupational Therapy,* 44(10), 931–934.

Ekman, P. (1976). Movements with precise meanings. *Journal of Communication, 26,* 14–26.

Ekman, P., & Friesen, W. (1969). The repertoire of nonverbal behavior: Categories, origin, usage, and coding. *Semiotica, 1,* 49–98.

Elder, P. S. (1977). Nonspeech visual symbol training. Paper presented at the annual meeting of the American Association of Mental Deficiency, New Orleans.

Elder, P. S. (1978). *Visual Symbol Communication Training. Part I: Receptive Instruction.* Wauconda, IL: Don Johnson Developmental Equipment.

Elder, P. S. (1980). A non-speech communication instruction strategy with multiply handicapped persons. Paper presented at the annual meeting of the American Speech-Language-Hearing Association, Detroit.

Elder, P. S., & Bergman, J. S. (1978). Visual symbol communication instruction with nonverbal multiply handicapped individuals. *Mental Retardation*, 16, 107–112.

Ellsworth, S., & Kotkin, R. (November/December, 1975). If only Jimmy could speak. *Hearing and Speech Action*, 43, 6–10.

Employment rights of people with communication disabilities (September 1992). *Asha*, 34, 56–57.

Enderby, P. (Ed.) (1987). *Assistive Communication Aids*. Edinburgh, Scotland: Churchill Livingstone, Robert Stevenson House.

Enderby, P., & Hamilton, G. (1981). Clinical trials for communication aids? A study provoked by the clinical trials of SPLINK. *International Journal of Rehabilitation Research*, 4(2), 181–195.

Enderby, P., & Hamilton, G. (1983). Communication aid and therapeutic tool: A report on the clinical trial using Splink with aphasic individuals. In C. Code & D. Muller (Eds.), *Aphasia Therapy*. London: Edward Arnold, pp. 187–193.

Enders, S. (1983). Funding for devices. *Rehabilitation Technology Review*, 2(4), 4–5.

Engineering a good deed (1964). *We*, 16(5), 34.

Englehart, T. W. (1971). A computerized typing system for the handicapped. M.S. thesis, University of Alberta, Alberta, Canada.

English, S. T., & Prutting, C. A. (1975). Teaching American Sign Language to a normally hearing infant with tracheostenosis: A case study. *Clinical Pediatrics* (Philadelphia), 14, 1141–1145.

Englander, D. (1980). *Computers in Medicine: An Introduction*. St. Louis: Mosby.

Enstrom, D. H. (1990). The Communication Resource Center: A service delivery model. *Augmentative and Alternative Communication*, 6, 142.

Enstrom, D. H. (1992). The Communication Resource Center: A New Jersey AAC service delivery model. *Augmentative and Alternative Communication*, 8, 234–242.

Enstrom, D. H., & Littman, M. G. (1992). Strategic alliance: Princeton University and New Jersey's Communication Resources Center. *Augmentative and Alternative Communication*, 8, 130.

Erickson, J. (1992). The AAC user traveling in Europe and the United States: Conversing and transversing. *Augmentative and Alternative Communication*, 8, 130.

Erickson, J., Duganne, J., Marshall, P., Millin, N., & Costello, J. (1992). Attending college: Experiences of consumers of augmentative communication. *Augmentative and Alternative Communication*, 8, 125–126.

Eriksson, B. (1985). *Headsticks and Optical Pointers*. Bromma, Sweden: Handicappinstitutet.

Esser, J. M., & Mizuko, M. I. (1989). Intervention effects on augmentative communication system (ACS) user's interaction skills. Paper presented at the annual meeting of the American Speech-Language-Hearing Association, St. Louis.

Eulenberg, J. B. (1990). Dynamic displays and the future of augmentative communication. *Communication Outlook*, 12(2), 21–23.

Eulenberg, J. B., Bridges, S. J., Blosser, S. R., Predny, R., & Predny, F. (1988). The coevolution of a communication system. *Augmentative and Alternative Communication*, 4, 152.

Eulenberg, J. B., & Rosenfeld, J. (1982). Vocaid—A new product from Texas Instruments. *Communication Outlook*, 3(3), 1, 3.

Evans, A. L., Gowdie, R. A., Keating, D., Smith, D. C., Wyper, D. J., & Cunningham, E.

(1985). A versatile speech output communication aid. *Journal of Medical Engineering and Technology*, 9(4), 180–182.

Everson, J. M., & Goodwyn, R. (1987). A comparison of the use of adaptive microswitches by students with cerebral palsy. *American Journal of Occupational Therapy*, 41, 739–744.

Ewing, A. M., & Thompson, M. (1980). Comuni-Kate: A way to talk. Paper presented at the annual meeting of the American Speech-Language-Hearing Association, Detroit.

Ezra, S. (1990). The development of an AAC resource library. *Augmentative and Alternative Communication*, 6, 142.

Fadman, A. (January 1980). The expanding world of Bill Rush. *Life*, 3(1), 90–98.

Fagerberg, G., & Raade, A. S. (1992). Icon access times in computer-based visual communication by aphasic clients. *Augmentative and Alternative Communication*, 8, 131.

Fahey, R., Zegarra, L., & Finch, A. (1990). Going on-line with and for individuals with communication disabilities. *Augmentative and Alternative Communication*, 6, 89.

Fairhurst, M. C., & Stephanidis, C. (1985). An interactive aid for expressive communication with pictographic symbols. *International Journal of Biomedical Computing*, 17(3–4), 177–184.

Fairhurst, M. C., & Stephanidis, C. (1988). An evaluation of the information interface in the design of computer-driven aids for expressive communication. *International Journal of Biomedical Computing*, 23(3–4), 177–189.

Fairhurst, M. C., & Stephanidis, C. (1989). A model-based approach to the specification of computer-based communication aids. *Journal of Medical Engineering and Technology*, 13(1–2), 13–17.

Fairweather, B. C., Haun, D. H., & Finkle, L. J. (1983). *Communication Systems for Severely Handicapped Persons*. Springfield, IL: Charles C. Thomas.

Farrier, L. D., Yorkston, K. M., Marriner, N. A., & Beukelman, D. R. (1985). Conversational control in nonimpaired speakers using an augmentative communication system. *Augmentative and Alternative Communication*, 1(2), 65–73.

Farwell, L. A., & Donchin, E. (1988). Talking off the top of your head: Toward a mental prosthesis utilizing event-related brain potentials. *Electroencephalography & Clinical Neurophysiology*, 70(6), 510–523.

Faw, J. D., Reid, D. H., Schepis, M. M. , Fitzgerald, J. R., & Welty, P. A. (1981). Involving institutional staff in the development and maintenance of sign language skills with profoundly retarded persons. *Journal of Applied Behavior Analysis*, 14, 411–423.

Fawcett, G. F., & Clibbens, J. S. (1983). The acquisition of signs by the mentally handicapped: Measurement criteria. *British Journal of Disorders of Communication*, 18(1), 13–21.

Fawcus, M. (1986). A study of the response to a signing system by a group of severe Broca's dysphasics. *Augmentative and Alternative Communication*, 2, 85.

Fawcus, R. (1986). A low-cost flexible interface system with choice of speech synthesis output modes. *Augmentative and Alternative Communication*, 2, 85.

Feallock, B. (1958). Communication for the nonverbal individual. *American Journal of Occupational Therapy*, 12, 60–63, 83.

Feeley, J., Brown, H. G., McNaughton, S., & Laughton, M. F. (1990). BlissTel Project: Status report. *Augmentative and Alternative Communication*, 6, 98.

Fell, A., Lynn, E., & Morrison, K. (1984). *Non-oral Communication Assessment*. Ann Arbor, MI: Alternatives to Speech, 1030 Duncan.

Fels, D., Shein, F., Chignell, M., & Milner, M. (1992). Taxonomy of device-independent information to provide multi-modal computer feedback. *Augmentative and Alternative Communication*, 8, 131.

Fenn, G., & Rowe, J. A. (1975). An experiment in manual communication. *British Journal of Disorders of Communication*, 10, 3–16.

Ferngren, H., & Ghisler, W. (1990). Stefan's communication 1985–1990. *Augmentative and Alternative Communication*, 6, 137.

Ferngren, H., & Sundberg, M. (1990). Sign language for habilitation of children with tracheotomies. *Augmentative and Alternative Communication*, 6, 105–106.

Ferrier, L. J. (1990). A procedure for evaluating intelligibility of synthetic speech versus voice. *Augmentative and Alternative Communication*, 6, 99.

Ferrier, L. J. (1991). Clinical study of a dysarthric adult using a touch talker with words strategy. *Augmentative and Alternative Communication*, 7, 266–274.

Ferrier, L. J., & Fell, H. J. (1992). The Baby-Babble-Blanket providing communication for severely impaired infants. Paper presented at the annual meeting of the American Speech-Language-Hearing Association, San Antonio.

Ferrier, L. J., Hanrahan, L. L., Stone, H. C., & Shane, H. C. (1986). Applications of augmentative communication systems to individuals with regressive disorders: A case study of Huntington's disease with juvenile onset. *Augmentative and Alternative Communication*, 2, 85.

Finkley, E. F., & Boysen, L. E. (1986). The role of physical and occupational therapy in augmentative communication. *Augmentative and Alternative Communication*, 2, 85–86.

Finkley, E. F., & Osborn, S. R. (1986). Progressive cause and effect augmentative communication strategies. *Augmentative and Alternative Communication*, 2, 86.

Finnegan, C. S., Bondy, A. S., & Wachowiak, J. (1989). Differential rates of acquisition for labelling versus requesting with pictures. Paper presented at the annual meeting of the American Speech-Language-Hearing Association, St. Louis.

Fiocca, G. (1981). Generally understood gestures: An approach to communication for persons with severe language impairments. Unpublished master's thesis, University of Illinois.

Fish, K. (May 27, 1969). Trying to break into "Their Own World." *Democrat and Chronicle* (Rochester, NY).

Fishman, I. R. (1987). *Electronic Communication Aids and Techniques: Selection and Use.* San Diego: College-Hill.

Fishman, I. R. (1988). Strategies for introducing speech output. *Augmentative and Alternative Communication*, 4, 170.

Fishman, S., Timler, G., & Yoder, D. E. (1985). Strategies for the prevention and repair of communication breakdown in interactions with communication board users. *Augmentative and Alternative Communication*, 1(1), 38–51.

Fitzgerald, J. R., Reid, D. H., Schepis, M. M., Faw, G. D. , Welty, P. A., & Pyfer, L. M. (1984). A rapid training procedure for teaching manual sign language skills to multidisciplinary institutional staff. *Applied Research in Mental Retardation*, 5(4), 451–469.

Flaherty, C., & Cook, S. (1981). Portable, inexpensive and individualized communication aids for the nonoral child. Paper presented at the annual meeting of the American Speech-Language-Hearing Association, Los Angeles.

Flaherty, C., & McDonald, C. (1989). Effective classroom services with computers for profoundly developmentally delayed students. Paper presented at the annual meeting of the American Speech-Language-Hearing Association, St. Louis.

Flensborg, C. (1988). *Snak med mig* [Talk with Me]. Socialstyrelsen, 2100 Copenhagen, Denmark.

Fletcher, E. C., & Havemeyer, S. (1977). Teaching sign language to severely retarded adults: Three case studies. Paper presented at the annual meeting of the American Speech-Language-Hearing Association, Chicago.

Flexner, S. B. (Ed.) (1987). *Random House Dictionary of the English Language.* New York: Random House.

Foldi, N., Gardner, H., Zurif, E., & Davis, L. (1976). Pragmatic use of gesture in aphasic communication. Paper presented at the Conference on Neurolinguistics and Sign, Rochester, NY.

Foley, B. E., & Davis, G. A. (1990). Phonological recording and congenital dysarthria: Implications for intervention. *Augmentative and Alternative Communication,* 6, 133.

Foley, B. E., & Eule, A. (1992). Literacy development in AAC users: Integrating analytic and holistic approaches. *Augmentative and Alternative Communication,* 8, 131.

Follansbee, R. A., Costello, J., & Corley, P. (1992). Comparison of encoding efficiency: Word prediction and semantic compaction. *Augmentative and Alternative Communication,* 8, 132.

Follansbee, R. A., & Sauer, M. (1990). Linking literacy and language: A cooperative model. *Augmentative and Alternative Communication,* 6, 150–151.

Follansbee, R. A., & Shane, H. (1992). Dictated composition using voice recognition technology for learning disabled individuals. *Augmentative and Alternative Communication,* 8, 132.

Follansbee, S., & Chambers, L. (1990). Equal access to curriculum with the Macintosh computer. *Augmentative and Alternative Communication,* 6, 134.

Fong, D., & Petty, L. (1990). The final touch—Mounting the communication aid. *Augmentative and Alternative Communication,* 6, 149.

Forest, M. (1988). *With a Little Help from My Friends* [videotape]. (Available from Expectations Unlimited, Box 655, Niwot, CO 80544; Centre for Integrated Education, 24 Thome Crescent, Toronto, Ont. M6H 2S5, Canada.)

Forsey, J. A., Bedrosian, J. L., & Bird, E. K. (1992). Input/output modality combinations: Language performance in individuals with autism. Paper presented at the annual meeting of the American Speech-Language-Hearing Association, San Antonio.

Fothergill, J., Vanderheiden, G. C., Holt, C., & Luster, M. J. (1978). Illustrated digest of nonverbal communication and writing aids for severely physically handicapped individuals. In Gregg C. Vanderheiden (Ed.), *Non-Vocal Communication Resourcebook.* Baltimore: University Park Press.

Foulds, R. A. (1972). The Tufts Interactive Communicator. Paper presented at the Carnahan Conference on Electronic Prosthesis, Lexington, KY. (Paper is published in the conference proceedings volume, pp. 16–24.)

Foulds, R. A. (1980). Communication rates for nonspeech expression as a function of manual tasks and linguistic constraints. In *Proceedings of the International Conference on Rehabilitation Engineering* (Toronto, June 16–20). Ottawa: National Speech Council of Canada.

Foulds, R. A. (1982). Applications of microcomputers in the education of the physically disabled child. *Exceptional Children,* 49(2), 155–162.

Foulds, R. A. (1985). Observations on interfacing in nonvocal communication. In C. Barry & M. Byrne (Eds.), *Proceedings of the Fourth International Conference on Communication Through Technology for the Physically Disabled.* London: International Cerebral Palsy Association, pp. 46–51.

Foulds, R. A. (1986). Telephone transmission of sign language for the deaf. *Augmentative and Alternative Communication,* 2, 87.

Foulds, R. A. (1987). Guest editorial. *Augmentative and Alternative Communication,* 3, 169.

Foulds, R. A., Baletsa, G., & Crochetiere, W. J. (1975). The effectiveness of language redundancy in non-verbal communication. Paper presented at the Seminar on Devices and Systems for the Disabled, Philadelphia. (Paper is published in seminar proceedings volume, pp. 82–86.)

Foulds, R. A., & Boubekker, M. (1986). Human quality synthetic speech using LPC diphones. *Augmentative and Alternative Communication*, 2, 86.

Foulds, R. A., & Gaddis, W. (1975). The practical application of an electronic communication device in a special needs classroom. Paper presented at the seminar on Devices and Systems for the Disabled, Philadelphia. (Paper is published in the Seminar proceedings volume, pp. 77–80.)

Foulds, R. A., & Galuska, S. (1990). Toward telephone transmission of manual communication via residential telephone. *Augmentative and Alternative Communication*, 6, 105.

Foulds, R. A., Soede, M., & van Balkom, H. (1987). Statistical disambiguation of multi-character keys applied to reduce motor requirements for augmentative and alternative communication. *Augmentative and Alternative Communication*, 3(4), 192–195.

Foxx, R. M., Kyle, M. S., Faw, G. D., & Bittle, R. G. (1988). Cues-pause-point training and simultaneous communication to teach the use of signed labeling repertoires. *American Journal on Mental Retardation*, 93(3), 305–311.

Francis, W. C. (1990). Clinical and research issues of vocabulary lists: Comments on Yorkston, Dowden, Honsinger, Marriner, and Smith (1988). *Augmentative and Alternative Communication*, 6, 275–276.

Francis, W., Nail, B., & Lloyd, L. (1990). Mentally retarded adults' perceptions of emotions represented by pictographic symbols. Paper presented at the annual meeting of the American Speech-Language-Hearing Association, Seattle.

Frankl, V. E. (1985). *Man's Search for Meaning.* New York: Washington Square Press.

Franklin, K. (1990). A comparison of five augmentative communication symbol assessment protocols. Paper presented at the annual meeting of the American Speech-Language-Hearing Association, Seattle.

Franklin, K., Phillips, G., & Mirenda, P. (1991). A comparison of five symbol assessment protocols. Unpublished manuscript, University of Nebraska, Lincoln.

Frattali, C., & Lynch, C. (April 1989). Functional assessment: Current issues and future challenges. *Asha*, 31, 70–74.

Frecks, K., & Beukelman, D. R. (1990). The comprehension of speech synthesized and natural voices by aphasic adults. Paper presented at the annual meeting of the American Speech-Language-Hearing Association, Seattle.

Freedman, S. L. (1992). The WOLF—A voice output communication aid costing only $400.00. Paper presented at the annual meeting of the American Speech-Language-Hearing Association, San Antonio.

Freeman, S. B., & Eulenberg, J. B. (1991). Children's attitudes toward synthesized speech varying in quality. Paper presented at the annual meeting of the American Speech-Language-Hearing Association, Atlanta.

Freiman, R., & Schlanger, P. H. (1977). Using pantomime therapy with aphasics. Paper presented at the annual meeting of the American Speech-Language-Hearing Association, Chicago. (Based on a M.A. thesis by R. Freiman, Herbert H. Lehman College, 1977.)

Freund, A., & Lenler, P. (1990). DAN BLISS 1. *Augmentative and Alternative Communication*, 6, 129.

Frey, M. R. (1992). Students, parents, teachers, therapists: Learning from each other. *Augmentative and Alternative Communication*, 8, 132.

Friedman, M., Kiliany, G., & Dzmura, M. (1984). An eye gaze controlled keyboard. *Proceedings of the Second International Conference on Rehabilitation Engineering*. Ottawa: Rehabilitation Engineering Society of North America (RESNA), pp. 446–447.

Friedman, R. B., Cheung, S., Entine, S., & Bartell, T. (1979). Verbal communication aid for nonvocal patients. *Medical and Biological Engineering and Computing*, 17, 103–106.

Fried-Oken, M. B. (1985). Voice recognition device as a computer interface for motor and speech impaired people. *Archives of Physical Medicine and Rehabilitation*, 66, 678–681.

Fried-Oken, M. B. (1987). Terminology in augmentative communication. *Language, Speech, and Hearing Services in Schools*, 18, 188–190.

Fried-Oken, M. B. (1989). Sentence recognition for auditory and visual scanning techniques in electronic augmentative communication devices. Paper presented at the RESNA/US-SAAC annual conference, New Orleans.

Fried-Oken, M. B. (1990). Comparing developmental language samples to vocabulary selected for nonspeaking children. *Augmentative and Alternative Communication*, 6, 148.

Fried-Oken, M. B., Goodenough-Trepagnier, C., & Galdieri, B. A. (1983). Progress report on the acquisition of preSPEEC. Paper presented at the annual meeting of the American Speech-Language-Hearing Association, Cincinnati.

Fried-Oken, M. B., Hamburg, D., & Baker, K. (1992). Twins and nonambulatory peers speak up for vocabulary selection research. *Augmentative and Alternative Communication*, 8, 132–133.

Fried-Oken, M. B., Howard, J. M., & Prillwitz, D. (1987). *Implementation Strategies for Improving the Use of Communication Aids in Schools Serving Handicapped Children*. Rockville, MD: American Speech-Language-Hearing Association.

Fried-Oken, M. B., Howard, J. M., & Prillwitz, D. (1988). Establishing initial communicative control with a loop-tape system. In S. Blackstone, E. Cassatt-James, & D. Bruskin (Eds.), *Augmentative Communication: Implementation Strategies*. Rockville, MD: American Speech-Language-Hearing Association, pp. 5.1-45–5.1-51.

Fried-Oken, M. B., Howard, J. M., & Stewart, S. R. (1988). Feedback on AAC intervention from patients with Guillain-Barré syndrome. *Augmentative and Alternative Communication*, 4, 141.

Fried-Oken, M. B., Howard, J. M., & Stewart, S. R. (1991). Feedback on AAC intervention from adults who are temporarily unable to speak. *Augmentative and Alternative Communication*, 7, 43–50.

Fried-Oken, M. B., & Kowalski, K. R. (1985). An auditory scanner for visually impaired nonspeaking persons. Paper presented at the annual meeting of the American Speech-Language-Hearing Association, Washington, DC.

Fried-Oken, M. B., & Minneman, S. L. (1988). Sentence recognition in electronic scanning devices: Three critical variables. *Augmentative and Alternative Communication*, 4, 165–166.

Fried-Oken, M. B., & More, L. (1992). An initial vocabulary for nonspeaking preschool children based on developmental and environmental language sources. *Augmentative and Alternative Communication*, 8, 41–56.

Friedrich, S. (1992). Facilitating communication for individuals with autism. *Augmentative and Alternative Communication*, 8, 133.

Friedrich, S., & Rom, M. (1992). The ever-changing role of a technical aids resource center. *Augmentative and Alternative Communication*, 8, 133.

Friedrich, S. S. (1988). Use of computer with two adult aphasic augmentative and alternative communication users. *Augmentative and Alternative Communication*, 4, 154.

Friedrich, S. S. (1990). Critical review of VOCA application with adults with acquired disorders. *Augmentative and Alternative Communication*, 6, 135.

Friedrich, S. S., Goldberg, S., Bialik, R., Yaniv, K., & Seligman-Wine, J. (1990). "The communication group": A multidisciplinary national service [in Israel]. *Augmentative and Alternative Communication*, 6, 120.

Friedrich, S. S., Salomon, D., & Katz, S. (1990). Roni speaks on the phone again: A case study. *Augmentative and Alternative Communication*, 6, 112.

Fristoe, M. (1976). *Language Intervention Systems for the Retarded*. Decatur, AL: L. B. Wallace Development Center.

Fristoe, M., & Bristow, D. (1982). Blissymbol translucency rating changes following three experimental manipulations. Paper presented at the annual meeting of the American Speech-Language-Hearing Association, Toronto.

Fristoe, M., & Lloyd, L. L. (1977). Manual communication for the retarded and others with severe communication impairments: A resource list. *Mental Retardation*, 15, 18–19.

Fristoe, M., and Lloyd, L. L. (1978). A survey of the use of non-speech systems with the severely communication impaired. *Mental Retardation*, 16(2), 99–103.

Fristoe, M., & Lloyd, L. L. (1979a). Nonspeech communication. In N. Ellis (Ed.), *Handbook of Mental Deficiency: Psychological Theory and Research*. 2nd ed. New York: Lawrence Erlbaum Associates, pp. 401–430.

Fristoe, M., & Lloyd, L. L. (1979b). Signs used in manual communication training with persons having severe communication impairments. *AAESPH Review*, 4, 364–373.

Fristoe, M., & Lloyd, L. L. (1980). Planning an initial expressive sign lexicon for persons with severe communication impairment. *Journal of Speech and Hearing Disorders*, 45, 170–180.

Frumkin, J. R. (1986a). Developing manual communication systems using Minspeak™ principles. Paper presented at the First Annual Minspeak Conference, Detroit.

Frumkin, J. R. (1986b). Enhancing interaction through role playing. In Sarah W. Blackstone (Ed.), *Augmentative Communication: An Introduction*. Rockville, MD: American Speech-Language-Hearing Association, pp. 329–335.

Frumkin, J. R. (1987). MINSPEAK remodeling. *Communication Outlook*, 9(1), 5–7.

Frumkin, J. R. (1990). Augmentative communication in New York State. Paper presented at the annual meeting of the American Speech-Language-Hearing Association, Seattle.

Frumkin, J. R., Geiger, C., Wilansky, L., & Cohen, C. (1984). *Magic Symbols*. Syracuse, NY: Schneier Communication Unit, Cerebral Palsy Center.

Fuller, D. R. (1987). Effects of translucency and complexity on the associative learning of Blissymbols by cognitively normal children and adults. Unpublished doctoral dissertation, Purdue University.

Fuller, D. R. (1988). Iconicity may not be everything, but it seems to be something: A comment on DePaul and Yoder (1966). *Augmentative and Alternative Communication*, 4, 123–125.

Fuller, D. R. (1992). Iconicity and Blissymbol learnability by persons with mental retardation. *Augmentative and Alternative Communication*, 8, 133.

Fuller, D. R., & Lloyd, L. L. (1987). A study of physical and semantic characteristics of a graphic symbol system as predictors of perceived complexity. *Augmentative and Alternative Communication*, 3(1), 26–35.

Fuller, D. R., & Lloyd, L. L. (1988). Generalizing adult-based translucency data to cognitively normal children. Paper presented at the annual meeting of the American Speech-Language-Hearing Association, Boston.

Fuller, D. R., & Lloyd, L. L. (1991). Toward a common usage of iconicity terminology. *Augmentative and Alternative Communication, 7,* 215–220.

Fuller, D. R., & Lloyd, L. L. (1992). Effects of configuration on the paired-associate learning of Blissymbols by preschool children with normal cognitive abilities. *Journal of Speech and Hearing Research, 35,* 1376–1383.

Fuller, D. R., Lloyd, L. L., & Schlosser, R. W. (1992). Further development of an augmentative and alternative communication symbol taxonomy. *Augmentative and Alternative Communication, 8,* 67–74.

Fuller, D. R., & Stratton, M. M. (1991). Representativeness versus translucency: Different theoretical backgrounds, but are they really different concepts? A position paper. *Augmentative and Alternative Communication, 7,* 51–58.

Fuller, P. (1990). Getting the message across: The work of the Ace Centre, Oxford. *Augmentative and Alternative Communication, 6,* 137.

Fuller, P., Donegan, M., & Jolleff, N. (1993). *The role of specialist AAC centres: Enablers or doers?* London: Wolfson Centre, Mecklenburgh Square.

Fuller, P., & Gray, C. (1992). Case study video of head injury project, ACE Centre. *Augmentative and Alternative Communication, 8,* 134.

Fuller, P., Newcombe, F., & Ounsted, C. (1983). Late language development in a child unable to recognize or produce speech sounds. *Archives of Neurology, 40,* 165–168.

Fuller, P., & Poon, P. (1990). Using microtechnology in the rehabilitation programs of children with head injury. *Augmentative and Alternative Communication, 6,* 106.

Fulwiler, R. L., & Fouts, R. S. (1976). Acquisition of American Sign Language by a noncommunicating autistic child. *Journal of Autism and Childhood Schizophrenia, 6,* 43–51.

Gaines, R., Leaper, C., Monahan, C., & Weickgenant, A. (1988). Language learning and retention in young language-disordered children. *Journal of Autism and Developmental Disorders, 18,* 281–296.

Galuska, S., Grove, T., Gray, J., & Founds, R. (1992). Design of visual communication devices for deaf persons. *Augmentative and Alternative Communication, 8,* 134.

Galyas, K. (1990). The multi-talk concept for efficient communication. *Augmentative and Alternative Communication, 6,* 95.

Galyas, K., Dahl, I., & Rosengren, E. (1988). Application of synthetic speech for communication, education, and training. *Augmentative and Alternative Communication, 4,* 139.

Galyas, K., Holmberg, S., & Sjöström, B. (1986). Experiences with the use of speech synthesizer in teaching nonvocal children reading and writing. *Augmentative and Alternative Communication, 2,* 87–88.

Galyas, K., & Hunnicutt, S. (1986). Recent developments with speech synthesis at the Royal Institute of Technology. *Augmentative and Alternative Communication, 2,* 88.

Galyas, K., Lundman, M., & Lagerman, U. (Eds.) (1982). *Kommunication for Gravt Talhandikappade* [Communication for Severely Speech Handicapped]. Bromma, Sweden: Handikappinstitutet.

Galyas, K., & Rosengren, E. (1988). An evaluation protocol for voice output communication aids (VOCAs). *Augmentative and Alternative Communication, 4,* 144.

Gandell, T. (1990). Telecommunication: Its effect on the reading skills of adults with multiple disabilities. *Augmentative and Alternative Communication, 6,* 133–134.

Gandell, T., & Head, H. (1990). Blissymbol telecommunications video: Report on a pilot project. *Augmentative and Alternative Communication*, 6, 117.

Gandell, T., & Sutton, A. (1990). Blissymbol telecommunications: Coding this new type of interaction. *Augmentative and Alternative Communication*, 6, 98.

Garcia, J. M., & Terrell, P. A. (1991). Communication competence: Including partner training in treatment of Broca's aphasia. Paper presented at the annual meeting of the American Speech-Language-Hearing Association, Atlanta.

Gardeazabal, L., Buldain, G., Gómez, E., & Arruabarrena, A. (1988). Commercial versus specific hardware to enhance communication for disabled people. *Augmentative and Alternative Communication*, 4, 152.

Gardner, H., Zurif, E. B., Berry, T., & Baker, E. (1976). Visual communication in aphasia. *Neuropsychologia*, 14, 275–292.

Gardner, R., & Gardner, B. (1969). Teaching sign language to a chimpanzee. *Science*, 165, 664–672.

Garrett, K. L., & Beukelman, D. R. (1992). Augmentative communication approaches for persons with severe aphasia. In K. Yorkston (Ed.), *Augmentative Communication in the Medical Setting*. Tucson, AZ: Communication Skill Builders, pp. 245–348.

Garrett, K. L., Beukelman, D. R., & Low, D. R. (1987). Case studies: Augmentative communication approaches for adult aphasics. Paper presented at the annual meeting of the American Speech-Language-Hearing Association, New Orleans.

Garrett, K. L., Beukelman, D. R., & Low-Morrow, D. R. (1989). A comprehensive augmentative communication system for an adult with Broca's aphasia. *Augmentative and Alternative Communication*, 5, 55–61.

Garrett, K. L., Schultz-Muehling, L., & Morrow, D. (1990). Low level head injury—A novel AAC approach. *Augmentative and Alternative Communication*, 6, 124.

Garrett, S. (1986). A case study in tactile Blissymbols. *Communicating Together*, 4(2), 16.

Garrison, J. H. (1982). Emergency signaling for a person with quadriplegia and extraordinary respiratory risk. *Archives of Physical Medicine and Rehabilitation*, 63, 180–181.

Gates, G. E. (1987). The acquisition of American Sign Language vs. Amerind signs by mentally retarded young adults. *Dissertation Abstracts International*, 48(6–B), 1800.

Gates, G. E., & Edwards, R. P. (1989). Acquisition of American Sign Language versus Amerind signs in a mentally retarded sample. *Journal of Communication Disorders*, 22(6), 423–435.

General reference source on aids for the severely handicapped (bibliography) (1974). In Keith Copeland (Ed.), *Aids for the Severely Handicapped*. New York: Grune & Stratton, pp. 141–144.

Gennaro, P. (1990). Teaching basic concepts of religion to nonspeaking children. *Augmentative and Alternative Communication*, 6, 147.

Gerber, S., & Kraat, A. (1992). Use of a developmental model of language acquisition: Applications to children using AAC systems. *Augmentative and Alternative Communication*, 8, 19–32.

Gertenrich, R. L. (August 1966). A simple mouth-held writing device for use with cerebral palsy patients. *Mental Retardation*, 4, 13–14.

Gethen, M. (1981). *Communicaid*. Cheltenham, Gloucestershire, England: M. Gethen, 173 Old Bath Road.

Getschow, C. O., Rosen, M. J., & Goodenough-Trepagnier, C. (1986). A systematic approach to design of a minimum distance alphabetical keyboard. *Proceedings of the Ninth Annual*

Conference on Rehabilitation Engineering. Washington, DC: Rehabilitation Engineering Society of North America, pp. 396–398.

Ghisler, W. (1990). Speeding up synthesized speech by using an optimized keyboard and abbreviations. *Augmentative and Alternative Communication*, 6, 89.

Gibbs, E. D., Sherman-Springer, A., & Cooley, W. C. (1990). Total communication for Down syndrome children: Patterns across six children. Paper presented at the annual meeting of the American Speech-Language-Hearing Association, Seattle.

Gibson, N., & McNaughton, S. (1990). The role of the teacher in augmentative education. *Augmentative and Alternative Communication*, 6, 100–101.

Gibson, N., Reid, B., & McCartney, N. (1990). Assessment in augmentative and alternative communication: Encompassing educational theory and practice. *Augmentative and Alternative Communication*, 6, 96.

Gibson, N., Reid, B., McCartney, N., & Watson,K. (1990). Easter Seal Communication Institute's educational service delivery model. *Augmentative and Alternative Communication*, 6, 142.

Gillette, Y. (1992). Communication contexts/strategies: Keys to using high tech interventions effectively. Paper presented at the annual meeting of the American Speech-Language-Hearing Association, San Antonio.

Girolametto, L. (1988). Improving the social-conversational skills of developmentally delayed children: An intervention study. *Journal of Speech and Hearing Disorders*, 53, 156–167.

Girolametto, L., Greenberg, J., & Manolson, A. (1986). Developing dialogue skills: The Hanen Early Language Parent Program. *Seminars in Speech and Language*, 7, 367–382.

Gitlis, K. R. (1975). Rationale and precedents for the use of simultaneous communication as an alternate system of communication for nonverbal children. Paper presented at the annual meeting of the American Speech-Language-Hearing Association, Washington, DC.

Glass, A. V., Gazzaniga, M. S., and Premack, D. (1973). Artificial language training in global aphasics. *Neuropsychologia*, 11, 95–103.

Glennen, S. L. (1992). Development of AAC skills in normal speakers and AAC users. *Augmentative and Alternative Communication*, 8, 134.

Glennen, S. L., & Calculator, S. N. (1985). Training functional communication board use: A pragmatic approach. *Augmentative and Alternative Communication*, 1(4), 134–142.

Glennen, S. L., Sharp, M. A., & Tullos, D. C. (1988). The effect of augmentative communication training on three communication modalities. Paper presented at the annual meeting of the American Speech-Language-Hearing Association, Boston.

Glennen, S. L., Sharp-Bittner, M. A., & Tullos, D. C. (1991). Augmentative and alternative communication training with a nonspeaking adult: Lessons from MH. *Augmentative and Alternative Communication*, 7, 240–247.

Glicksman, M. A., Duganne, III, J. A., & DeRuyter, F. (1990). Consumer, family, professional collaboration: Finding solutions together. *Augmentative and Alternative Communication*, 6, 130.

Glusker, P., Curtiss, S., Dronkers, N., Howard, F., Moilanen, N., Neville, H., Reisman, C. O., Ervin-Tripp, S., & Yancey, V. (1990). The Chelsea Project. *Augmentative and Alternative Communication*, 6, 97.

Goddard, C. (1977). Application of symbols with deaf children. *Blissymbol Communication Institute Newsletter, No. 3*. Toronto: Blissymbolics Communication Institute.

Goehl, H. (1986). An alternative to alternative communication. *Augmentative and Alternative Communication*, 2, 88.

Goehl, H. (1990). Is there really a role for speech in augmentative communication? *Augmentative and Alternative Communication*, 6, 123.

Goetz, L., Gee, K., & Sailor, W. (1983). Crossmodal transfer of stimulus control: Preparing students with severe multiple disabilities for audiological assessments. *Journal of the Association for Persons with Severe Handicaps*, 8, 3–13.

Goetz, L., Gee, K., & Sailor, W. (1985). Using a behavior train interruption strategy to teach communication skills to students with severe disabilities. *Journal of the Association for Persons with Severe Handicaps*, 10, 21–30.

Goldberg, H. R., & Fenton, J. (1960). *Aphonic Communication for those with Cerebral Palsy: Guide to the Development and Use of a Conversation Board*. New York: United Cerebral Palsy of New York State.

Goldenberg, E. P., Russell, S. J., & Carter, C. J. (1984). *Computers, Education and Special Needs*. Reading, MA: Addison-Wesley.

Goldojarb, M. F. (1976). The use of video confrontation in teaching AMERIND to aphasic adults. Videotape presented at the annual meeting of the American Speech-Language-Hearing Association, Houston.

Goldstein, H., & Cameron, H. (1952). A new method of communication for the aphasic patient. *Arizona Medicine*, 8, 17–21.

Golin, A., & Ducanis, A. (1981). *The Interdisciplinary Team*. Rockville, MD: Aspen Systems.

González-Abasacal, J., Gómez, E., Buldain, G., & Gardeazabal, L. (1990). A software tool to evaluate methods of enhancing communication speed. *Augmentative and Alternative Communication*, 6, 94.

Goodenough-Trepagnier, C. (1978). Language development of children without articulate speech. In R. Campbell & P. Smith (Eds.), *Recent Advances in the Psychology of Language: Part A, Language and Mother-Child Interaction*. New York: Plenum Press, pp. 421–426.

Goodenough-Trepagnier, C., Askey, D., & Koeppel, B. (1992). ACTOR, A "virtual environment" for communication in aphasia: Preliminary results. *Augmentative and Alternative Communication*, 8, 134–135.

Goodenough-Trepagnier, C., & Deser, T. (1980). Rate of output with a SPEEC non-vocal communication board. Paper presented at the International Conference on Rehabilitation Engineering, Toronto.

Goodenough-Trepagnier, C., Hochheiser, H., & Rosen, M. J. (1992). Tools for predictive assessment of speech recognition accuracy. *Augmentative and Alternative Communication*, 8, 135.

Goodenough-Trepagnier, C., & Prather, P. (1981). Communication systems for the nonvocal based on frequent phoneme sequences. *Journal of Speech and Hearing Research*, 24, 322–329.

Goodenough-Trepagnier, C., & Prather, P. (1982). *Manual for Teachers of SPEEC*. Boston: Biomedical Engineering Center, Tufts-New England Medical Center.

Goodenough-Trepagnier, C., & Rosen, M. J. (1888). Predictive assessment for communication aid prescription: Motor-determined maximum communication rate. In L. Bernstein (Ed.), *The Vocally Impaired: Clinical Practice and Research*. Needham Heights, MA: Allyn & Bacon.

Goodenough-Trepagnier, C., Tarry, E., & Prather, P. (1982). Derivation of an efficient nonvocal communication system. *Human Factors,* 24, 163–172.

Goodman, J., & Remington, B. (1993). Acquisition of expressive signing: Comparison of reinforcement strategies. *Augmentative and Alternative Communication,* 9, 26–35.

Goodman, L., Wilson, P. S., & Bornstein, H. (1978). Results of a national survey of sign language programs in special education. *Mental Retardation,* 16(2), 104–106.

Goodwin, M., & Goodwin, T. C. (1969). In a dark mirror. *Mental Hygiene,* 53, 550–563.

Goold, L. (1992). Individualized gestures: Personalized manual signs for individuals with severe impairments. *Augmentative and Alternative Communication,* 8, 135.

Goold, L., Mendelson, V., Borbilas, P., & Yates, J. (1992). Communication for individuals with severe impairments: The story "down under." *Augmentative and Alternative Communication,* 8, 135.

Goolsby, E., & Porter, P. (1984). Augmentative communication: The team approach. *North Carolina Augmentative Communication Association Newsletter.* 2(2), 3–4.

Goossens', C. A. (1983). The relative iconicity and learnability of verb referents represented in Blissymbolics, rebus symbols, and manual signs: An investigation with moderately retarded individuals. Unpublished doctoral dissertation, Purdue University.

Goossens', C. A. (1989). Aided communication intervention before assessment: A case study of a child with cerebral palsy. *Augmentative and Alternative Communication,* 5, 14–26.

Goossens', C., & Crain, S. (1985). *Eye-gaze Communication Systems: Assessment and Intervention.* Birmingham, AL: Authors, Sparks Center for Developmental and Learning Disorders, 1720 Seventh Avenue South.

Goossens'. C., & Crain, S. (Eds.) (1986a). *Augmentative Communication Assessment Resource.* Wauconda, IL: Don Johnson Developmental Equipment.

Goossens', C., & Crain, S. (Eds.) (1986b). *Augmentative Communication Intervention Resource.* Wauconda, IL: Don Johnson Developmental Equipment.

Goossens', C., & Crain, S. (1986c). Establishing multiple communication displays. In Sarah W. Blackstone (Ed.), *Augmentative Communication: An Introduction.* Rockville, MD: American Speech-Language-Hearing Association, pp. 337–343.

Goossens', C. A., & Crain, S. S. (1987a). Guidelines for customizing Minspeak based communication in a time and cost efficient manner. *Minspeak Conference Proceedings,* New Orleans.

Goossens', C. A., & Crain, S. S. (1987b). Overview of nonelectronic eye-gaze communication techniques. *Augmentative and Alternative Communication,* 3, 77–89.

Goossens', C. A., & Crain, S. S. (1992). *Utilizing Switch Interfaces with Children Who Are Severely Physically Challenged.* Austin, TX: Pro-Ed.

Goossens', C. A., Crain, S. S., Bergman, J., & Barnacastle, N. (1986). Customizing formats for hand activated switches. *Augmentative and Alternative Communication,* 2, 88–89.

Goossens', C. A., Elder, P. S., & Bray, N. W. (1990). Validity of the semantic compaction competency profile in normally developing preschool children. Paper presented at the Fifth Annual Minspeak Conference.

Goossens', C. A., Elder, P. S., Caldwell, M. A., & Page, J. L. (1988). Long range planning: A continuum of semantic compaction overlays. *Proceedings of the Third Annual Minspeak Conference,* Anaheim, CA, pp. 1–24.

Goossens', C. A., Elder, P. S., & Crain, S. (1988). Engineering the preschool classroom environment for interactive symbolic communication. *Augmentative and Alternative Communication,* 4, 166.

Goossens', C. A., Heine, K., Crain, S., & Burke, C. (1987). *Modifying Piagetian Tasks for Use with Physically-Challenged Individuals.* Birmingham, AL: Sparks Center for Developmental and Learning Disorders, University of Alabama.

Goossens', C. A., & Kraat, A. (1985). Technology as a tool for conversation and language learning for the physically handicapped. *Topics in Language Disorders*, 6, 56–70.

Gordan, W. L., Johnson, C. B., & Montague, J. L. (1979). Speech pathologist's role in the treatment of ventilator-dependent quadriplegic patients. Paper presented at the annual meeting of the American Speech-Language-Hearing Association, Atlanta.

Gordon, C. E., Lafontaine, L. M., DeRuyter, F., & Lehman, M. (1985). Swing-away picture communication board. Paper presented at the annual meeting of the American Speech-Language-Hearing Association, Washington, DC.

Gordon, J. (1975). Symbol communication system. B.S. thesis, University of Manitoba, Winnipeg.

Gordon, K. C., & Hyta, M. B. (1977). Assessment of nonverbal gestures in language-disabled children. Paper presented at the annual meeting of the American Speech-Language-Hearing Association, Chicago.

Gorenflo, C. W., Eulenberg, J. B., & Casby, M. W. (1987). Effects of augmentative communication technique on attitudes toward non-speaking individuals. Paper presented at the annual meeting of the American Speech-Language-Hearing Association, New Orleans.

Gorenflo, C. W., & Gorenflo, D. W. (1991). The effects of information and augmentative communication technique on attitudes toward nonspeaking individuals. *Journal of Speech and Hearing Research*, 34, 19–26.

Gorenflo, C. W., Gorenflo, D. W., & Santer, S. A. (1994). Effects of synthetic voice output on attitudes toward the augmented communicator. *Journal of Speech and Hearing Research*, 37, 64–68.

Grabowski, K., & Shane, H. (1986). *Communication Profile for Severe Expressive Impairment.* Boston: Communication Enhancement Clinic, Children's Hospital.

Graff, L. L., & Wotus, M. (1985). A categorical training protocol for the ACS Speech PAC. Paper presented at the annual meeting of the American Speech-Language-Hearing Association, Washington, DC.

Graham, L. W. (1976). Language programming and intervention. In Lyle L. Lloyd (Ed.), *Communication Assessment and Intervention Strategies.* Baltimore: University Park Press, pp. 371–422.

Grandin, T. (1989). An autistic person's view of holding therapy. *Communication*, 23, 75–78.

Granlund, M., & Olsson, C. (1987). *Talspraksalternativ Kommunikation och Begavningshandikapp* [Alternative Communication and Mental Retardation]. Stockholm, Sweden: Stiftelsen ALA.

Granlund, M., & Olsson, C. (1988). *Kommunicera Mera* [Communicate More]. Stockholm, Sweden: Stiftelsen ALA.

Granlund, M., Strom, E., and Olsson, C. (1989). Iconicity and productive recall of a selected sample of signs from signed Swedish. *Augmentative and Alternative Communication*, 5, 173–182.

Granlund, M., & Terneby, J. (1990). Creating communicative opportunities through inservice training of direct care staff. *Augmentative and Alternative Communication*, 6, 103.

Grattan, K. T., & Palmer, A. W. (1984). Interrupted reflection fibre optic communication device for the severely disabled. *Journal of Biomedical Engineering*, 6(4), 321–322.

Grattan, K. T., Palmer, A. W., & Mason, M. (1987). Communication by eye-closure. II—New hardware for optical switching. *IEEE Transactions on Biomedical Engineering*, 34(3), 255–257.

Grecco, R. (1972). *Manual Language Program*. Available from the Mansfield Training School, Mansfield Depot, CT.

Green, C. N. (1977). A signal system of communication. *Hearing and Speech Action*, 45(4), 22–23.

Green, L. C. (1975). Acquisition of words versus signs in receptive language therapy with severely retarded, institutionalized children. Paper presented at the annual meeting of the American Speech-Language-Hearing Association, Washington, DC.

Green, S. M., Newhoff, M., & Raney, S. (1985). Revision strategies via communication boards. Paper presented at the annual meeting of the American Speech-Language-Hearing Association, Washington, DC.

Green, S. M., & Scherer, N. J. (1985). Pragmatic intervention in augmentative communication: A case study. Paper presented at the annual meeting of the American Speech-Language-Hearing Association, Washington, DC.

Gregory, C. (1992). Toward realistic AAC objectives: Comment on Calculator and Jorgensen (September 1991). *Augmentative and Alternative Communication*, 8, 71–75.

Griffin, H. C., & Gerber, P. J. (1980). Non-verbal communication alternatives for handicapped individuals. *Journal of Rehabilitation*, 46(4), 36–39.

Griffith, P. L., & Robinson, J. H. (1980). Influence of iconicity and phonological similiarity on sign learning by mentally retarded children. *American Journal of Mental Deficiency*, 85(3), 291–298.

Grimmel, M., DeLamore, K., & Lippke, B. (Spring 1976). Sign it successfully—Manual English encourages successful communication. *Teaching Exceptional Children*, 123–124.

Grove, N. (1990). Developing intelligible signs with learning-disabled students: A review of the literature and an assessment procedure. *British Journal of Disorders of Communication*, 25(3), 265–293.

Grove, N., & McDougall, S. (1990). First steps in the evaluation of signing environments. *Augmentative and Alternative Communication*, 6, 109.

Grove, N., & McDougall, S. (1991). Exploring sign use in two settings. *British Journal of Special Education*, 18(4), 149–156.

Grove, N., & Walker, M. (1990). The Makaton vocabulary: Using manual signs and graphic symbols to develop interpersonal communication. *Augmentative and Alternative Communication*, 6, 15–28.

Guenet, L. (1986). P.D.C.O. Projectiur à Diapositives Contrôlé par Ordinateur: Incorporation of the slide projector as part of your computer hardware. *Augmentative and Alternative Communication*, 2, 89.

Guess, D., Sailor, W., & Baer, D. (1974–1978). *Functional Speech and Language Training for the Severely Handicapped*. Austin, TX: Pro-Ed. [An intervention program composed of four books.]

Guess, D., Sailor, W., & Baer, D. (1977). A behavioral-remedial approach to language training for the severely handicapped. In S. Sontag & N. Certo (Eds.), *Educational Programming for the Severely and Profoundly Handicapped*. Reston, VA: Division on Mental Retardation, Council for Exceptional Children, pp. 307–308.

Guess, D., Sailor, W., & Baer, D. (1978). Children with limited language. In R. Schiefelbusch (Ed.), *Language Intervention Strategies*. Baltimore: University Park Press.

Guilford, A. M., Scheuerle, J., & Shirek, P. G. (1982). Manual communication skills in aphasia. *Archives of Physical Medicine and Rehabilitation*, 63, 601–604.

Gutmann, M. L. (1990). Mobile adult augmentative communication services: Innovative service delivery in Ontario. Paper presented at the annual meeting of the American Speech-Language-Hearing Association, Seattle.

Guttman, K. (1990). A follow-up study of nonspeaking pupils who communicate with Blissymbols. *Augmentative and Alternative Communication*, 6, 108.

Hadjian, S. (1990). A statewide enabling technology collaborative consultation delivery system: Follow-up study. Paper presented at the annual meeting of the American Speech-Language-Hearing Association, Seattle.

Hadjian, S., Heiner, D., & Mefford, G. I. (1989). Augmentative-alternative communication: A state-wide collaborative consultation delivery system. Paper presented at the annual meeting of the American Speech-Language-Hearing Association, St. Louis.

Hagen, C., Porter, W., & Brink, J. (1973). Nonverbal communication: An alternative mode of communication for the child with severe cerebral palsy. *Journal of Speech and Hearing Disorders*, 38, 448–455.

Haight, C. (1975). Modification of signs to maximize the learning of concepts. In M. P. Creedon (Ed.), *Appropriate Behavior Through Communication: A New Program in Simultaneous Language*. Chicago: Dysfunctioning Child Center, pp. 74–84.

Haight, P. L. (1992). Comparison of communication interactions: Communication board versus electronic communication system. *Augmentative and Alternative Communication*, 8, 135–136.

Haight, P. L., & Mentch, M. W. (1990). AAC services in Ohio: The public/private initiative. Paper presented at the annual meeting of the American Speech-Language-Hearing Association, Seattle.

Haight, P. L., Nisenboum, J., White, L. C., & Dobres, R. (1992). Comparing encoding system learning by adults with acquired neurological impairment. *Augmentative and Alternative Communication*, 8, 136.

Haines, K. B., & Cartwright, L. R. (1992). Augmentative and alternative communication in West Virginia public schools. Paper presented at the annual meeting of the American Speech-Language-Hearing Association, San Antonio.

Hall, S. M., & Talkington, L. W. (1970). Evaluation of a manual approach to programming for deaf retarded. *American Journal of Mental Deficiency*, 75, 378–380.

Halle, J. W. (1982). Teaching functional language to the handicapped: An integrative model of natural environment teaching techniques. *Journal of the Association for Persons with Severe Handicaps*, 7, 27–37.

Halle, J. W., Alpert, C., & Anderson, S. (1984). Natural environment language assessment and intervention with severely impaired preschoolers. *Topics in Early Childhood Special Education*, 4(2), 35–56.

Halle, J. W., Baer, D., & Spradlin, J. (1981). Teachers' generalized use of delay as a stimulus control procedure to increase language use by handicapped children. *Journal of Applied Behavior Analysis*, 14, 389–409.

Halle, J. M., Marshall, A., & Spradlin, J. (1979). Time delay: A technique to increase language use and facilitate generalization in retarded children. *Journal of Applied Behavior Analysis*, 12, 431–439.

Hammond, J., & Bailey, P. (1976). An experiment with Blissymbolics. *Special Education Forward Trends*, 3(3), 21–22.

Hammons, J., Yager, B. E., & Swindell, C. S. (1989). Minspeak in the treatment of severe Broca's aphasia. Paper presented at the annual meeting of the American Speech-Language-Hearing Association, St. Louis.

Hamre-Nietupski, S., Fullerton, P., Holtz, K., Ryan-Flottum, M., Stoll, A., & Brown, L. (1977). Curricular strategies for teaching selected nonverbal communication skills to nonverbal and verbal severely handicapped students. In L. Brown, J. Nietupski, S. Lyon, S. Hamre-Nietupski, T. Crowner, & L. Gruenewald (Eds.), *Curriculum Strategies for Teaching Nonverbal Communication, Functional Object Use, Problem Solving, and Mealtime Skills to Severely Handicapped Students (Volume III, Part I)*. Madison: University of Wisconsin-Madison and Madison Metropolitan School District.

Hanagan, K. (1992). Let's keep real AAC users in studies about AAC users: Comments on Doss et al. (1991). *Augmentative and Alternative Communication, 8*, 251.

Handicapped youth "talks" with eyes (October 22, 1974). *News Journal* (Mansfield, OH).

Haney, C. A. (1986). 70 augmentative communication system users: Patterns of usage and implications. *Augmentative and Alternative Communication, 2*, 89–90.

Haney, C. A. (1988a). 400 systems later: Outcomes of the Pennsylvania Project. *Augmentative and Alternative Communication, 4*, 170.

Haney, C. A. (1988b). Maintaining short- and long-term loan programs for assistive devices. *Augmentative and Alternative Communication, 4*, 138.

Haney, C. A. (1990a). 100 local augmentative specialists respond to statewide survey. *Augmentative and Alternative Communication, 6*, 120.

Haney, C. A. (1990b). 600 systems later: Augmentative and alternative communication in Pennsylvania. *Augmentative and Alternative Communication, 6*, 120.

Haney, C. A. (1990c). The Augmentative Communication Profile revised: Results of the past six years. *Augmentative and Alternative Communication, 6*, 142–143.

Haney, C. A. (1990d). Implementing technology in the classroom. *Augmentative and Alternative Communication, 6*, 112.

Haney, C. A. (1990e). Parents/students/teachers and therapists learning from each other: Pennsylvania's model. *Augmentative and Alternative Communication, 6*, 87.

Haney, C. A. (November 1992). The place for assistive technology. *Asha, 34*, 47–48.

Haney, C. A., & Quinlisk-Gill, S. (1988). Monitoring change through the augmentative communication profile. *Augmentative and Alternative Communication, 4*, 167.

Hanrahan, L., & Odykirk, B. (1992). A handshape strategy for teaching children with apraxia to speak. *Augmentative and Alternative Communication, 8*, 136.

Hanrahan, L. L., & Chin, J. (1986). A reversal design study of the effect of verbal prompting on nonverbal communication. *Augmentative and Alternative Communication, 2*, 90.

Hanrahan, L. L., & Finn, W. (1990). From switch activation to communication: What's in between? *Augmentative and Alternative Communication, 6*, 147.

Hanrahan, L. L., Jolie, K. R., & Fishman, S. (1989). A categorical analysis of augmentative technology needs for school aged children. Paper presented at the annual meeting of the American Speech-Language-Hearing Association, St. Louis.

Hanson, W. R. (1976). Measuring gestural communication in a brain- injured adult. Videotape presented at the annual meeting of the American Speech-Language-Hearing Association, Houston.

Harding, P. J. R., Kingman, V. J., Kozak, A. J., Storemore, K. A., & Vaneldik, J. F. (1973). Typewriter for teaching severely handicapped children. Paper presented at the Carnahan Conference on Electronic Prosthetics, Lexington, KY. (Paper is published in the conference proceedings volume, pp. 43–46.)

Haring, T., Neetz, J., Lovinger, L., Peck, C., & Semmel, M. (1987). Effects of four modified incidental teaching procedures to create opportunities for communication. *Journal of the Association for Persons with Severe Handicaps*, 12, 218–226.

Harlan, C. L. (1988). Customized computer augmentative communication via HyperCard. Paper presented at the annual meeting of the American Speech-Language-Hearing Association, Boston.

Harlan, N. T., Blackstone, S. W., Cassatt-James, E. L., Trefler, E., & Flexer, C. (1992). Technology in classroom: A self-instructional program. *Augmentative and Alternative Communication*, 8, 136–137.

Harmon, G. M. (March 31, 1974). He'll huff and puff, turn his TV set on, thanks to space device. *Times-Picayune* (New Orleans).

Harmuth, P. (1990). Outreach: Developing educational curriculum for students with multiple severe disabilities. *Augmentative and Alternative Communication*, 6, 127.

Harmuth, P., Batstone, S., & Batstone, D. (1990). Yes? No? Maybe so. *Augmentative and Alternative Communication*, 6, 140.

Harrington, K. (1988). A letter from Annie. *Communicating Together*, 6(4), 5–7.

Harrington, K., & Harrington, R. (1986). Kari: Communicating, creating, and learning. *Augmentative and Alternative Communication*, 2, 90.

Harris, D. (1978). Descriptive analysis of communication interaction processes involving nonvocal severely handicapped children. Unpublished doctoral dissertation, University of Wisconsin, Madison.

Harris, D. (1982). Communicative interaction processes involving nonvocal physically handicapped children. *Topics in Language Disorders*, 2, 21–37.

Harris, D., & Vanderheiden, G. C. (1980). Enhancing the development of communicative interaction. In R. L. Schiefelbusch (Ed.), *Nonspeech Language and Communication: Analysis and Intervention*. Baltimore: University Park Press, pp. 227–257.

Harris, G., Batstone, S., & Harmuth, P. (1990). Oh say, can you see? *Augmentative and Alternative Communication*, 6, 96.

Harris, O. L. (1992). The social context of literacy development with an augmentative communicator. Paper presented at the annual meeting of the American Speech-Language-Hearing Association, San Antonio.

Harris, S. (1976). Teaching language to nonverbal children—With emphasis on problems of generalization. *Psychological Bulletin*, 82, 565–585.

Harris-Vanderheiden, D. (1975). *A Survey of Critical Factors in Evaluating Communication Aids*. Madison: Trace Research and Development Center for the Severely Communicatively Handicapped. University of Wisconsin.

Harris-Vanderheiden, D. (1976a). Blissymbols and the mentally retarded. In Gregg C. Vanderheiden & Kate Grilley (Eds.), *Non-vocal Communication Techniques and Aids for the Severely Physically Handicapped*. Baltimore: University Park Press, pp. 120–131.

Harris-Vanderheiden, D. (1976b). Field evaluation of the Auto-Com. In Gregg C. Vanderheiden & Kate Grilley (Eds.), *Non-vocal Communication Techniques and Aids for the Severely Physically Handicapped*. Baltimore: University Park Press, pp. 144–151.

Harris-Vanderheiden, D., & DePape, D. J. (1977). *Review of Common Symbol Systems for Use with Communication Aids: Preliminary Notes*. Madison: Trace Research and Development Center for the Severely Communicatively Handicapped, University of Wisconsin.

Harris-Vanderheiden, D., Lippert, J. C., Yoder, D. E., & Vanderheiden, G. C (1978). Bliss Symbols: An augmentative symbol/communication system for non-vocal severely handicapped children. In R. York and E. Edgar (Eds.), *Teaching the Severely Handicapped*.

Vol. 4. Seattle: American Association for the Education of the Severely Physically Handicapped.

Harris-Vanderheiden, D., McNaughton, S., & McDonald, E. T. (1976). Some remarks on assessment. In Gregg C. Vanderheiden & Kate Grilley (Eds.), *Non-vocal Communication Techniques and Aids for the Severely Physically Handicapped*. Baltimore: University Park Press, pp. 152–158.

Harris-Vanderheiden, D., Speilman, M., Valley, V., & Geisler, C. (1973). *A Preliminary Evaluation of the Auto-Com as an Aid to the Education and Communication of the Non-vocal Physically Handicapped Child*. Madison: Trace Research and Development Center for the Severely Communicatively Handicapped, University of Wisconsin.

Harris-Vanderheiden, D., & Vanderheiden, G. C. (1980). Augmentative communication techniques. In R. L. Schiefelbusch (Ed.), *Nonspeech Language and Communication: Analysis and Intervention*. Baltimore: University Park Press, pp. 259–301.

Harris-Vanderheiden, D., & Vanderheiden, G. C. (1977). Basic considerations in the development of communicative and interactive skills for non-vocal severely handicapped children. In S. Sontag & N. Certo (Eds.), *Educational Programming for the Severely and Profoundly Handicapped*. Reston, VA: Division on Mental Retardation, Council for Exceptional Children.

Harris-Vanderheiden, D., & Vanderheiden, G. C. (1980). Enhancing the development of communicative interaction in non-vocal severely physically handicapped children. In R. Schiefelbusch (Ed.), *Non-speech Language Intervention Processes*. Baltimore: University Park Press, pp. 227–257.

Harrison, Jr., E., and Vise, Jr., G. T. (1984). Simple devices for the physically disabled. *Paraplegia*, 22(3), 182–193.

Hart, B. (1985). Naturalistic language training techniques. In S. Warren & A. Rogers-Warren (Eds.), *Teaching Functional Language*, Austin, TX: Pro-Ed, pp. 63–88.

Hart, B., & Risley, T. (1982). *How to Use Incidental Teaching for Elaborating Language*. Austin, TX: Pro-Ed.

Hartley, N. (1974). Symbols for diplomats used for children. *Special Education Canada*, 48(2), 5–7.

Hartsell, K., & Romski, M. A. (1992). Implementing a statewide AAC technical assistance program: The Georgia model. *Augmentative and Alternative Communication*, 8, 137.

Harvie, L. (1992). Watch your tone of voice. *Augmentative and Alternative Communication*, 8, 137.

Harwin, W. S., & Jackson, R. D. (1986). Computer recognition of head gestures. *Augmentative and Alternative Communication*, 2, 90.

Harwin, W. S., & Jackson, R. D. (1990). Analysis of intentional head gestures to assist computer access by physically disabled people. *Journal of Biomedical Engineering*, 12(3), 193–198.

Hayes, H. T. P. (June 12, 1977). The pursuit of reason. *The New York Times Magazine*.

Haynes, C. W., & Quist, R. W. (1992). Computer-assisted teaching versus "live" presentation for Blissymbol learning. *Augmentative and Alternative Communication*, 8, 137.

He puffs past his handicap (March 21, 1974). *The News and Observer* (Raleigh, NC).

Head, H. (1926). *Aphasia and Kindred Disorders of Speech*. 2 vols. New York: Macmillan.

Heaton, E. M. (1986). Technology—The normalization dilemma. *Augmentative and Alternative Communication*, 2, 91.

Heckathorne, C. W., Leibowitz, L., & Strysik, J. (1983). Microdec II—Anticipatory computer input aid. *Proceedings of the Sixth Annual Conference on Rehabilitation Engineering.* Rehabilitation Engineering Society of North America.

Heckathorne, C. W., Voda, J. A., & Leibowitz, L. J. (1987). Design rationale and evalution of the Portable Anticipatory Communication Aid—PACA. *Augmentative and Alternative Communication*, 3(4), 170–180.

Hedbring, C. (1985). Computers and autistic learners: An evolving technology. *Australian Journal of Human Communication Disorders*, 13, 169–194.

Hedrick, D., Prather, E., & Tobin, A. (1984). *Sequenced Inventory of Communication Development.* rev. ed. Seattle: University of Washington Press.

Hehner, B. (1980). *Blissymbols for Use.* Toronto: Blissymbolics Communication Institute.

Heim, M. (1990). Communication skills of nonspeaking children with cerebral palsy: A study on interaction. *Augmentative and Alternative Communication*, 6, 92.

Heim, M. J. M., & Mills, A. E. (1992). Effects of partner instruction on the communication development of nonspeaking toddlers with cerebral palsy. *Augmentative and Alternative Communication*, 8, 138.

Helfrich, K. R. (1976). Total communication with an oral apractic child. Videotape presented at the annual meeting of the American Speech-Language-Hearing Association, Houston.

Helm-Estabrooks, N., & Walsh, M. J. (1982). The response of aphasic patients to an electronic communication system. Paper presented at the annual meeting of the American Speech-Language-Hearing Association, Toronto.

Help for patients with language and visual problems (1974). *Physical Therapy*, 54, 69.

Henderson, J. (1992). Get ready for ABC'S with AAC—A preschool AAC checklist. *Augmentative and Alternative Communication*, 8, 138.

Henderson, J., & Barker, M. R. (1988). Multidisciplinary team evaluation and implementation strategies for augmentative and alternative communication systems. *Augmentative and Alternative Communication*, 4, 164.

Henderson, J., & Deegan, M. (1988). The Augmentative Communication Panel: A local inter-agency resource. *Augmentative and Alternative Communication*, 4, 173.

Henkle, J. E. (1977). A micro-processor-based gesture entry non-vocal communication system. Paper presented at the Fourth Annual Conference on Systems and Devices for the Disabled, Seattle. (Paper is published in conference proceedings volume, distributed by Continuing Medical Education, University of Washington School of Medicine.)

Hershberger, D., & Patterson, J. (1992). How to get clinical knowledge implemented into assistive devices. *Augmentative and Alternative Communication*, 8, 138.

Hickey, M., Page, C., & Falkner, T. (1992). Using text retrieval techniques in an AAC system. *Augmentative and Alternative Communication*, 8, 138-139.

Higginbotham, D. J. (1986). Message formulation using augmentative communication systems: A study of social communication and interaction. *Augmentative and Alternative Communication*, 2, 91.

Higginbotham, D. J. (1989). The interplay of communication device output mode and interaction style between nonspeaking persons and their speaking partners. *Journal of Speech and Hearing Disorders*, 54, 320–333.

Higginbotham, D. J. (1990a). An assessment of keystroke efficiency for five augmentative communication technologies. Paper presented at the annual meeting of the American Speech-Language-Hearing Association, Seattle.

Higginbotham, D. J. (1990b). The evaluation of keystroke efficiency for five augmentative and alternative communication technologies. *Augmentative and Alternative Communication*, 6, 94.

Higginbotham, D. J. (1992). Evaluation of keystroke savings across five assistive communication technologies. *Augmentative and Alternative Communication*, 8, 258–272.

Higginbotham, D. J., Mathy-Laikko, P., & Yoder, D. (1988). Studying conversations of augmentative communication system users. In L. E. Bernstein (Ed.), *The Vocally Impaired: Clinical Practice and Research*. Philadelphia: Grune & Stratton, pp. 265–294.

Higginbotham, D. J., & Yoder, D. (1982). Communication within natural conversational interaction: Implications for severe communicatively impaired persons. *Topics in Language Disorders*, 2, 1–19.

Higgins, J., & Mills, J. (1986). Communication training in real environments. In Sarah W. Blackstone (Ed.), *Augmentative Communication: An Introduction*. Rockville, MD: American Speech-Language-Hearing Association, pp. 345–351.

Higgins, J., Romich, B., & Baker, B. (1988). A preservice/continuing education unit on vocabulary selection and organization. *Augmentative and Alternative Communication*, 4, 145.

Hildén, A. (1990). Using the computer with severely and profoundly retarded, disabled children. *Augmentative and Alternative Communication*, 6, 140.

Hill, S. D., Campagna, J., Long, D., Munch, J., & Naecher, S. (1968). An explanation of the use of a two-response keyboard as a means of communication for the severely handicapped child. *Perceptual and Motor Skills*, 26, 699–704.

Hilling, S. (1990). 15 month development in half a year. *Augmentative and Alternative Communication*, 6, 146.

Hind, M. (1988). Using a computer to help teach correct sequencing of Blissymbols. *Augmentative and Alternative Communication*, 4, 152.

Hind, M. (1989). Synrel: Programs to teach sequencing of Blissymbols. *Communication Outlook*, 10, 6–9.

Hind, M. (1990). Motivation to use switches. *Augmentative and Alternative Communication*, 6, 135.

Hinderscheit, L. R., & Reichle, J. (1987). Teaching direct selection color encoding to an adolescent with multiple handicaps. *Augmentative and Alternative Communication*, 3(3), 137–142.

Hinerman, P. S., Jenson, W. R., Walker, G. R., & Peterson, P. B. (1982). Positive practice overcorrection combined with traditional procedures to teach signed words to an autistic child. *Journal of Autism and Developmental Disorders*, 12(3), 253–263.

Hjelmquist, E., Benedetto, A. D., & Hedelin, L. (1990). Conceptions of linguistic and alternative communication among communicatively handicapped children. *Augmentative and Alternative Communication*, 6, 133.

Hoag, L. A., & Bedrosian, J. L. (1992). Effects of speech output type, message length, and reauditorization on perceptions of the communicative competence of an adult AAC user. *Journal of Speech and Hearing Research*, 35, 1363–1366.

Hoag, L. A., Bedrosian, J. L., & Calculator, S. N. (1990). Variables influencing listeners' judgments of communicative competence. *Augmentative and Alternative Communication*, 6, 135–136.

Hoag, L. A., Bedrosian, J. L., Molineux, B. R., & Calculator, S. N. (1992). Variables affecting perceptions of social competence in AAC users. *Augmentative and Alternative Communication*, 8, 139.

Hobson, P. A., & Duncan, P. (1979). Sign learning and profoundly retarded people. *Mental Retardation*, 17(1), 33–37.

Hodges, P. M., & Deich, R. F. (1978). Teaching an artificial language system to nonverbal retardates. *Behavior Modification*, 2, 489–509.

Hodges, P. M., & Schwethelm, B. (1984). A comparison of the effectiveness of graphic symbol and manual sign training with profoundly retarded children. *Applied Psycholinguistics*, 5, 223–253.

Hodgetts, M., Beard, J., & Hobson, D. (1980). Electronic device control using retroflective concept. *Proceedings of the International Conference on Rehabilitation Engineering*. Toronto: Rehabilitation Engineering Society of North America, pp. 242–243.

Hofman, A. C. (1988). *The Many Faces of Funding*. (Available from Phonic Ear, 3380 Cypress Drive, Petaluma, CA 94954.)

Hoffmeister, R. J., & Farmer, A. (1972). The development of manual sign language in mentally retarded deaf individuals. *Journal of Rehabilitation of the Deaf*, 6, 19–26.

Hoit-Dalgaard, J., Newhoff, M., & Barnes, G. J. (1981). Enhancing verbal interaction through pantomime: A gestural protocol for aphasia. *Texas Journal of Audiology and Speech Pathology*, 6(1), 4–7.

Holbrook, A., & Hardiman, C. J. (1977). Nonverbal communication systems for the severely handicapped. Paper presented at the annual meeting of the American Speech-Language-Hearing Association, Chicago.

Hollander, F. M., & Juhrs, P. D. (1974). Orff-Schulwerk, an effective treatment tool for autistic children. *Journal of Music Therapy*, 11, 1–12.

Hollis, J. H., & Carrier, Jr., J. K. (1975). Research implications for communication deficiencies. *Exceptional Children*, 41, 405–412.

Hollis, J. H., Carrier, Jr., J. K., & Spradlin, J. E. (1976). An approach to remediation of communication and learning deficiencies. In Lyle L. Lloyd (Ed.), *Communication Assessment and Intervention Strategies*. Baltimore: University Park Press, pp. 265–294.

Holmlund, B., & Kavanagh, R. (1976). Communication aids for the handicapped. *American Journal of Occupational Therapy*, 21, 357–361.

Holmquist, E. (1984). I am my own person. *Conversations with Non-speaking People*. Toronto: Canadian Rehabilitation Council for the Disabled.

Holst, A., & Holmberg, S. (1990). Developing pictogram materials for persons with moderate and severe mental retardation. *Augmentative and Alternative Communication*, 6, 108.

Holt, C., Buelow, D., & Vanderheiden, G. (1976). *Interface Switch Profile and Annotated List of Commercial Switches*. Madison: Trace Research and Development Center for the Severely Communicatively Handicapped, University of Wisconsin.

Holt, C., Raitzer, G. A., Harris-Vanderheiden, D., & Vanderheiden, G. (1976). *Formative Evaluation/Design of a Low Cost Scanning Aid*. Madison: Trace Research and Development Center for the Severely Communicatively Handicapped, University of Wisconsin.

Holt, C., & Vanderheiden, G. (1974). *Master Chart of Communication Aids*. Madison: Trace Research and Development Center for the Severely Communicatively Handicapped, University of Wisconsin.

Holton, R. A. (1990). Eye gaze communication systems: Unlocking "locked-in syndrome." Paper presented at the annual meeting of the American Speech-Language-Hearing Association, Seattle.

Homan, R. W., Criswell, E., Wada, J. A., & Ross, E. D. (1982). Hemispheric contributions to manual communication (signing and finger-spelling). *Neurology*, 32, 1020–1023.

Honsinger, M. J. (1989). Midcourse intervention in multiple sclerosis: An inpatient model. *Augmentative and Alternative Communication*, 5, 71–73.

Honsinger, M. J., Yorkston, K., & Dowden, P. (May–June 1987). Communication options for intubated patients. *Respiratory Management*, 45–52.

Hooper, C. R., Maklouf, M., Wayda, E., and Holden, M. (1991). Dental communication symbols in special care clinics. Paper presented at the annual meeting of the American Speech-Language-Hearing Association, Atlanta.

Hooper, H., & Bowler, D. M. (1991). Peer-tutoring of manual signs by adults with mental handicaps. *Mental Handicap Research*, 4(2), 207–215.

Hooper, J., Connell, T. M., & Flett, P. J. (1987). Blissymbols and manual signs: A multimodality approach to intervention in a case of multiple disability. *Augmentative and Alternative Communication*, 3(2), 68–76.

Hoover, J., Reichle, J., Van Tassell, D., & Cole, D. (1987). The intelligbility of synthesized speech: Echo II versus Votrax. *Journal of Speech and Hearing Research*, 30, 425–431.

Hopkins, J., & Woolfe, L. (1986). Critical issues in the use of switch technology for establishing prelinguistic communication. *Augmentative and Alternative Communication*, 2, 91–92.

Hopper, C., & Hemlick, R. (1977). Nonverbal communication and the severely handicapped: Some considerations. *American Association for the Education of the Severely/Profoundly Handicapped Review*, 2, 47–52.

Horner, R., Sprague, J., O'Brien, M., & Heathfield, L. (1990). The role of response efficiency in the reduction of problem behaviors through functional equivalence training: A case study. *Journal of the Association for Persons with Severe Handicaps*, 15, 91–97.

Horner, R. H., & Budd, C. M. (1985). Acquisition of manual sign use: Collateral reduction of maladaptive behavior and factors limiting generalization. *Education and Training of the Mentally Retarded*, 20, 39–47.

Horstmann, H. M., & Levine, S. P. (1990). Modeling of user performance with computer access and augmentative communication systems for handicapped people. *Augmentative and Alternative Communication*, 6, 231–241.

Hough, S. D. (1992). Augmentative communication for an Amish child. Paper presented at the annual meeting of the American Speech-Language-Hearing Association, San Antonio.

Hough, S. D., & St. Louis, K. W. (1992). Case studies using WOLF technology. Paper presented at the annual meeting of the American Speech-Language-Hearing Association, San Antonio.

Hough, S. O. (1992). Computerized language assessments for individuals wih physical disabilities. *Augmentative and Alternative Communication*, 8, 139.

Houghton, J., Bronicki, B., & Guess, D. (1987). Opportunities to express preferences and make choices among students with severe disabilities in classroom settings. *Journal of the Association for Persons with Severe Handicaps*, 11, 255–265.

House, B. J., Hanley, M. J., & Magid, D. F. (1980). Logographic reading by TMR adults. *American Journal of Mental Deficiency*, 85(2), 161–170.

House, L., & Rogerson, B. (1984). *Comprehensive Screening Tool for Determining Optimal Communication Mode*. East Aurora, NY: United Educational Services.

Howard, G. (Ed.) (1974). *Helping the Handicapped*. New York: Telephone Pioneers of America.

Howlin, P. (1989). Changing approaches to communication training with autistic children. *British Journal of Disorders of Communication*, 24(2), 151–168.

Hubbard, B. (1987). Implementing a computerized data system for a communication aids program. Intervention strategy developed under Contract No. 300-85-0139 (*Implementation Strategies for Improving the Use of Communication Aids in Schools Serving Handicapped Children*) from the U.S. Department of Education distributed by the American Speech-Language-Hearing Association.

Hubbard, B. (1987). Implementing a system for acquiring, disseminating, maintaining, and monitoring high-tech communication aids. Intervention strategy developed under Contract No. 300-85-0139 (*Implementation Strategies for Improving the Use of Communication Aids in Schools Serving Handicapped Children*) from the U.S. Department of Education distributed by the American Speech-Language-Hearing Association.

Hudson, A., Melita, B., & Arnold, N. (1993). Brief report: A case study assessing the validity of facilitated communication. *Journal of Autism and Developmental Disorders*, 23(1), 165–173.

Huer, M. B. (1983). *The Nonspeech Test*. Lake Zurich, IL: Don Johnson Developmental Equipment.

Huer, M. B. (1986). White's gestural system for lower extremities. *Augmentative and Alternative Communication*, 2, 92.

Huer, M. B. (1987). White's gestural system for the lower extremeties. *Communicating Together*, 5, 3–4.

Huer, M. B. (1990). University disabled student services programs: A survey of AAC services. *Augmentative and Alternative Communication*, 6, 121.

Huer, M. B. (1991). University students using augmentative and alternative communication in the USA: A demographic study. *Augmentative and Alternative Communication*, 7, 231–239.

Huer, M. B., Balmer, L., & Klink, P. (1989). A survey of test taking assistance for disabled university students. Paper presented at the annual meeting of the American Speech-Language-Hearing Association, St. Louis.

Huer, M. B., Balmer, L., Klink, P., Simon, L., & Vogel, L. (1990). Augmentative and alternative communication in Wisconsin: University, hospital, school activities. Paper presented at the annual meeting of the American Speech-Language-Hearing Association, Seattle.

Huer, M. B., Bosanko, M., & Bustos, J. (1992). AAC student's perceived decision-making matrix: Options beyond high school. Paper presented at the annual meeting of the American Speech-Language-Hearing Association, San Antonio.

Huer, M. B., Kempka, D., Schmidt, J., & Stewart, K. P. (1988). AAC users on university campuses: State of the art report. *Augmentative and Alternative Communication*, 4, 136.

Huer, M. B., & Lloyd, L. L. (1988). Perspectives of AAC users. *Communication Outlook*, 9(2), 10–18.

Huer, M. B., & Lloyd, L. L. (1990). AAC users' perspectives on augmentative and alternative communication. *Augmentative and Alternative Communication,* 6, 242–249.

Huer, M. B., & West, R. L. (1989). University disabled student services programs: A survey of AAC services. Paper presented at the annual meeting of the American Speech-Language-Hearing Association, St. Louis.

Hughes, J. (1974/5). Acquisition of a non-verbal "language" by aphasic children. *Cognition*, 3, 41–55.

Hughes, M. J. (1979). Sequencing of visual and auditory stimuli in teaching words and Blissymbols to the mentally retarded. *Australian Journal of Mental Retardation*, 5, 298–302.

Hunnicutt, S. (1988). Word prediction: Two programs and experiences with their use. *Augmentative and Alternative Communication*, 4, 152.

Hunnicutt, S. (1990). Word prediction: Exploring the use of semantic and syntactic information. *Augmentative and Alternative Communication, 6,* 148–149.

Hunnicutt, S., & Mossberg, K. (1992). Lexical access in aphasia rehabilitation. *Augmentative and Alternative Communication, 8,* 139–140.

Hunnicutt, S., Rosengren, W., & Baker, B. (1990). Development of the Swedish Language Minspeak words strategy. *Augmentative and Alternative Communication, 6,* 115–116.

Hunt, P., Alwell, M., & Goetz, L. (1988). Acquisition of conversational skills and the reduction of inappropriate interaction behaviors. *Journal of the Association for Persons with Severe Handicaps, 13,* 20–27.

Hunt, P., Alwell, M., & Goetz, L. (1990). *Teaching Conversational Skills to Individuals with Severe Disabilities with a Communication Book Adaptation.* (Available from P. Hunt, San Francisco State University, 14 Tapia Street, San Francisco, CA 94132.)

Hunt, P., Alwell, M., & Goetz, L. (1991a). Establishing conversational exchanges with family and friends: Moving from training to meaningful communication. *Journal of Special Education, 25,* 305–319.

Hunt, P., Alwell, M., & Goetz, L. (1991b). Interacting with peers through conversation turn-taking with a communication book adaptation. *Augmentative and Alternative Communication, 7,* 117–126.

Hunt, P., & Goetz, L. (1988a). Teaching simultaneous communication in natural settings through interrupted behavior chains. *Topics in Language Disorders, 9*(1), 58–71.

Hunt, P., & Goetz, L. (1988b). *Using the Interrupted Behavior Chain Strategy to Teach Initial Communication Skills to Learners with Severe Disabilities.* (Available from P. Hunt, San Francisco State University, 14 Tapia Street, San Francisco, CA 94132.)

Hunt, P., Goetz, L., Alwell, M., & Sailor, W. (1986). Using an interrupted behavior chain strategy to teach generalized communication responses. *Journal of the Association for Persons with Severe Handicaps, 11,* 196–204.

Hunt-Berg, M. M., Kaiser, H. W., & Wiesner, C. R. (1990). Now what's shakin' in California? Paper presented at the annual meeting of the American Speech-Language-Hearing Association, Seattle.

Huntress, L., Lee, L., Creaghead, N., Wheeler, D., & Braveman, K. (1990). Aphasic subjects' comprehension of synthetic and natural speech. *Journal of Speech and Hearing Disorders, 55,* 21–27.

Hurlbut, B. I., Iwata, B. A., & Green, J. D. (1982). Nonvocal language acquisition in adolescents with severe physical disabilities: Blissymbol versus iconic stimulus formats. *Journal of Applied Behavior Analysis, 15*(2), 241–258.

Hurlburt, M., & Ottenbacher, K. J. (1992). An examination of direct selection typing rate and accuracy for persons with high-level spinal cord injury using QWERTY and default on-screen keyboards. *Journal of Rehabilitation Research and Development, 29*(4), 54–63.

Hussey, I. (1991). Beginning AAC in Zimbabwe. *Communicating Together, 9*(1), 19–20.

Hux, K., Beukelman, D. R., Rankin, J., Simpson, K., Hahn, D., Snyder, B., & Dombrovskis, M. (1992). Semantic organization research: Implications for augmentative and alternative (AAC) message coding. *Augmentative and Alternative Communication, 8,* 140.

Iacono, T., & Balandin, S. (1992). AAC for writing and conversational participation in an academic setting. *Augmentative and Alternative Communication, 8,* 140.

Iacono, T. A. (1991). A comparison of unimodal and multimodal augmentative communication language intervention techniques for children with intellectual disabilities. *Dissertation Abstracts International, 51*(8–B), 3805.

Iacono, T. A. (1992). Individual language learning styles and augmentative and alternative communication. *Augmentative and Alternative Communication*, 8, 33–40.

Iacono, T. A., Franklin, K., & Mathy-Laikko, P. (1990). A comparison of unimodal and multimodal AAC language interventions. Paper presented at the annual meeting of the American Speech-Language-Hearing Association, Seattle.

Iacono, T. A., & Parsons, C. (1986a). A comparison of techniques for teaching signs to intellectually disabled individuals using an alternating treatment design. *Australian Journal of Human Communication Disorders*, 14, 23–34.

Iacono, T. A., & Parsons, C. (1986b). A survey of the use of signing with the intellectually disabled. *Australian Communication Quarterly*, 2, 21–25.

Iles, G. H. (1974). Interfaces for the C.P. Paper presented at the Seminar on Electronic Controls for the Severely Handicapped, Vancouver, British Columbia. (Paper published in seminar proceedings volume, pp. 71–82.)

Imhoff, T. E., & McMillen, M. H. (1984). The transparency of Amer-Ind and S.E.E. to untrained peers. Paper presented at the annual meeting of the American Speech-Language-Hearing Association, San Francisco.

Intellectual Disability Review Panel (1989). *Report to the Director-General on the Reliability and Validity of Assisted [Facilitated] Communication*. Melbourne, Australia: Author.

Interdisciplinary Working Party on Issues of Severe Communication Impairment (1988). *DEAL Communication Center Operations. A Statement of Concern*. Melbourne, Australia: Author. [Deals with facilitated communication]

Irwin, D. L. (1977). Amerind. *Asha*, 19, 746.

Israel, B. L. (1969). *Responsive Environment Program, Brooklyn, New York*. Springfield, VA: U.S. Department of Commerce, Institute of Applied Technology.

Itoh, H. (March 1991). Augmentative nonspeech communication systems and application for autistic disorders [title translated from Japanese]. *Tokushu Kyoiku Kenkyu Shisetsu Hokoku/RLIEEC Report*, 40, 83–93.

Jack H. Eichler: Builds communication device (June, 1973). *Case Alumnus*. Publication of Case Institute of Technology Alumni Association, Cleveland, OH.

Jackson, L. B. (1988). Assessing the communicative competence of persons with multiple impairments. *Augmentative and Alternative Communication*, 4, 163.

Jackson, S. A., Stirling, J. M. M., & Dixon, C. R. (1983). A speech-prompted communication aid for the severely handicapped. *Journal of Medical Engineering and Technology*, 7(2), 88–91.

Jadd, E. B., Farr, S. D., Stein, R. H., & Higginbotham, D. J. (1988). Morsewriter augmentative and alternative communication system. *Augmentative and Alternative Communication*, 4, 160–161.

Jadd, E. B., & Weitzner-Lin, B. (1992). Using EZ Keys: A case study with a dysgraphic adolescent. *Augmentative and Alternative Communication*, 8, 140–141.

Jardine, P., Jerman, S., Seddon, N., & Rees, J. A. (1984). A communication aid for the physically handicapped. *Journal of Biomedical Engineering*, 6(3), 230–236.

Jaroma, M., Cregan, A., & Taipale, E. (1990). Real-life results?—Multi-system support for dysphasic children. *Augmentative and Alternative Communication*, 6, 108.

Jarrell, N. F., & Shane, H. (1990). Technical considerations and application of the interactive phonetic screen keyboard. *Augmentative and Alternative Communication*, 6, 95.

Jefcoate, R. (December 1970). Possum—Its significance to multiple sclerosis patients. *M.S. News*.

Jefcoate, R. (1974). New independence for the disabled. In Keith Copeland (Ed.), *Aids for the Severely Handicapped*. New York: Grune & Stratton, pp. 129–136.

Jefcoate, R. (1981). Supplying electronic aids to disabled people. *Physiotherapy*, 67(2), 45–46.

Jeffree, D. (1981). A bridge between pictures and print. *Special Education Forward Trends*, 8 (1), 28–31.

Jenkins, R. (1967). Possum, a new communication aid. *Special Education* (Great Britain), 56, 9–11.

Jenkins, S., Efrom, M., & Ginsberg, A. (1986). Teaching reliable eye tracking skills to the multihandicapped/visually impaired. *Augmentative and Alternative Communication*, 2, 92.

Jenkins-Peters, S. (1992). Grass roots advocacy: Starting an AAC association for your state. *Augmentative and Alternative Communication*, 8, 141.

Jennische, M. (1988). Alternative and augmentative routes used by a nonspeaking autistic boy. *Augmentative and Alternative Communication*, 4, 149–150.

Jensen, M. H. (1986). A microcomputer aided communication system. *Augmentative and Alternative Communication*, 2, 92–93.

Jensen, M. H., & Hansen, S. R. (1990). A play and communication device for handicapped infants. *Augmentative and Alternative Communication*, 6, 112.

Jewell, K. H. (1989). A custom-made head pointer for children. *American Journal of Occupational Therapy*, 43(7), 456–460.

Jim Brooks system: A foot-operated portable communication (1980). *Communication Outlook*, 2(2), 11.

Jinks, A., & Pashek, G. (1992). Conversational applications of AAC systems in aphasia. Paper presented at the annual meeting of the American Speech-Language-Hearing Association, San Antonio.

Jodock-King, S., & King, A. (1992). How our thoughts are heard. *Augmentative and Alternative Communication*, 8, 141.

Jodock-King, S., King, A., & Campbell, D. (1990). A real home at last. *Augmentative and Alternative Communication*, 6, 143.

Johannsen-Horbach, H., Cegla, B., Mager, U., Schempp, B., & Wallesch, C.W. (1985). Treatment of chronic global aphasia with a nonverbal communication system. *Brain and Language*, 24(1), 74–82.

Jonansson, I. (1990). Contributions of language to cognitive development. *Augmentative and Alternative Communication*, 6, 147.

Johnsen, B. (1990). Acquisition of reading and writing: A neurolinguistic approach. *Augmentative and Alternative Communication*, 6, 132–133.

Johnson, D. W., & Wolf, P. (1988). Telecommunications for the communicatively impaired: A Minnesota interdisciplinary effort. Paper presented at the annual meeting of the American Speech-Language-Hearing Association, Boston.

Johnson, H., & Bloomberg, K. P. (1986). Severe communication impairment in Victoria, Australia. *Augmentative and Alternative Communication*, 2, 93.

Johnson, H., & Bloomberg, K. P. (1988). Teaching the teachers: Outreach work in Australia. *Augmentative and Alternative Communication*, 4, 137.

Johnson, J. (1986). *Self-Talk: Communication Boards for Children and Adults*. Tucson, AZ: Communication Skill Builders.

Johnson, J. (1988). *Self-Talk Stickers: Pictures and Words for Augmentative Communication Boards*. Tucson, AZ: Communication Skill Builders.

Johnson, J. M. (1989). Comment on terminology. *Augmentative and Alternative Communication*, 5, 74.

Johnson, P. L. (1987). *Express Yourself: Communication Disabilities Need Not Be Handicaps.* Richfield, MN: Pegijohn, 6432 Fifth Avenue.

Johnson, P. L., & Cramer, J. D. (1992). Your Expressive Society (YES): An AAC users support group. *Augmentative and Alternative Communication*, 8, 141.

Johnson, R. (1981). *The Picture Communication Symbols.* Salana Beach, CA: Mayer-Johnson.

Johnson, R. (1985a). *The Picture Communication Symbols: Book II.* Salana Beach, CA: Mayer-Johnson.

Johnson, R. (1985b). Picture communication symbols. *Communicating Together*, 3(3), 23.

Johnson-Martin, N., Wolters, P., & Sowers, S. (1987). Psychological assessment of the nonvocal, physically handicapped child. *Physical and Occupational Therapy in Pediatrics*, 7(2), 23–28.

Johnston, H. B., Manning, R. P., & Lappin, J. S. (1972). A communications prosthesis for a quadraplegic. Paper presented at the Carnahan Conference on Engineering Devices in Rehabilitation, Lexington, KY. (Paper is published in conference proceedings volume.)

Johnston, J. (1990). Classroom participation of a mainstreamed AAC user. *Augmentative and Alternative Communication*, 6, 127.

Johnston, R. G., & Lange, T. A. (1992). Communication programming for the MR group home population. Paper presented at the annual meeting of the American Speech-Language-Hearing Association, San Antonio.

Jolie, K. (1985). On peer interaction. *Communicating Together*, 3(1), 18–19.

Jolie, K. R., & Hall, M. (1988). A statewide augmentative communication service delivery system. *Augmentative and Alternative Communication*, 4, 137.

Jolleff, N., & Clayton, C. (1992). Database in AAC: What can it tell us? *Augmentative and Alternative Communication*, 8, 141–142.

Jolleff, N., & McConachie, H. (1992). Communication aids—Who, what, why and how? Paper presented at the fourth meeting of the European Academy of Childhood Disability, Jesolo, Italy.

Jolleff, N., McConachie, H., Winyard, S., Jones, S., Wisbeach, A., & Clayton, C. (1992). Communication aids for children: Procedures and problems. *Developmental Medicine and Child Neurology*, 34, 719–730.

Jones, D. (1981). Computers revolutionize aids for nonspeakers. *Asha*, 23, 555–557.

Jones, K. (1979). A rebus system of non-fade visual language. *Child Care, Health, and Development*, 5, 1–7.

Jones, K., & Cregan, A. (1986). *Sign and Symbol Communication for Mentally Handicapped People.* Beckenham, England: Croom Helm.

Jones, M. V. (1961). Electronic communication devices. *American Journal of Occupational Therapy*, 15, 110–111.

Jones, S., Jolleff, N., McConachie, H., & Wisbeach, A. (1990). A model for assessment of children for augmentative communication systems. *Child Language Teaching and Therapy*, 6, 305–321.

Jonker, V. M., & Heim, M. J. M.(1992). A communication program for nonspeaking children and their partners. *Augmentative and Alternative Communication*, 8, 142.

Joseph, D. (1986). The morning. *Communication Outlook*, 8(2), 8.

Joseph, R. (1992). Los Angeles County California Children Services augmentative and alternative communication (AAC) program. *Augmentatve and Alternative Communication*, 8, 142.

Joubert, Z. F. (1979). Fingercom—An electronic communicator for the disabled. *Medical and Biological Engineering and Computing,* 17, 489–491.

Joyce, M. (1992). Expanding awareness in the realm of public speaking. *Augmentative and Alternative Communication,* 8, 142.

Justice, F. L., & Wilke, R. A. (1992). Using a continuum model for augmentative and alternative communication (AAC) assessment and training. *Augmentative and Alternative Communication,* 8, 142.

Kafafian, H. (1970–1973). *A Study of Man-Machine Communication Systems for the Handicapped.* 3 vols. Washington, DC: Cybernetics Research Institute.

Kahn, J. V. (1977). A comparison of manual and oral training with mute retarded children. *Mental Retardation,* 15(3), 21–23.

Kahn, J. V. (1981). A comparison of sign and verbal language training with nonverbal retarded children. *Journal of Speech and Hearing Research,* 24, 113–119.

Kalimikerakis, C. (1983). Training mentally handicapped children to use Blissymbolics. Unpublished master's thesis, University of London, Institute of Education.

Kamp, L., & O'Dornan, S. (1992). Centralized assessments for assistive devices: Reactions from the community. *Augmentative and Alternative Communication,* 8, 142–143.

Kamphuis, H. (1990). Enhancing communication rate: Two input systems for augmentative communication aids. *Augmentative and Alternative Communication,* 6, 95.

Kangas, K. A. (1992). Comparison of familiar and unfamiliar listeners' perceptions of communicative competence. *Augmentative and Alternative Communication,* 8, 143.

Kangas, K. A., & Allen, D. W. (1992). Consultative diagnostic evaluations for augmentative and alternative communication. Paper presented at the annual meeting of the American Speech-Language-Hearing Association, San Antonio.

Kangas, K. A., & Lloyd, L. L. (1988a). Effects of sign knowledge on perceived translucency of Sigsymbols. *Augmentative and Alternative Communication,* 4, 145–146.

Kangas, K. A., & Lloyd, L. L. (1988b). Early cognitive skills as prerequisites to augmentative and alternative communication use: What are we waiting for? *Augmentative and Alternative Communication,* 4, 211–221.

Kannenberg, P., Marquardt, T. P., & Larson, J. (1988). Speech intelligibility of two voice output communication aids. *Journal of Communication Disorders,* 21(1) 11–20.

Kaplan, J. (1984). Additional information on battery-operated toys. *Language, Speech, and Hearing Services in Schools,* 15, 221.

Karjalainen, M. A., Laine, U. K., & Rahko, T. (1980). Speech synthesizer in the Finnish language. *Folia Phoniatrica,* 32, 309–314.

Karlan, G. R. (1991a). Implementing environmental communication teaching with severely disabled students. Paper presented at the annual meeting of the American Speech-Language-Hearing Association, Atlanta.

Karlan, G. R. (1991b). Manual communication with those who can hear. In H. Bornstein (Ed.), *Manual Communication: Implications for Education.* Washington, DC: Gallaudet University Press, pp. 151–185.

Karlan, G. R. (1992). Environmental communication teaching for severely disabled students who use AAC. *Augmentative and Alternative Communication,* 8, 143.

Karlan, G. R., Brenn-White, B., Lentz, A., Hodur, P., Egger, D., & Frankoff, D. (1982). Establishing generalized, productive verb-noun phrase usage in a manual language system with moderately handicapped children. *Journal of Speech and Hearing Disorders,* 47, 31–42.

Karlan, G. R., & Lloyd, L. L. (1983). Considerations in the planning of communication intervention: Selecting a lexicon. *Journal of the Association for the Severely Handicapped*, 8, 13–25.

Karlan, G. R., & Lloyd, L. L. (198?). *Communication Intervention for the Moderately and Severely Handicapped*. Austin, TX: Pro-Ed.

Karlan, G. R., McEwen, I. R., Ward, M. F., Swanson, L. A., & Kongas, K. (1989). Classroom-based interactions of young children with severe disabilities. Paper presented at the annual meeting of the American Speech-Language-Hearing Association, St. Louis.

Karlan, G. R., & McNaughton, S. (1986). Toward a multidimensional model of graphic system effects. *Augmentative and Alternative Communication*, 2, 93.

Kates, B., & McNaughton, S. (1975). The first application of Blissymbolics as a communication medium for non-speaking children: History and development, 1971–1974. Distributed by Blissymbolics Communication Foundation. 862 Eglinton Avenue East, Toronto, Ont., Canada.

Kates, B., McNaughton, S., & Silverman, H. (1977). *Handbook for Instructors, Users, Parents, and Administrators*. Toronto: Blissymbolics Communication Institute.

Kaul, S. (1990). Sounds of silence. *Communication Outlook*, 11(3), 6–9.

Kavanagh, R. N., Holmlund, B. A., & Krause, A. E. (1966). Communications systems for the physically handicapped. Paper presented at the Canadian Medical and Biological Engineering Conference. (Paper is published in the conference digest volume.)

Kearns, T. (1990). Training families as effective sign communication partners and teachers. *Augmentative and Alternative Communication*, 6, 103–104.

Keating, D., Evans, A. L., Smith, D. C., Wyper, D. J., Cunningham, E., & Bone, I. (1986). Text-to-speech using LPC synthesiser. *Augmentative and Alternative Communication*, 2, 93–94.

Keating, D., Smith, D. C., Evans, A. L., Wyper, D. J., & Cunningham, E. (1989). The pocket speech aid. *Medical and Biological Engineering and Computing*, 27(3), 288–290.

Keirn, Z. A., & Aunon, J. I. (1990). A new mode of communication between man and his surroundings. *IEEE Transactions on Biomedical Engineering*, 37(12), 1209–1214.

Kelford, A., Thurston, S., Light, J., Parnes, P., & O'Keefe, B. (1986). A model for the assessment of written communication via microcomputers of nonspeaking physically disabled individuals. *Augmentative and Alternative Communication*, 2, 94.

Kelford-Smith, A., Thurston, S., Light, J., Parnes, P., & O'Keefe, B. (1989). The form and use of written communication produced by physically disabled individuals using microcomputers. *Augmentative and Alternative Communication*, 5, 115–124.

Kennedy, G. H., Horner, R. H., & Newton, J. S. (1989). Social contacts of adults with severe disabilities living in the community: A descriptive analysis of relationship patterns. *Journal of the Association for Persons with Severe Handicaps*, 14(3), 190–196.

Kent, L. (1974). *Language Acquisition Program for the Severely Retarded*. Champaign, IL: Research Press.

Kent-Udolf, L. (1986). Facilitating communication with severely speech-impaired children with abnormal socialization patterns. In Sarah W. Blackstone (Ed.), *Augmentative Communication: An Introduction*. Rockville, MD: American Speech-Language-Hearing Association, pp. 353–367.

Keogh, D., Whitman, T. L., Beeman, D., Halligan, K., & Starzynski, T. (1987). Teaching interactive signing in a dialogue situation to mentally retarded individuals. *Research in Developmental Disabilities*, 8(1), 39–53.

Keogh, W., & Reichle, J. (1985). Communication intervention for the "difficult to teach" severely handicapped. In S. F. Warren & A. K. Rogers-Warren (Eds.), *Teaching Functional Language*. Austin, TX: Pro-Ed, pp. 157–194.

Kibitlewski, R. (1978). Communication enhancement: A parent's view. *Communication Outlook*, 1(2), 1.

Kiernan, C. (1977). Alternatives to speech: A review of research on manual and other forms of communication with mentally handicapped and other noncommunicating populations. *Journal of Mental Subnormality*, 23, 6–28.

Kiernan, C. (1980). Communication for the handicapped: The hands say it all. *Nursing Mirror*, 151(13), 16–20.

Kiernan, C. (1983). The use of nonvocal communication techniques with autistic individuals. *Journal of Child Psychology and Psychiatry*, 24(3), 339–375.

Kiernan, C., & Jones, M. (1985). The heuristic programme: A combined use of signs and symbols with severely mentally retarded, autistic children. *Australian Journal of Human Communication Disorders*, 13(2), 153–168.

Kiernan, C., & Reid, B. (1984). The use of augmentative communication systems in schools and units for autistic and aphasic children in the United Kingdom. *British Journal of Disorders of Communication*, 19(1), 47–61.

Kiernan, C., & Reid, B. (1987). *Pre-verbal Communication Schedule*. Windsor: NFER-Nelson.

Kiernan, C., Reid, B., & Jones, L. (1982). *Signs and Symbols: Use of Non-Vocal Communication Systems*. London: Heinemann.

Kiernan, S. C., Anderson, P. M., & Ashida, K. (1988). Creative approaches to the use of auditory scanning. *Augmentative and Alternative Communication*, 4, 171.

Kiesow, J. (n.d.). *Effective Communication Training for the Profoundly Retarded*. Chippewa Falls, WI: Northern Wisconsin Center for the Developmentally Disabled.

Kilgallon, M. J., Roberts, D. P., & Miller, S. (1987). Adapting personal computers for use by high-level quadriplegics. *Medical Instrumentation*, 21(2), 97–102.

Kimble, S. L. (1975). A language teaching technique with totally nonverbal, severely mentally retarded adolescents. Paper presented at the annual meeting of the American Speech-Language-Hearing Association, Washington, DC.

Kimura, D., Davidson, W., & McCormick, C. W. (1982). No impairment in sign language after right-hemisphere stroke. *Brain and Language*, 17, 359–362.

King, B. (1983). Me and my Handivoice. *Communication Outlook*, 4(3), 10.

King, T. W. (1990). An improvised eye-pointing communication system for temporary use. *Language, Speech, and Hearing Services in Schools*, 21, 116–117.

King, T. W. (1991). A signalling device for non-oral communicators. *Language, Speech, and Hearing Services in Schools*, 22, 277–282.

Kirk, S., McCarthy, J., & Kirk, W. (1968). *Illinois Test of Psycholinguistic Abilities*. Urbana: University of Illinois Press.

Kirkebaek, B. (1987). *Handicappede Smaborn—Kan De Snakke?* [Handicapped infants—Can they talk?]. Kobenhavns Amtskommune, Box 1341, 2600 Glostrup, Denmark.

Kirschner, A. E. (1977). A comparison of two manual communication systems: Implications for training the nonverbal mentally retarded. Unpublished M.A. thesis, University of Florida.

Kirschner, A. E., Algozzine, B., & Abbott, T. (1977). Manual communication systems. *Education and Training of the Mentally Retarded*, 14, 5–10.

Kirshner, H. S., & Webb, W. G. (1981). Selective involvement of the auditory-verbal modality in an acquired communication disorder: Benefit from sign language therapy. *Brain and Language*, 13, 161–170.

Kirstein, I. J. (1981). *Oakland Schools Picture Dictionary*. Wauconda, IL: Don Johnson Developmental Equipment.

Kirstein, I. J., & Peters, N. A. (1987). Establishing an equipment library. Intervention strategy developed under Contract No. 300-85-0139 (*Implementation Strategies for Improving the Use of Communication Aids in Schools Serving Handicapped Children*) from the U.S. Department of Education distributed by the American Speech-Language-Hearing Association.

Kirstein, I. J., & Bernstein, C. (1981). *Oakland Schools Picture Dictionary*. Pontiac, MI: Oakland Schools Communication Enhancement Center.

Kissick, L. (1984). Communication devices and an enriched life: An autobiography. *The Exceptional Parent*, 14, 9–14.

Klein, M. (1988). *Pre-sign Language Motor Skills*. Tucson, AZ: Communication Skill Builders.

Kladde, A. G. (1974). Nonoral communication techniques: Project summary no. 1, August 1967. In Beverly Vicker (Ed.), *Nonoral Communication System Project 1964/1973*, Iowa City: University of Iowa, pp. 57–104.

Knight, S., Poon, P., & Ringrose, I. (1986). The development and use of a hardware keyboard emulation facility. *Augmentative and Alternative Communication*, 2, 94.

Knox, D. (1971). *Portrait of Aphasia*. Detroit: Wayne State University Press.

Kobacker, N., & Todaro, M. P. (1992). Use of an assistive device by a preschooler with autism. *Augmentative and Alternative Communication*, 8, 143–144.

Koehler, L. J. S., & Lloyd, L. L. (1986). The use of fingerspelling and manual sign to facilitate reading and spelling. *Augmentative and Alternative Communication*, 2, 94–95.

Koehler, L. J. S., Lloyd, L. L., & Swanson, L. (1990). Promoting phonological awareness with manual alphabet letters. *Augmentative and Alternative Communication*, 6, 151–152.

Koehler, L. J. S., Lloyd, L. L., & Swanson, L. (1992). Metalinguistic features of manual communication that facilitate literacy. *Augmentative and Alternative Communication*, 8, 144.

Koerselman, E., & Burger, J. (1992). Every human being is unique. *Augmentative and Alternative Communication*, 8, 144.

Kohl, F. L. (1981). Effects of motoric requirements on the acquisition of manual sign responses by severely handicapped students. *American Journal of Mental Deficiency*, 85(4), 396–403.

Koivikko, M., & Korpela, R. (1990). Survey of technical aids for severely disabled children. *Augmentative and Alternative Communication*, 6, 99–100.

Kojima, T. (1990). One year follow-up of VOCA use by a retarded child. *Augmentative and Alternative Communication*, 6, 137.

Kojima, T., Iwatate, S., Hayashi, K., & Matsumoto, Y. (1988). Application of Japanese-based graphic symbol system with a nonspeaking boy. *Augmentative and Alternative Communication*, 4, 143.

Koke, S., & Neilson, J. (1987). *The Effect of Auditory Feedback on the Spelling of Nonspeaking Physically Disabled Individuals Who Use Microcomputers*. Toronto: University of Toronto.

Koko: The signs of language (1977). *Science News*, 111, 172.

Koller, J. J., Schlanger, P. H., & Geffner, D. S. (1975). Identification of action words and activity pantomimes by aphasics. Paper presented at the annual meeting of the American Speech-Language-Hearing Association, Washington, DC.

Kollinzas, G. (1983). The communication record: Sharing information to promote sign language generalization. *Journal of the Association for Persons with Severe Handicaps*, 8, 49–55.

Kolstoe, B. J. (1976). Assisting the non-verbal to talk. *Journal of Physically Handicapped, Homebound, and Hospitalized*, 3, 18–21.

Konstantareas, M. M. (1984). Sign language as a communication prosthesis with language-impaired children. *Journal of Autism and Developmental Disorders*, 14(1), 9–25.

Konstantareas, M. M. (1985). Review of evidence on the relevance of sign language in early communication training of autistic children. *Australian Journal of Human Communication Disorders*, 13(2), 77–97.

Konstantareas, M. M. (1987). Autistic children exposed to simultaneous communication training: A follow-up. *Journal of Autism and Developmental Disorders*, 17, 115–132.

Konstantareas, M. M., Hunter, D., & Sloman, L. (1982). Training a blind autistic child to communicate through signs. *Journal of Autism and Developmental Disorders*, 12, 1–11.

Konstantareas, M. M., Oxman, J., & Webster, C. D. (1977). Spontaneous communication with autistic and other severely dysfunctional nonverbal children. *Journal of Communication Disorders*, 10, 267–282.

Konstantareas, M. M., Oxman, J., & Webster, C. D. (1978). Iconicity: Effects on the acquisition of sign language by autistic and other severely dysfunctional children. In P. Siple (Ed.), *Understanding Language Through Sign Language Research*. New York: Academic Press, pp. 213–237.

Konstantareas, M. M., Oxman, J., Webster, C., Fischer, H., & Miller, K. (1975). *A Five Week Simultaneous Communication Programme for Severely Dysfunctional Children: Outcome and Implications for Future Research*. Distributed by Clarke Institute of Psychiatry, Toronto.

Konstantareas, M. M., Webster, C. D., & Oxman, J. (1979). Manual language acquisition and its influence on other areas of functioning in four autistic and autistic-like children. *Journal of Child Psychology and Psychiatry*, 20, 337–350.

Kopchick, Jr., G. A., & Lloyd, L. L. (1976). Total communication programming for the severely language impaired—A 24-hour approach. In Lyle L. Lloyd (Ed.), *Communication Assessment and Intervention Strategies*. Baltimore: University Park Press, pp. 501–521.

Kopchick, Jr., G. A., Romback, D. W., & Smilovitz, R. (1975). A total communication environment in an institution. *Mental Retardation*, 13(3), 22–23.

Koppenhaver, D. A., Hedrick, W. B., Abraham, L. M., & Yoder, D. E. (1992). Social and academic organization of literacy lessions for AAC users. *Augmentative and Alternative Communication*, 8, 144.

Koppenhaver, D. A., Evans, D. A., & Yoder, D. E. (1991). Childhood reading and writing experiences of literate adults with severe speech and motor impairments. *Augmentative and Alternative Communication*, 7, 20–33.

Koppenhaver, D. A., & Yoder, D. (1988). Literacy and the augmentative and alternative communication user. *Augmentative and Alternative Communication*, 4, 156–157.

Koppenhaver, D. A., & Yoder, D. (1990a). A descriptive analysis of classroom reading and writing instruction for adolescents with severe speech and physical impairments. Paper presented at the International Special Education Conference, Cardiff, Wales.

Koppenhaver, D. A., & Yoder, D. (1990b). Classroom interaction, literacy acquisition, and nonspeaking children with physical impairments. *Augmentative and Alternative Communication*, 6, 152.

Koppenhaver, D. A., & Yoder, D. (1990c). Facilitating literacy learning in children with speech and physical impairments. *Augmentative and Alternative Communication*, 6, 107–108.

Koppenhaver, D. A., & Yoder, D. (1992). Literacy issues in persons with severe physical and speech impairments. In R. Gaylord-Ross (Ed.), *Issues and Research in Special Education*. Vol. 2. New York: Teachers College Press, pp. 156–201.

Korabic, E. W., Silverman, F. H., & Rosa M. (1987). An inexpensive single-switch scanning communication aid. *Journal for Computer Users in Speech and Hearing*, 3(1), 34–38.

Korzybski, A. (1933). *Science and Samity: An Introduction to Non-Aristotelian Systems and General Semantics*. Lakeville, CT: Institute of General Semantics.

Kose, G., Beilin, H., & O'Connor, J. M. (1983). Children's comprehension of actions depicted in photographs. *Developmental Psychology*, 19, 636–643.

Koselka, M. J., Hannah, E. P., Gardner, J. O., & Reagan, W. (1975). Total communication therapy for a nondeaf child and his family. Paper presented at the annual meeting of the American Speech-Language-Hearing Association, Washington, DC.

Kostraba, J., Sauer, M., Brown, C., Frische, E., & Wyatt, C. (1992). Research on efficacy of eyegaze/headpointing technology and mental retardation. *Augmentative and Alternative Communication*, 8, 144–145.

Kotkin, R. A., Simpson, S. B., & Desanto, D. (1978). The effect of sign language on picture naming in two retarded girls possessing normal hearing. *Journal of Mental Deficiency Research*, 22, 19–25.

Koul, R. K., & Allen, G. D. (1992). Segmental intelligibility of high-quality synthetic speech in the presence of speech noise. *Augmentative and Alternative Communication*, 8, 145.

Kouri, T. A. (1988). Effects of simultaneous communication in a child-directed treatment approach with preschoolers with severe disabilities. *Augmentative and Alternative Communication*, 4, 222–232.

Kouri, T. A. (1989). How manual sign acquisition relates to the development of spoken language: A case study. *Language, Speech, and Hearing Services in Schools*, 20, 50–62.

Kovach, T. M. (1990). Collaboration in Colorado for augmentative/alternative communication. Paper presented at the annual meeting of the American Speech-Language-Hearing Association, Seattle.

Kovach, T. M., Donaldson, C. A., & Bodine, C. (1992). Talking with technology camp. *Augmentative and Alternative Communication*, 8, 145.

Kovach,T. M., Grady, A. P., & Shannon, L. (1990). Technology for living and learning. *Augmentative and Alternative Communication*, 6, 143.

Kovach, T. M., Sementelli, C. A., McCord, G. S., & Moore, S. M. (1990). Toddlers talk with technology: Application of the storybook curriculum. *Augmentative and Alternative Communication*, 6, 146.

Kovarik-Kuhlmeier, A. M. (1990). Rett syndrome: A case study. Paper presented at the annual meeting of the American Speech-Language-Hearing Association, Seattle.

Kowalski, K., & Carlson, C. (1990). An admissions screening tool for identification of potential AAC users. *Augmentative and Alternative Communication*, 6, 112.

Kozleski, E. B. (1991). Expectant delay procedure for teaching requests. *Augmentative and Alternative Communication*, 7, 11–19.

Kraat, A. W. (1982). Training augmentative communication use: Clinical and research issues.

In K. Galyas, M. Lundman, & U. Lagerman (Eds.), *Communication for the Severely Handicapped*. Bromma, Sweden: Swedish Institute for the Handicapped, pp. 76–93.

Kraat, A. W. (1985a). *Communication Interaction Between Aided and Natural Speakers: A State of the Art Report*. Toronto: Canadian Rehabilitation Council for the Disabled.

Kraat, A. W. (1985b). The jump from language boards to electronic/computerised devices: Some critical training issues. *Proceedings of the Fourth International Conference, Communication Through Technology for the Physically Disabled*. Dublin, Ireland: Central Remedial Clinic, pp. 58–63.

Kraat, A. W. (1986). Developing intervention goals. In Sarah W. Blackstone (Ed.), *Augmentative Communication: An Introduction*. Rockville, MD: American Speech-Language-Hearing Association, pp. 197–265.

Kraat, A. W. (1988). Comparison of augmentative rate enhancement techniques from a user's perspective. Paper presented at the annual meeting of the American Speech-Language-Hearing Association, Boston.

Kraat, A. W., & Potter, C. (1988). "Hey big ears!"—Playful teasing in the social interactions of children using aided communication. *Augmentative and Alternative Communication, 4,* 136.

Kraat, A. W., & Sitver-Kogut, M. (1984). *Features of Commercially Available Communication Aids*. Wooster, OH: Prentke Romich Co.

Kraat, A. W., & Sitver-Kogut, M. (1991). *Features of Portable Communication Devices* [wall-chart]. Wilmington: Applied Science and Engineering Laboratories, University of Delaware/A. I. duPont Institute.

Kravitz, E. (1986a). The amount of intervention time needed to adequately serve communication device users. *Augmentative and Alternative Communication, 2,* 95.

Kravitz, E. (1986b). Training individuals with mental retardation to use augmentative communication devices. *Augmentative and Alternative Communication, 2,* 95–96.

Kravitz, E., & Littman, S. (1990). A communication system for a nonspeaking person with hearing and cognitive impairments. *Augmentatve and Alternative Communication, 6,* 100.

Kravitz, E., Littman, S., & Cassidy, K. (1992). Meeting the communication needs of nonspeaking adults with mental retardation. *Augmentative and Alternative Communication, 8,* 145–146.

Kreb, R. (1991). *Third Party Payment for Funding Special Education and Related Services*. Horsham, PA: LRP Publications.

Krichbaum, S., & Ellis, L. (1992). Increasing interaction skills of preschool augmentative and alternative communication (AAC) users. *Augmentative and Alternative Communication, 8,* 146.

Kriegsmann, E., Gallagher, J. C., & Meyers, A. (1982). Sign programs with nonverbal hearing children. *Exceptional Child, 48*(5), 436–445.

Krolikowski, D. M. (1992). Getting the word out to those in the trenches. *Augmentative and Alternative Communication, 8,* 146.

Krolikowski, D. M., & Hollman, D. (1992). Automatic processing in augmentative and alternative communication (AAC) access. *Augmentative and Alternative Communication, 8,* 146.

Kuntz, J. B. (1974). A nonvocal communication development program for severely retarded children. Unpublished doctoral dissertation, Kansas State University.

Kuntz, J. B., Carrier, J., & Hollis, J. (1978). A nonvocal system for teaching retarded children to read and write. In C. Meyers (Ed.), *Quality of Life in Severely and Profoundly Mentally*

Retarded People: Research Foundations for Improvement. Washington, DC.: American Association on Mental Deficiency, pp. 145–191.

Kurzweil, R. (1986). The technology of the Kurzweil voice writer. *Byte*, March, 177–186.

LaCourse, J. R., & Hludik, F. C., Jr. (1990). An eye movement communication-control system for the disabled. *IEEE Transactions on Biomedical Engineering*, 37(12), 1215–1220.

Ladd, D., & McCartney, N. (1988). Service delivery in augmentative and alternative communication: Implications for education. *Augmentative and Alternative Communication*, 4, 138.

Ladtkow, M., & Culp, D. (1992). Augmentative communication with traumatic brain injury. In K. Yorkston (Ed.), *Augmentative Communication in the Medical Setting*. Tucson, AZ: Communication Skill Builders, pp. 139–244.

Lafontaine, L. M., & DeRuyter, F. (1987). The nonspeaking cerebral palsied: A clinical and demographic database report. *Augmentative and Alternative Communication*, 3(3), 153–162.

Lagerman, U., & Höök, O. (1982). Communication aids for patients with dys/anathria. *Scandinavian Journal of Rehabilitation Medicine*, 14, 155–158.

Lahey, M., & Bloom, L. (1977). Planning a first lexicon: Which words to teach first. *Journal of Speech and Hearing Disorders*, 42, 340–349.

Laine, C., & Follansbee, R. (1992). Improving the writing of low-functioning hearing-impaired students. *Augmentative and Alternative Communication*, 8, 146–147.

Lake, S. J. (1976). *The Hand-Book*. Tucson, AZ: Communication Skill Builders.

Lakkanna, S., & Kravitz, E. (1992). A mechanical versus nonmechanical communication aid for an individual with autism. *Augmentative and Alternative Communication*, 8, 147.

Landman, C., & Schaeffler, C. (1986). Object communication boards. *Communication Outlook*, 8(1), 7–8.

Landry, S. H., & Loveland, K. A. (1988). Communication behaviors in autism and developmental language delay. *Journal of Child Psychology, Psychiatry, and Allied Disciplines*, 29(5), 621–634.

Lane, V. W., & Samples, J. M. (1981). Facilitating communication skills in adult apraxics: Application of Blissymbols in a group setting. *Journal of Communication Disorders*, 14, 157–167.

Langley, B. (1980). *Functional Vision Inventory for the Multiply and Severely Handicapped*. Chicago: Stoelting Co.

Lapidus, D., Adler, N., & Modugno, P. (1984). The use of communication boards with the autistic population: A training workshop for educators and parents. Paper presented at the annual meeting of the Council for Exceptional Children, Washington, DC.

Larcher, J. M., Banks, J., & Fisher, D. (1990). Communication for independence: A group training package. *Augmentative and Alternative Communication*, 6, 96.

Lariviere, J. (1992). Draw, write, and play games: Simply talk to your computer. *Augmentative and Alternative Communication*, 8, 147.

Larson, J., & Woodfin, S. T. (1986). Training communication partners of augmentative communication users. *Augmentative and Alternative Communication*, 2, 96.

Larson, J., & Woodfin, S. T. (1990). Technological assistance in adaptative technology assessment: A developmental levels framework. Paper presented at the annual meeting of the American Speech-Language-Hearing Association, Seattle.

Larson, T. (1971). Communications for the nonverbal child. *Academic Therapy Quarterly*, 6, 305–312.

Larson, T. (1975). *Communication for the Non-verbal Child.* Johnstown, PA: Mafex Associates.

Larson, V., & Steiner, S. (1985). Language intervention using microcomputers. *Topics in Language Disorders,* 6(1), 41–55.

Launonen, K., & Kokkonen, K. (1990). Using sign in the early intervention of children with Down syndrome. *Augmentative and Alternative Communication,* 6, 110.

Laurent, D. L., & Cascella, P. W. (1989). Intervention using an electronic communication device with profoundly retarded adults. Paper presented at the annual meeting of the American Speech-Language-Hearing Association, St. Louis.

Laurent, D. L., & Spencer, A. R. (1990). Where to turn in Connecticut for augmentative communication services. Paper presented at the annual meeting of the American Speech-Language-Hearing Association, Seattle.

Lavoy, R. W. (1957). Rick's communicator. *Exceptional Child,* 23, 338–340.

Lawrence, P. D., & Horne, S. J. (1979). Input modes: Their importance in the clinical application of electronic aids for disabled persons. *Archives of Physical Medicine and Rehabilitation,* 60, 516–521.

Lawrence-Dederich, S. M., Kelly, C., McNaughton, S., & Higginbotham, D.J. (1992). A case study of assessment and transition issues. Paper presented at the annual meeting of the American Speech-Language-Hearing Association, San Antonio.

Layton, T. L. (1988). Language training with autistic children using four different modes of presentation. *Journal of Communication Disorders,* 21(4), 333–350.

Layton, T. L., & Baker, P. S. (1981). Description of semantic-syntactic relations in an autistic child. *Journal of Autistic and Developmental Disorders,* 11, 385–399.

Leathers, D. (1986). *Successful Nonverbal Communication: Principles and Applications.* New York: Macmillan.

Lebeis, S., & Lebeis, R. F. (1975). The use of signed communication with the normal-hearing, nonverbal mentally retarded. *Bureau Memorandum* (Wisconsin Department of Public Instruction), 17(1), 28–30.

Le Cardinal, G., Legrand, C., & Guyonnet, J.-F. (1986). Systematic model of interpersonal communication applied to analyze the communication problems of handicapped persons. *Augmentative and Alternative Communication,* 2, 96–97.

Lee, B. E., & Fina, R. B. (1985). Augmentative communication systems for tracheostomy patients. Paper presented at the annual meeting of the American Speech-Language-Hearing Association, Washington, DC.

Lee, K., & Thomas D. (1990). *Control of Computer-based Technology for People with Physical Disabilities: An Assessment Manual.* Toronto: University of Toronto Press.

Lee, K., Thomas, D., Balfour, L., & Parnes, P. (1988). Selecting access systems for persons with disabilities. *Augmentative and Alternative Communication,* 4, 162.

Legrand, C., & Le Cardinal, G. (1986). Proposition for a diagrammatic assessment of augmentative and alternative communication of a user's daily life. *Augmentative and Alternative Communication,* 2, 97.

Leibel, J., Pettet, A., & Webster, C. D. (1974). *Two Behavior Modification Approaches to the Treatment of Autistic Children: Simultaneous Communications vs. Vocal Imitation* (Substudy 74-7). Distributed by Clarke Institute of Psychiatry, Toronto.

Leins, J. D., & Coleman, C. L. (1950). Interaction/training construction set. *Augmentative and Alternative Communication,* 4, 150.

Leite, J., & Hotchkiss, K. (1988). Of dreams and discoveries. *Augmentative and Alternative Communication,* 4, 161.

Lennon, A., DeBaun, P., Reeves, R., & Romski, M. A. (1990). Augmentative communication programs in Georgia. Paper presented at the annual meeting of the American Speech-Language-Hearing Association, Seattle.

Leonhart, W., & Maharaj, S. (1979). A comparison of initial recognition and rate of acquisition of pictogram ideogram communication (PIC) and Bliss symbols with institutionalized severely retarded adults. Unpublished manuscript.

Le Prevost, P. (1983). Using the Makaton Vocabulary in early language training with a Down's baby: A case study. *Mental Handicap*, 11, 28–29.

Lestz, N. M., Constance, J. E., Davies, P. L., & Noller, K. M. (1985). Augmentative communication evaluation: An integrated team approach. Paper presented at the annual meeting of the American Speech-Language-Hearing Association, Washington, DC.

Levett, L. M. (1969). A method of communication for nonspeaking, severely subnormal children. *British Journal of Disorders of Communication*, 4, 64–66.

Levett, L. M. (1971a). Discovering how mime can help. *Special Education*, 60, 17–19.

Levett, L. M. (1971b). A method of communication for nonspeaking, severely subnormal children—Trial results. *British Journal of Disorders of Communication*, 6, 125–128.

Levin, J., & Scherfenberg, L. (1988). *Selection and Use of Simple Technology in Home, School, Work, and Community Settings*. Wauconda, IL: Don Johnson Developmental Equipment.

Levine, S. H., & Goodenough-Trepagnier, C. (1990). Customized text-entry devices for motor-impaired users. *Applied Ergonomics*, 23(1), 55–62.

Levine, S. P., Gauger, J. R. D., Bowers, L. D., & Khan, K. J. (1986). A comparison of mouth-stick and Morse code text inputs. *Augmentative and Alternative Communication*, 2(2), 51–55.

Lidén, M., & Olsson, C. (1990). The symbol bank. *Augmentative and Alternative Communication*, 6, 148.

Light, J. (1984). The communicative interaction patterns of young nonspeaking physically disabled children and their primary caregivers. Master's thesis, University of Toronto.

Light, J. (1988). Interaction involving individuals using augmentative and alternative communication systems: State of the art and future directions. *Augmentative and Alternative Communication*, 4, 66–82.

Light, J. (1989a). Encoding techniques for augmentative communication systems: An investigation of the recall performance of nonspeaking physically disabled adults. Unpublished doctoral dissertation, University of Toronto.

Light, J. (1989b). Toward a definition of communicative competence for individuals using augmentative and alternative communication systems. *Augmentative and Alternative Communication*, 5, 137–144.

Light, J., Beesley, M., & Collier, B. (1988). Transition through multiple augmentative and alternative communication systems: A three-year case study of a head injured adolescent. *Augmentative and Alternative Communication*, 4, 2–14.

Light, J., & Binger, C. (1992). Story reading experiences of preschoolers using AAC systems. *Augmentative and Alternative Communication*, 8, 148.

Light, J., & Collier, B. (1986). Facilitating the development of effective intervention strategies by nonspeaking, physically disabled children. In Sarah W. Blackstone (Ed.), *Augmentative Communication: An Introduction*. Rockville, MD: American Speech-Language-Hearing Association, pp. 369–375.

Light, J., Collier, B., & Parnes, P. (1985a). Communicative interaction between young non-speaking physically disabled children and their primary caregivers: Part I. Discourse patterns. *Augmentative and Alternative Communication*, 1(2), 74–83.

Light, J., Collier, B., & Parnes, P. (1985b). Communicative interaction between young non-speaking physically disabled children and their primary caregivers: Part II. Communicative function. *Augmentative and Alternative Communication*, 1(3), 98–107.

Light, J., Collier, B., & Parnes, P. (1985c). Communicative interaction between young non-speaking physically disabled children and their primary caregivers: Part III. Modes of communication. *Augmentative and Alternative Communication*, 1(4), 125–133.

Light, J., Collier, B., Smith, A. K., Norris, L., Parnes, P., Rothschild, N., & Woodall, S. (1988). Developing the foundations of communicative competence with users of augmentative and alternative communication systems. *Augmentative and Alternative Communication*, 4, 148.

Light, J., Dattilo, J., English, J., Gutierrez, L., & Hartz, J. (1992). Instructing facilitators to support the communication of people who use augmentative communication systems. *Journal of Speech and Hearing Research*, 35, 865–875.

Light, J., Dattilo, J., & St. Peters, S. (1992). Leisure and social participation patterns of youth using AAC systems. *Augmentative and Alternative Communication*, 8, 147–148.

Light, J., Johnston, K. A., Lordo, L., & Schober, M. A. (1992). Interaction between peers using AAC systems. *Augmentative and Alternative Communication*, 8, 148.

Light, J., & Kelford-Smith, A. (in press). The home literacy experiences of preschoolers who use augmentative communication systems and their nondisabled peers. *Augmentative and Alternative Communication*.

Light, J., & Lindsay, P. (1991a). Cognitive science and augmentative and alternative communication. *Augmentative and Alternative Communication*, 7, 186–203.

Light, J., & Lindsay, P. (1991b), Developing a research base for understanding the demands of message encoding techniques: A response to Bray and Goossens' (1991). *Augmentative and Alternative Communication*, 7, 293–294.

Light, J., & Lindsay, P. (1992). Message-encoding techniques for augmentative communication systems: The recall performances of adults with severe speech impairments. *Journal of Speech and Hearing Research*, 35, 853–864.

Light, J., Lindsay, P., Siegel, L., & Parnes, P. (1990). The effects of message encoding techniques on recall by literate adults using AAC systems. *Augmentative and Alternative Communication*, 6, 184–201.

Light, J., McNaughton, D., & Parnes, P. (1986a). A communication assessment profile for nonspeaking severely and profoundly developmentally handicapped adults and their facilitators. *Augmentative and Alternative Communication*, 2, 97.

Light, J., McNaughton, D., & Parnes, P. (1986b). *A Protocol for the Assessment of the Communication Interaction Skills of Nonspeaking Severely Handicapped Adults and Their Facilitators*. Toronto: Augmentative Communication Service, Hugh MacMillan Medical Centre.

Light, J., Parnes, P., Lindsay, P., & Siegel, L. (1988). The information processing demands for message encoding techniques. *Augmentative and Alternative Communication*, 4, 158.

Light, J., Rothschild, N., & Parnes, P. (1985). The effect of communication interaction with nonspeaking physically disabled children. Paper presented at the annual meeting of the American Speech-Language-Hearing Association, Washington, DC.

Light, J., & Smith, A. K. (1993). Home literacy experiences of preschoolers who use AAC systems and of their nondisabled peers. *Augmentative and Alternative Communication*, 9, 10–25.

Light, J., Smith, A. K., & McNaughton, D. (1990). The literacy experiences of preschoolers who use augmentative and alternative communication systems. *Augmentative and Alternative Communication*, 6, 132.

Light, P., Watson, J., & Remington, B. (1990). Beyond the single sign: The significance of sign order in a matrix-based approach to teaching productive sign combinations. *Mental Handicap Research*, 3(2), 161–178.

Lindblom, B. (1990). On the communication process: Speaker-listener interaction and the development of speech. *Augmentative and Alternative Communication*, 6, 220–230.

Lindberg, B., & Hook, O. (1974). Communication aid for patients with anarthria. *Scandinavian Journal of Rehabilitation Medicine*, 6, 102–103.

Lindsay, P. H., Cambria, R. J., & McNaughton, S. (1986). The educational needs of nonspeaking students and their teachers or primary caregivers. *Augmentative and Alternative Communication*, 2, 97–98.

Lindsay, P. H., Cambria, R. J., McNaughton, S., & Warrick, A. (1986). The educational needs of nonspeaking students and their teachers. Paper presented at the fourth biennial conference of the International Society for Augmentative and Alternative Communication, Cardiff, Wales.

Lindsay, P. H., McNaughton, S., & Gibson, N. (1990). Developing support services for educating nonspeaking students. *Augmentative and Alternative Communication*, 6, 114.

Lindsay, P. H., McNaughton, S., Vanderveiden, M., Ellis, V., Krogh, K., & McNamara, A. (1992). A model of literacy acquisition in the AAC user. *Augmentative and Alternative Communication*, 8, 148–149.

Linville, S. E. (1977). Signed English: A language teaching technique with totally nonverbal severely mentally retarded adolescents. *Language, Speech, and Hearing Services in Schools*, 8, 170–175.

Lipinski, J. P., Hoodin, R. B., & Gorenflo, C. W. (1991). Effectiveness of a communication in nonfluent aphasia. Paper presented at the annual meeting of the American Speech-Language-Hearing Association, Atlanta.

Lipschultz, R. W., & Shane, H. C. (1981). Characterizing institutionalized nonspeaking persons: Identifying potential augmentative communication users. Paper presented at the annual meeting of the American Speech-Language-Hearing Association, Los Angeles.

Lipschultz, S., & Shane, H. C. (1980). *Assessment Procedures for Nonspeaking Persons* (Experimental Edition). Boston: Communication Enhancement Clinic, Children's Hospital.

Lister, P. F., Calder, D. J., & Watson, J. D. M. (1986). Large vocabulary synthesized speech aids for the vocally handicapped. *Augmentative and Alternative Communication*, 2, 98.

Livesay, L. L., Friedman-Hanna, K., & Seigel-Hershfield, K. (1989). Augmentative communication in TBI: A diagnostic-therapeutic approach. Paper presented at the annual meeting of the American Speech-Language-Hearing Association, St. Louis.

Lloyd, L. L. (Ed.) (1976). *Communication Assessment and Intervention Strategies*. Baltimore: University Park Press.

Lloyd, L. L. (1980a). Nonspeech communication: Discussant's comments. In B. Urban (Ed.), *Proceedings of the 18th Congress of the International Association of Logopedics and Phoniatrics*. Vol. II. Rockville, MD: American Speech-Language-Hearing Association, pp. 43–48.

Lloyd, L. L. (1980b). Unaided nonspeech communication for severely handicapped individuals: An extensive bibliography. *Education and Training of the Mentally Retarded*, 15, 15–34.

Lloyd, L. L. (1982). Symbol and initial lexicon selection. *Proceedings of the Second Interna-*

tional Conference on Non-Speech Communication. Toronto: Ontario Institute for Studies in Education, pp. 9–15.

Lloyd, L. L. (1985). Comments on terminology. *Augmentative and Alternative Communication*, 1, 95–97.

Lloyd, L. L. (1986). Augmentative/alternative communication symbols: Recent developments and research issues. *Augmentative and Alternative Communication*, 2, 99.

Lloyd, L. L., & Blischak, D. M. (1992). AAC terminology policy and issues update. *Augmentative and Alternative Communication*, 8, 104–109.

Lloyd, L. L., & Cregan, A. (1984). Sigsymbols: Simplified graphic symbols conceptually linked with manual signs. *Asha*, 26 (10), 90.

Lloyd, L. L., & Daniloff, J. K. (1983). Issues in using Amer-Ind Code with retarded persons. In T. Gallagher & C. Prutting (Eds.), *Pragmatic Issues: Assessment and Intervention.* Houston: College Hill Press.

Lloyd, L. L., & Fuller, D. R. (1986). Toward an augmentative and alternative communication symbol taxonomy: A proposed superordinate classification. *Augmentative and Alternative Communication*, 2(4), 165–171.

Lloyd, L. L., & Fuller, D. R. (1990). The role of iconicity in augmentative and alternative communication-symbol learning. In W. I. Fraser (Ed.), *Key Issues in Mental Retardation Research.* London: Routledge.

Lloyd, L. L., & Kangas, K. A. (1988a). AAC terminology policy and issues. *Augmentative and Alternative Communication*, 4, 54–57.

Lloyd, L. L., & Kangas, K. A. (1988b). To print or not to print: Writing for AAC. *Augmentative and Alternative Communication*, 4, 147.

Lloyd, L. L., & Kangas, K. A., (1990). AAC policy and issues update. *Augmentative and Alternative Communication*, 6, 167–170.

Lloyd, L. L., & Karlan, G. R. (1984). Non-speech communication symbols and systems: Where have we been and where are we going? *Journal of Mental Deficiency Research*, 28 (Part 1), 3–20.

Lloyd, L. L., Quist, R. W., & Windsor, J. (1990). A proposed augmentative and alternative communication model. *Augmentative and Alternative Communication*, 6, 172–183.

Lloyd, L. L., van Balkom, H., Cregan, A., Fuller, D. R., Jennische, M., Johnsen, B., Lindsay, P. H., McNaughton, S., Schlosser, R. W., Steele, R., & Donker-Gimbrere, M. W. (1992). Graphic symbols: Clinical/educational and research issues. *Augmentative and Alternative Communication*, 8, 149.

Locke, P. A., & Feeley, K. (1992). Effects of voice output on symbol acquisition. *Augmentative and Alternative Communication*, 8, 149.

Locke, P. A., & Mirenda, P. (1988). A computer-supported communication approach for a child with severe communication, visual, and cognitive impairments: A case study. *Augmentative and Alternative Communication*, 4, 15–22.

Locke, P. A., & Mirenda, P. (1992). Roles and responsibilities of special education teachers serving on teams delivering AAC services. *Augmentative and Alternative Communication*, 8, 200–214.

Loeding, B. L. (1988). A scoring system for evaluation of manual sign production. *Augmentative and Alternative Communication*, 4, 149.

Loeding, B. L. (1989). Effects of symmetry and associative stories on manual sign acquisition. Paper presented at the annual meeting of the American Speech-Language-Hearing Association, St. Louis.

Loeding, B. L., Zangari, C., & Lloyd, L. L. (1990). A "working party" approach to planning inservice training in manual communication for an entire public school staff. *Augmentative and Alternative Communication*, 6, 38–49.

Logan, J., Pisoni, D., & Greene, B. (1985). Measuring the segmental intelligibility of synthetic speech: Results from eight text-to-speech systems. *Research on Speech Perception. Progress Report No. 11.* Bloomington: Indiana University.

Lohr, M. J. (1992). Assisting the transition from spelling to speed enhancement software. *Augmentative and Alternative Communication*, 8, 149.

Lombardino, L., & Langley, M. B. (1989). Strategies for assessing severely multihandicapped children for augmentative and alternative communication. *European Journal of Special Needs Education*, 4, 157–170.

Lombardino, L. J., Willems, S., & MacDonald, J. D. (1981). Critical considerations in total communication and an environmental intervention model for the developmentally delayed. *Exceptional Children*, 47(6), 455–461.

Loncke, F., Nijs, M., & Smet, L. (1992). Modality influences in AAC using manual signs. *Augmentative and Alternative Communication*, 8, 149–150.

Lopes, C. M., & Launer, P. B. (1986). For all intents and purposes: Functional communication in nonspeaking children. *Augmentative and Alternative Communication*, 2, 99–100.

Lorencic, M. (1990). Alternative modes of communication [in Yugoslavia]. *Augmentative and Alternative Communication*, 6, 117.

Lorowitz, L., Plotnick, C., & Belloff, T. (1992). Facilitating communication in the home: A parent-child approach. *Augmentative and Alternative Communication*, 8, 150.

Lossing, C. (1981). A technique for the quantification of non-vocal communicative performance by listeners. Unpublished master's thesis, University of Washington.

Lossing, C., Yorkston, K., & Beukelman, D. (1985). Communication augmentation systems: Quantification in natural settings. *Archives of Physical Medicine and Rehabilitation*, 66, 380–384.

Lowe, H., Churchill, T., Gosling, T., & Battison, D. (1974). Lightwriter. In Keith Copeland (Ed.), *Aids for the Severely Handicapped.* New York: Grune & Stratton, pp. 109–115.

Lowman, E. W., & Klinger, J. A. (1969). *Aids to Independent Living: Self-Help for the Handicapped.* New York: McGraw-Hill.

Lubinski, R. (Ed.) (1991). *Dementia and Communication.* Philadelphia: B. C. Decker.

Lubinski, R., & Frattali, C. (January 1993). Nursing home reform: The Resident Assessment Instrument. *Asha*, 35(1), 59–62.

Lucas, E. V., & Dean, M. B. (1976). An alternative approach to oral communication for an autistic child. Videotape presented at the annual meeting of the American Speech-Language-Hearing Association, Houston.

Luftig, R. L. (1982). Increasing probability of sign language learning by severely mentally retarded individuals: A discussion of learner, sign production, and linguistic variables. *Applied Research in Mental Retardation*, 3(1), 81–97.

Luftig, R. L. (1983). Manual sign translucency and referential concreteness in the sign learning of moderately/severely mentally retarded students. *American Journal of Mental Deficiency*, 88, 279–286.

Luftig, R. L. (1984). An analysis of initial sign lexicons as a function of eight learnability variables. *Journal of the Association for Persons with Severe Handicaps.* 9, 193–200.

Luftig, R. L., & Bersani, H. A. (1985a). An initial investigation of the effects of translucency, transparency, and component complexity of Blissymbolics. *Journal of Childhood Communication Disorders*, 8, 191–209.

Luftig, R. L., & Bersani, Jr., H. A. (1985b). An investigation of two variables influencing

Blissymbol learnability with nonhandicapped adults. *Augmentative and Alternative Communication*, 1(1), 32–37.

Luftig, R. L., Gauthier, R. A., Freeman, S. A., & Lloyd, L. L. (1980). Modality preference and facilitation of learning using mixed and pure sign, oral and graphic inputs. *Sign Language Studies*, 28, 255–266.

Luftig, R. L., & Lloyd, L. L. (1981), Manual sign translucency and referential concreteness in the learning of signs. *Sign Language Studies*, 30, 49–60. √

Luftig, R. L., Lloyd, L. L., & Page, J. L. (1982). Ratings of sign translucency and gloss concreteness of two grammatical classes of signs. *Sign Language Studies*, 37, 305–343.

Luftig, R. L., Page, J. L., & Lloyd, L. L. (1983). Ratings of perceived translucency in manual signs as a predictor of sign learnability. *Journal of Childhood Communication Disorders*, 6, 117–134.

Lundälv, M., & Olsson, E. (1990). Exercises with "PLOCKA": A demonstration of and discussion around the possibilities offered by an authoring and enabling tool aimed at severely handicapped children. *Augmentative and Alternative Communication*, 6, 125.

Lundälv, M., & Poon, P. (1990). The Comspec Project: Specifications for a versatile communication aid. *Augmentative and Alternative Communication*, 6, 149.

Lundman, M. (1990). Electronic mail and computer conferencing: Close contact through distant means? *Augmentative and Alternative Communication*, 6, 128–129.

Lundman, M., & Magnusson, M. (1988). Computer conferencing—A new medium for nonspeakers. *Augmentative and Alternative Communication*, 4, 142.

Lundman, M., Teneholtz, E., & Galyas, K. (1978). *Technical Aids for the Speech-Impaired: Proposal for Research and Development Activities*. Bromma, Sweden: Handikappinstitute.

Luster, M. J. (1974). *Preliminary Selected Bibliography of Articles, Brochures, and Books Related to Communication Techniques and Aids for the Severely Handicapped*. Madison, WI: Trace Research and Development Center for the Severely Communicatively Handicapped, University of Wisconsin.

Luster, M. J., & Vanderheiden, G. C. (1974a). *Preliminary Annotated Bibliography of Communication Aids*. Madison, WI: Trace Research and Development Center for the Severely Communicatively Handicapped, University of Wisconsin.

Luster, M. J., & Vanderheiden, G. C. (1974b). *Preliminary Annotated Bibliography of Researchers and Institutions*. Madison: Trace Research and Development Center for the Severely Communicatively Handicapped, University of Wisconsin.

Lykos, C. M. (1971). *Cued Speech: Handbook for Teachers*. Washington, DC: Gallaudet College Cued Speech Program.

Lyon, J., & Helm-Estabrooks, N. (1987). Drawing: Its communicative significance for expressively restricted aphasic adults. *Topics in Language Disorders*, 8, 61–71.

Lyon, S. R., & Ross, L. E. (1984). Comparison scan training and the matching and scanning performance of severely and profoundly mentally retarded students. *Applied Research in Mental Retardation*, 5, 439–449.

Lytton, R. (1992). Informed consent: Role of the consumer in AAC evaluations. *Augmentative and Alternative Communication*, 8, 150.

Lytton, R., Carlson, J. H., De Silva, A., Glass, J., Lake, K., & Pensa, D. (1987). Fostering child-adult communicative interaction in the classroom. Intervention strategy developed under Contract No. 300-85-0139 (*Implementation Strategies for Improving the Use of Communication Aids in Schools Serving Handicapped Children*) from the U.S. Department of Education distributed by the American Speech-Language-Hearing Association.

Lytton, R., Carlson, J. H., De Silva, A., Glass, J., Lake, K., & Pensa, D. (1987). Fostering child-child communicative interaction in the classroom. Intervention strategy developed under Contract No. 300-85-0139 (*Implementation Strategies for Improving the Use of Communication Aids in Schools Serving Handicapped Children*) from the U.S. Department of Education distributed by the American Speech-Language-Hearing Association.

Lywood, D. W., & Vasa, J. J. (1974). A brief survey and classification of available systems. Paper presented at the Seminar on Electronic Controls for the Severely Disabled, Vancouver, British Columbia. (Paper is published in the seminar proceedings volume, pp. 7–11.)

MacDonald, A. (1990). Enhancing the social skills of Blissymbolics users through Minspeak. *Augmentative and Alternative Communication*, 6, 104.

MacDonald, B.-J., & Olynyk, P. (1986), A model for software development. *Augmentative and Alternative Communication*, 2, 101.

MacDonald, J. (1985). Language through conversation: A model for intervention with language-delayed persons. In S. Warren & A. Rogers-Warren (Eds.), *Teaching Functional Language: Generalization and Maintenance of Language Skills*. Austin, TX: Pro-Ed, pp. 89–122.

MacDonald, J., & Gillette, Y. (1986a). Communicating with persons with severe handicaps: Role of parents and professionals. *Journal of the Association for Persons with Severe Handicaps*, 11, 255–265.

MacDonald, J., & Gillette, Y. (1986b). *Ecological Communication Systems (ECO)*. Columbus: Nisonger Center, Ohio State University.

MacDonald, J., Gillette, Y., Bickley, M., & Rodrigues, C. (1984). *Conversation Routines*. Columbus: Ohio State University.

MacDonald, S., & Howey, A. (1992). Education in isolation. *Augmentative and Alternative Communication*, 8, 150–151.

MacGillivray, J., Del, P. C., Evans, A. L., & Smith, D. C. (1984). An aid to visual pointing for children with severe physical handicap. *Journal of Medical Engineering and Technology*, 8(4), 184–185.

MacKinnon, E. (1990). Considerations for mounting communication systems: Customizing and compromising! *Augmentative and Alternative Communication*, 6, 149.

MacKinnon, E., & Elder, S. B. (1988). Staying current in augmentative and alternative communication. *Augmentative and Alternative Communication*, 4, 141.

MacKinnon, E., & King, J. S. (1992). Service delivery via electronic mail for individuals with physical disabilities. *Augmentative and Alternative Communication*, 8, 151.

Macleod, I. (1981). Information processing aids for physically handicapped people. *Australian Nurses Journal*, 10(6), 46–53.

MacNeela, J. C. (1987). An overview of therapeutic positioning for multiply-handicapped persons, including augmentative communication users. *Physical and Occupational Therapy in Pediatrics*, 7(2), 39–60.

Magnuson, T., & Hunnicutt, S. (1990). Measuring the effect of a word processor with prediction. *Augmentative and Alternative Communication*, 6, 94–95.

Magnuson, T., & Hunnicutt, S. (1992). Swedish word prediction: A follow-up investigation. *Augmentative and Alternative Communication*, 8, 151.

Magnússon, J. H. (1990). Experience with the ISBLISS symbolic-processing program as a written communication aid. *Augmentative and Alternative Communication*, 6, 129.

Magnússon, M. (1982). Mina ord i bild-fallstudie av Blis [My words in pictures: Case study in Bliss]. Broma, Sweden: Handikappinstitutet.

Maharaj, S. (1980). *Pictogram Ideogram Communication*. Regina, Canada: George Reed

Foundation for the Handicapped. [May be obtained from the Pictogram Centre, Saskatchewan Association of Rehabilitation Centres, Saskatoon, Sask., Canada.]

Makarushka, M. (October 6, 1991). The words they can't say. *New York Times Magazine*, pp. 32, 33, 36, 70. [Deals with facilitated communication.]

Makohon, L., & Fredericks, H. (1985). *Teaching Expressive and Receptive Language to Students with Moderate and Severe Handicaps*. Austin, TX: Pro-Ed.

Malanga, P., & Poling, A. (1992). Letter recognition by adults with mental handicaps: Improving performance through differential outcomes. *Developmental Disabilities Bulletin*, 20(2), 39–48.

Maling, R. G. (1974). Control systems—Concept and development (POSSUM). In Keith Copeland (Ed.), *Aids for the Severely Handicapped*. New York: Grune & Stratton, pp. 22–30.

Maling, R. G., & Clarkson, D. C. (1963). Electronic controls for the tetraplegic (Possum) (patient operated selector mechanism—P.O.S.M.). *Paraplegia*, 1, 161–174.

Manji, S. (1992). Educating partners in strategies for interacting with AAC users: Training videotape. *Augmentative and Alternative Communication*, 8, 151.

Manji, S., McGinnis, J., & Warrick, A. (1992). Effect of a voice output communication aid on interaction patterns and partners. *Augmentative and Alternative Communication*, 8, 152.

Mann, A., Morroni, K., Gamber, A., Vernion, J., & Pighetti, C. D. (1986). The assessment and functional use of four augmentative communication devices—A video presentation. *Augmentative and Alternative Communication*, 2, 103.

Mann, K. (1988). Accessing literacy: A whole language approach for augmentative and alternative communicators. *Augmentative and Alternative Communication*, 4, 164.

Marriner, N., Beukelman, D., Wilson, W., & Ross, A. (1988). Implementing Morse code in an augmentative communication system for ten nonspeaking individuals. Unpublished manuscript, University of Washington, Seattle.

Marshall, N. R., & Hegrenes, J. (1972). The use of written language as a communication system for an autistic child. *Journal of Speech and Hearing Disorders*, 37, 258–261.

Marvin, C., Beukelman, D., & Vanderhoof, D. (1991). Vocabulary use patterns by preschool children in home and school contexts. Unpublished manuscript, University of Washington, Seattle.

Massey, H. (1988). Language-impaired children's comprehension of synthetic speech. *Language, Speech, and Hearing Services in Schools*, 19, 401–409.

Matas, J. A., & Beukelman, D. (1989). Teaching Morse code as an augmentative communication technique: Learner and instructor performance. Unpublished manuscript, University of Washington, Seattle.

Matas, J. A., Mathy-Laikko, P., Beukelman, D. R., & Legresley, K. (1985). Identifying the nonspeaking population: A demographic study. *Augmentative and Alternative Communication*, 1(1), 17–31.

Matas, J. A., White, K. M., & Watson, L. (1988). Implementing microcomputers in the schools: One district's solution. *Augmentative and Alternative Communication*, 4, 171–172.

Mathy-Laikko, P. A. (1992). Comprehensibility of AAC output methods. Paper presented at the annual meeting of the American Speech-Language-Hearing Association, San Antonio.

Mathy-Laikko, P. A., & Coxson, L. (1984). Listener reactions to augmentative communication system output modes. Paper presented at the annual meeting of the American Speech-Language-Hearing Association, San Francisco.

Mathy-Laikko, P. A., & Iacono, T. A. (1988). Training a deaf-blind multihandicapped child to use a tactile augmentative and alternative communication device. *Augmentative and Alternative Communication*, 4, 163.

Mathy-Laikko, P. A., Iacono, T. A., Ratcliff, A., Villarruel, F., Yoder, D., & Vanderheiden, G. (1989). Teaching a child with multiple disabilities to use a tactile augmentative communication device. *Augmentative and Alternative Communication*, 5, 249–256.

Mathy-Laikko, P. A., Ratcliff, A. E., Villarruel, F., & Yoder, D. E. (1987). Augmentative communication systems. In M. Bullis (Ed.), *Communication Development in Young Children with Deaf-Blindness: Literature Review III*. Monmouth, OR: Communication Skills Center for Young Children with Deaf-Blindness, Teaching Research Division, Oregon State System of Higher Education, pp. 205–241.

Mathy-Laikko, P. A., & Yoder, D. E. (1986). Future needs and directions in augmentative communication. In Sarah W. Blackstone (Ed.), *Augmentative Communication: An Introduction*. Rockville, MD: American Speech-Language-Hearing Association, pp. 471–493.

Mathy-Laikko, P. A., Zellhofer, C. M., & Jones, R. S. (1990). Comparison of two keystroke saving strategies. Paper presented at the annual meeting of the American Speech-Language-Hearing Association, Seattle.

Matson, J. L., Manikam, R., Doe, D., Raymond, K. & Taras, M. (1988). Training social skills to severely mentally retarded multiply handicapped adolescents. *Research in Developmental Disabilities*, 9(2), 195–208.

Mayberry, R. (1976). If a chimp can learn sign language, surely my nonverbal client can too. *Asha*, 18, 223–228.

Mayer-Johnson Co. (1989). *Boardmaker*. Solana Beach, CA: Author.

Mayer-Johnson Co. (1990). *Talking Symbols*. Solana Beach, CA: Author.

McAfee, P. H., Napper, S.A., & Robey, B. L. (1988). An expert system for prescription of augmentative and alternative communication devices. *Augmentative and Alternative Communication*, 4, 155.

McBride, T., & Blau, A. (1985). A letter to our nonspeaking friends. *Communicating Together*, 3(3), 4–6.

McCartney, N., Odell, S., & McNaughton, S. (1988). Blissymbol strategies as the relate to voice output communication aids. *Augmentative and Alternative Communication*, 4, 168.

McCarus, C. J. (1986). Teaching awareness of feelings in mentally impaired students via augmentative communication systems. *Augmentative and Alternative Communication*, 2, 100.

McClennen, S., & Gabel, S. (1992). Family use of facilitated communication following introduction. *Augmentative and Alternative Communication*, 8, 152.

McCormack, J. E., & Chalmers, A. J. (1978). *Early Cognitive Instruction for the Moderately and Severely Handicapped*. Champaign, IL: Research Press.

McDonald, A. (1984). Blissymbolics and manual sign: A combined approach. *Communicating Together*, 2(4), 20–21.

McDonald, E. T. (1976a). Conventional symbols of English. In Gregg C. Vanderheiden and Kate Grilley (Eds.), *Non-vocal Communication Techniques and Aids for the Severely Physically Handicapped*. Baltimore: University Park Press, pp. 77–84.

McDonald, E. T. (1976b). Design and application of communication boards. In Gregg C. Vanderheiden & Kate Grilley (Eds.), *Non-vocal Communication Techniques and Aids for the Severely Physically Handicapped*. Baltimore: University Park Press, pp. 105–119.

McDonald, E. T. (1976c). Identification of children at risk. In Gregg C. Vanderheiden & Kate Grilley (Eds.), *Non-vocal Communication Techniques and Aids for the Severely Physically Handicapped*. Baltimore: University Park Press, pp. 12–15.

McDonald, E. T. (1980a). Early identification and treatment of children at risk for speech development. In R. L. Schiefelbusch (Ed.), *Nonspeech Language and Communication: Analysis and Intervention*. Baltimore: University Park Press, pp. 49–79.

McDonald, E. T. (1980b). *Teaching and Using Blissymbolics*. Toronto: Blissymbolics Communication Institute.

McDonald, E. T. (1984). Blissymbolics and manual signing. *Communicating Together*, 2(4), 20–21.

McDonald, E. T. (1987). *Treating Cerebral Palsy: For Clinicians by Clinicians*. Austin, TX: Pro-Ed.

McDonald, E. T., & Schultz, A. R. (1973). Communication boards for cerebral palsied children. *Journal of Speech and Hearing Disorders*, 38, 73–78.

McDonald, J., Schwejda, P., Marriner, N., Wilson, W., & Ross, A. (1982). Advantages of Morse code as a computer input for school-aged children with physical disability. *Computers and the Handicapped*. Ottawa: National Research Council of Canada, pp. 95–106.

McEntee, M. K. (1985). The sign parameters and sign acquisition in the mentally retarded. Paper presented at the annual meeting of the American Speech-Language-Hearing Association, Washington, DC.

McEwen, I. R. (1992). Positioning for optimal AAC use: Practical application of the research. *Augmentative and Alternative Communication*, 8, 152–153.

McEwen, I. R., & Karlan, G. R. (1988). Effect of position on communication board use. *Augmentative and Alternative Communication*, 4, 157.

McEwen, I. R., & Karlan, G. R. (1989). Assessment of effects of position on communication board access by individuals with cerebral palsy. *Augmentative and Alternative Communication*, 5, 235–242.

McEwen, I. R., & Karlan, G. R. (1990). Case studies: Why and how. *Augmentative and Alternative Communication*, 6, 69–75.

McEwen, I. R., & Lloyd, L. L. (1990a). Positioning students with cerebral palsy to use augmentative and alternative communication. *Language, Speech, and Hearing Services in Schools*, 21, 15–21.

McEwen, I. R., & Lloyd, L. L. (1990b). Some considerations about the motor requirements of manual signs. *Augmentative and Alternative Communication*, 6, 207–216.

McFadden, G., & Rothschild, N. (1986). The Prism Communication Device—One solution to increasing vocabulary space. *Augmentative and Alternative Communication*, 2, 101.

McCormack, D. J. (1990). The effects of keyguard use and pelvic positioning on typing speed and accuracy in a boy with cerebral palsy. *American Journal of Occupational Therapy*, 44, 312–315.

McGaffey, C., Wolfus, B., & McPhail, P. (1988). An augmentative and alternative training methodology with a multihandicapped adult. *Augmentative and Alternative Communication*, 4, 162.

McGann, W. M., & Paslawski, T. M. (1991). Incomplete locked-in syndrome: Two cases with successful communication outcomes. *American Journal of Speech-Language Pathology*, 1(1), 32–37.

McGinnis, J. S. (1991). Development of two source lists for vocabulary selection in augmentative communication: Documentation of the spoken and written vocabulary of third grade students. Unpublished doctoral dissertation, University of Nebraska, Lincoln.

McGinnis, J. S., & Beukelman, D. R. (1989). Vocabulary requirements for writing activities for the academically mainstreamed student with disabilities. *Augmentative and Alternative Communication*, 5, 183–191.

McGregor, A., & Alm, N. (1953). Thoughts of a nonspeaking member of an AAC research team. *Augmentative and Alternative Communication*, 8, 153.

McGregor, G., & Fraser, B. A. (1992). Physical characteristics assessment: Computer access for individuals with cerebral palsy. *Augmentative and Alternative Communication*, 8, 153.

McGregor, G., Young, J., Gerak, J., Thomas, B., & Vogelsberg, R. T. (1992). Increasing functional use of an assistive communication device by a student with severe disabilities. *Augmentative and Alternative Communication*, 8, 243–250.

McGuire, M. P., Wegner, J., & Molineaux, B. (1992). The communicative competence of augmentative device users with different partners. Paper presented at the annual meeting of the American Speech-Language-Hearing Association, San Antonio.

McGuire, T. J., Palaganas-Tosco, A., & Redford, J. B. (1988). Dystonia musculorum deformans: Three cases treated on a rehabilitation unit. *Archives of Physical Medicine and Rehabilitation*, 69(5), 373–376.

McIlvane, W. J., Bass, R. W., O'Brien, J. M., Gerovac, B. J., & Stoddard, L. T. (1984). Spoken and signed naming of foods after receptive exclusion training in severe retardation. *Applied Research in Mental Retardation*, 5, 1–27.

McKenna, P. S. (1990). Normalization/communication in a progressive democracy: What we learn from Sweden. *Augmentative and Alternative Communication*, 6, 102.

McKinlay, A., & Newell, A. F. (1992). Dialogue structures in an AAC device. *Augmentative and Alternative Communication*, 8, 153.

McLean, J. E. (1992). Facilitated communication: Some thoughts on Biklen's and Calculator's interaction. *American Journal of Speech-Language Pathology*, 1(2), 25–27.

McLean, J. E. (1993). Assuring best practices in communication for children and youth with severe disabilities. *Clinics in Communication Disorders*, 3(2), 1–6.

McLean, L. K., & McLean, J. E. (1974). A language training program for nonverbal autistic children. *Journal of Speech and Hearing Disorders*, 39, 186–194.

McLean, J. E., McLean, L. K. S., Brady, N. C., & Morris, K. (1992). Communication of individuals with severe mental retardation: Phase II direct testing. Paper presented at the annual meeting of the American Speech-Language-Hearing Association, San Antonio.

McLean, J. E., McLean, L. K. S., Brady, N. C., & Etter, R. (1991). Communication profiles of two types of gesture using nonverbal persons with severe to profound mental retardation. *Journal of Speech and Hearing Research*, 34, 294–308.

McLean, J. E., & Snyder-McLean, L. (1988). Application of pragmatics to severely mentally retarded children and youth. In R. L. Schiefelbusch & L. L. Lloyd (Eds.), *Language Perspectives: Acquisition, Retardation, and Intervention*. Austin, TX: Pro-Ed, pp. 255–288.

McNairn, P., & Shioleno, C. (1992). Literacy skills for nonspeaking childen. *Augmentative and Alternative Communication*, 8, 153.

McNaughton, D. (1988). The development of multi-component communication systems for nonspeaking children. Paper presented at the annual meeting of the American Speech-Language-Hearing Association, Boston.

McNaughton, D. (1992). Spelling instruction for adults who use AAC. *Augmentative and Alternative Communication*, 8, 153–154.

McNaughton, D., & Drynan, D. (1990). Assessment and intervention issues in written communication: A case study. *Augmentative and Alternative Communication*, 6, 137–138.

McNaughton, D., & Light, J. (1986). Strategies to facilitate communication. *Communicating Together*, 4(1), 10–11.

McNaughton, D., & Light, J. (1989). Teaching facilitators to support the communication skills of an adult with severe cognitive disabilities: A case study. *Augmentative and Alternative Communication*, 5, 35–41.

McNaughton, D., Winer, F., & Neisworth, J. (1992). Repeated listening experiences and the intellibility of synthesized speech. *Augmentative and Alternative Communication*, 8, 154.

McNaughton, S. (1975). *Symbol Secrets*. Toronto: Blissymbolics Communication Institute.

McNaughton, S. (1976a). Blissymbolics—An alternative symbol system for the non-vocal prereading child. In Gregg C. Vanderheiden & Kate Grilley (Eds.), *Non-vocal Communication Techniques and Aids for the Severely Physically Handicapped*. Baltimore: University Park Press, pp. 85–104.

McNaughton, S. (1976b). Symbol Communication Programme at OCCC. In Gregg C. Vanderheiden & Kate Grilley (Eds.), *Non-vocal Communication Techniques and Aids for the Severely Physically Handicapped*. Baltimore: University Park Press, pp. 132–143.

McNaughton, S. (1978). Electronic aids in Blissymbol communications. In P. Nelson (Ed.), *Proceedings of the Workshop on Communication Aids*. Ottawa: Canadian Medical and Biological Engineering Society, National Research Council.

McNaughton, S. (1981). *Personal Computers and Blissymbolics*. Toronto: Blissymbolics Communication International.

McNaughton, S. (1982). Augmentative communication system: Blissymbolics. In Bleck & Nagel (Eds.), *Physically Handicapped Children —A Medical Atlas for Teachers*. New York: Grune & Stratton.

McNaughton, S. (Ed.) (1985). *Communicating with Blissymbolics*. Toronto: Blissymbolics Communication International.

McNaughton, S. (1986a). An educational model relating to the graphic symbol system within augmentative communication. *Augmentative and Alternative Communication*, 2, 101–102.

McNaughton, S. (1986b). Toward an understanding of graphic system effects: An introduction. *Augmentative and Alternative Communication*, 2, 102.

McNaughton, S. (1990a). Gaining the most from AAC's growing years. *Augmentative and Alternative Communication*, 6, 2–14.

McNaughton, S. (1990b). Introducing Access Bliss. *Communicating Together*, 8(2), 12–13.

McNaughton, S. (1990c). Literacy and Blissymbolics. *Augmentative and Alternative Communication*, 6, 122.

McNaughton, S. (1990d). StoryBliss. *Communicating Together*, 8(1), 12–13.

McNaughton, S., & Kates, B. (1974). Visual symbols: Communication system for the prereading physically handicapped child. Paper presented at the annual meeting of the American Association on Mental Deficiency, Toronto.

McNaughton, S., & Kates, B. (1980). The application of Blissymbolics. In R. L. Schiefelbusch (Ed.), *Nonspeech Language and Communication: Analysis and Intervention*. Baltimore: University Park Press, pp. 303–321.

McNaughton, S., Kates, B., & Silverman, H. (1975). *Teaching Guidelines*. Toronto: Blissymbolics Communication Foundation.

McNaughton, S., Kates, B., & Silverman, H. (1976). *Provisional Dictionary: Revised Edition.* Toronto: Blissymbolics Communication Institute.

McNaughton, S., Kates, B., & Silverman, H. (1978). *Handbook of Blissymbolics.* Toronto: Blissymbolics Communication Institute.

McNaughton, S., Mann, G., Harrington, K., & Harrington, R. (1988). Learning from those who know. *Augmentative and Alternative Communication*, 4, 141.

McNaughton, S., Reid, B., Odell, S., & Harrington, K. (1988). Selecting graphics for communication boards. *Augmentative and Alternative Communication*, 4, 156.

McNaughton, S., & Seybold, K. (1990). Blissymbolics and technology. *Augmentative and Alternative Communication*, 6, 117.

McNaughton, S., & Warrick, A. (1984). Picture your Blissymbols. *Canadian Journal of Mental Retardation*, 34(4), 1–7.

McNaughton, S., & Warrick, A. (1986). An educational model for service delivery of alternative and augmentative communication in education. *Augmentative and Alternative Communication*, 2, 102–103.

McNaughton, S., & Wood, C. (1986). Blissymbol use—1986. *Augmentative and Alternative Communication*, 2, 103.

Meador, D., Rumbaugh, D., Tribble, M., & Thompson, S. (1984). Facilitating visual discrimination learning of moderately and severely mentally retarded children through illumination of stimuli. *American Journal of Mental Deficiency*, 89, 313–316.

Meir, M. (1990). HANDYCOM—A new approach to communication. *Augmentative and Alternative Communication*, 6, 125.

Meline, T. J. (1980). Teaching gestural communication to the cerebral palsied child. Paper presented at the annual meeting of the American Speech-Language-Hearing Association, Detroit.

Mendoza, A. K., & Damico, J. S. (1991). Locked-in syndrome: Implications for successful augmentation. Paper presented at the annual meeting of the American Speech-Language-Hearing Association, Atlanta.

Menyuk, P. (1974). The bases of language acquisition: Some questions. *Journal of Autism and Childhood Schizophrenia*, 4, 325–345.

Mercaitis, P. A. (1987). Clinical training issues in augmentative communication. Paper presented at the annual meeting of the American Speech-Language-Hearing Association, New Orleans.

Merchant, M. F., & Skarakis-Doyle, E. (1988). Communication board use by aphasics: A follow-up study. Paper presented at the annual meeting of the American Speech-Language-Hearing Association, Boston.

Metz, G., Horst, D., & Kruger, H. (1984). [An electronic communication aid with a large keyboard for artificial respiration patients in the intensive care unit.] *Anasth-Intensivther-Notfallmed.*, 19 (4), 204–205.

Meyer, L., Peck, C., & Brown, L. (Eds.) (1991). *Critical Issues in the Lives of People with Severe Disabilities.* Baltimore: Paul H. Brookes.

Meyers, L. F. (1983). The use of microprocessors to promote acquisition of beginning language and literacy skills in young handicapped children. *Proceedings of the American Association for the Advancement of Science Conference on Computers and the Handicapped.* Washington, DC: American Association for the Advancement of Science.

Meyers, L. F. (Ed.) (1984a). *Augmenting Language Skills with Microcomputers.* New York: Thieme-Stratton.

Meyers, L. F. (1984b). Use of microprocessors to initiate language use in young non-oral children. In W. Perkins (Ed.), *Current Therapy of Communication Disorders*. New York: Thieme-Stratton.

Meyers, L. F. (1990). Technology: A powerful tool for children learning language. *OSERS News in Print*, 3(2), 2–7.

Meyers, L. F., Grows, N., Coleman, C., & Cook, M. (1980). *An Assessment Battery for Assistive Device Systems Recommendations: Part 1*. Sacramento: Assistive Device Center, California State University.

Microprocessor based voice synthesizer puts speech at its user's fingertips (March 1977). *Digital Design*, 15–16.

Millar, S., & Joss, A. (1990). Scottish Minspeak holiday for adults—1990. *Augmentative and Alternative Communication*, 6, 150.

Miller, A., & Miller, E. E. (1973). Cognitive-developmental training with elevated boards and sign language. *Journal of Autism and Childhood Schizophrenia*, 3, 65–85.

Miller, J., & Carpenter, C. (1964). Electronics for communication. *American Journal of Occupational Therapy*, 18, 20–23.

Miller, J. F., Sedey, A., Miolo, G., Rosin, M., & Murray-Branch, J. (1991). Spoken and sign vocabulary acquisition in children with Down syndrome. Paper presented at the annual meeting of the American Speech-Language-Hearing Association, Atlanta.

Miller, L., Demasco, P., Mineo, B., & Gilliam, D. (1992). GRAPHCOM—An AAC system based on computerized photographic quality images. *Augmentative and Alternative Communication*, 8, 154.

Miller, M. S. (1987). Sign iconicity: Single-sign receptive vocabulary skills of nonsigning hearing preschoolers. *Journal of Communication Disorders*, 20, 359–365.

Miller, S. B., & Toca, J. M. (1979). Adapted melodic intonational therapy: A case study of an experimental language program for an autistic child. *Journal of Clinical Psychiatry*, 40(4), 201–203.

Mills, A. E., & van den Bogaerde, B. (1992). Input and interaction in the visual modality: Evidence from SLN. *Augmentative and Alternative Commuication*, 8, 154.

Mills, J., & Higgins, J. (1983). *Non-oral Communication Assessment and Training Guide*. Encinitas, CA: Author.

Mineo, B. A. (1988). What do symbols really symbolize? *Augmentative and Alternative Communication*, 4, 163.

Mineo, B. A. (1990a). AAC systems: Where are we and where are we going? *Augmentative and Alternative Communication*, 6, 150.

Mineo, B. A. (1990b). Augmentative communication in Delaware. Paper presented at the annual meeting of the American Speech-Language-Hearing Association, Seattle.

Mineo, B. A. (1990c). A feature-based approach to the evaluation of representational capabilities. *Augmentative and Alternative Communication*, 6, 93.

Mineo, B. A., Foulds, R. A., Demasco, P. W., Miller, L. J., & Yarrington, D. (1990). The Rehabilitation Engineering Center on Augmentative Communication. Paper presented at the annual meeting of the American Speech-Language-Hearing Association, Seattle.

Minneman, S. L. (1986). Optimization of key layouts for use with a single digit. *Augmentative and Alternative Communication*, 2, 103–104.

Minneman, S. L., & Demasco, P. W. (1986). Computer access using a multitasking approach. *Augmentative and Alternative Communication*, 2, 104–105.

Minor, E., & Robison, A. (1988). Statewide augmentative and alternative communication teams in Colorado: An innovative approach. *Augmentative and Alternative Communication, 4,* 140.

Mirenda, P. (1985). Designing pictorial communication systems for physically able-bodied students with severe handicaps. *Augmentative and Alternative Communication,* 1(2), 58–64.

Mirenda, P. (1988). Synthetic speech: Intelligibility and listener preferences across the age range. *Augmentative and Alternative Communication, 4,* 160.

Mirenda, P. (1990). Communication access for students with severe intellectual disabilities. *Augmentative and Alternative Communication, 6,* 97.

Mirenda, P. (1991). Terminology about people: Comments on Lloyd and Kangas (1990). *Augmentative and Alternative Communication, 7,* 59–60.

Mirenda, P. (1991). Communication approaches to challenging behavior: Functional communication instruction. *Augmentative and Alternative Communication, 8,* 155.

Mirenda, P. (1993). AAC: Bonding the uncertain mosaic. *Augmentative and Alternative Communication, 9,* 3–9.

Mirenda, P., & Beukelman, D. R. (1987). A comparison of speech synthesis intelligibility with listeners from three age groups. *Augmentative and Alternative Communication,* 3(3), 120–128.

Mirenda, P., & Beukelman, D. R. (1990). A comparison of intelligibility among natural speech and seven speech synthesizers with listeners from three age groups. *Augmentative and Alternative Communication, 6,* 61–68.

Mirenda, P., & Dattilo, J. (1987). Instructional techniques in alternative communication for students with severe intellectual handicaps. *Augmentative and Alternative Communication,* 3(3), 143–152.

Mirenda, P., & Donnellan, A. (1986). Effects of adult interaction style on conversational behavior in students with severe communication problems. *Language, Speech, and Hearing Services in Schools, 17,* 126–141.

Mirenda, P., Eicher, D., & Beukelman, D. (1989). Synthetic and natural speech preferences of make and female listeners in four age groups. *Journal of Speech and Hearing Research, 32,* 175–183, 703.

Mirenda, P., & Iacono, T. (1988). Strategies for promoting augmentative and alternative communication in natural contexts with students with autism. *Focus on Autistic Behavior,* 3(4), 1–16.

Mirenda, P., Iacono, T., & Williams, R. (1990). Communication options for persons with severe and profound disabilities: State of the art and future directions. *Journal of the Association for Persons with Severe Handicaps, 15,* 3–21.

Mirenda, P., & Locke, P. A. (1989). A comparison of symbol transparency in nonspeaking persons with intellectual disabilities. *Journal of Speech and Hearing Disorders, 54,* 131–140.

Mirenda, P., & Mathy-Laikko, P. (1989). Augmentative and alternative communication applications for persons with severe congenital communication disorders: An introduction. *Augmentative and Alternative Communication, 5,* 3–13.

Mirenda, P., & Santogrossi, J. (1985). A prompt-free strategy to teach pictorial communication system use. *Augmentative and Alternative Communication,* 1(4), 143–150.

Mirenda, P., & Schuler, A. L. (1988a). Augmenting communication for persons with autism: Issues and strategies. *Topics in Language Disorders,* 9(1), 24–43.

Mirenda, P., & Schuler, A. L. (1988b). Teaching individuals with autism and related disorders to use visual-spatial symbols to communicate. In S. Blackstone, E. Cassatt-James, & D. Bruskin (Eds.), *Augmentative Communication: Intervention Strategies*. Rockville, MD: American Speech-Language-Hearing Association, pp. 5.1-17–5.1-25.

Mitchell, J., & Cobb, J. A. (1989). Assessment and communication program for students with autism. Paper presented at the annual meeting of the American Speech-Language-Hearing Association, St. Louis.

Mitchell, P. R., & Atkins, C. P. (1988). A comparison of the single word intelligibility of two voice output communication aids. *Augmentative and Alternative Communication, 4*, 84–88.

Mitchell, P. R., & Atkins, C. P. (1989). Comparison of synthesized speech intelligibility to child and adult listeners. Paper presented at the annual meeting of the American Speech-Language-Hearing Association, St. Louis.

Mitsuda, P., Baarslag-Benson, R., Hazel, K., & Therriault, T. (1992). Augmentative communication in intensive and acute care unit settings. In Y. Yorkston (Ed.), *Augmentative Communication in the Medical Setting*. Tucson, AZ: Communication Skill Builders, pp. 5–58.

Mizuko, M. I. (1986). Iconicity and initial learning of three symbol systems in normal three-year-old children. *Augmentative and Alternative Communication, 2*, 105.

Mizuko, M. I. (1987a). Iconicity and initial learning of three symbol systems. Paper presented at the annual meeting of the American Speech-Language-Hearing Association, New Orleans.

Mizuko, M. I. (1987b). Transparency and ease of learning of symbols represented by Blissymbols, PCS, and Picsyms. *Augmentative and Alternative Communication, 3*(3), 129–136.

Mizuko, M. I. (1988). An introduction to the Adaptive Firmware Card. *Augmentative and Alternative Communication, 4*, 173.

Mizuko, M. I. (1991). Simulation of a communication device on the Macintosh. Paper presented at the annual meeting of the American Speech-Language-Hearing Association, Atlanta.

Mizuko, M. I. (1993). Personal computers as augmentative and alternative communication aids. *American Journal of Speech-Language Pathology, 2*(3), 8–10.

Mizuko, M. I., Benoit, C. S., & Esser, J. M. (1990). The comparison of recall between Blissymbols and enhanced Blissymbols. Paper presented at the annual meeting of the American Speech-Language-Hearing Association, Seattle.

Mizuko, M. I., & Esser, J. M. (1989). The effect of direct selection and scanning on visual recall. Paper presented at the annual meeting of the American Speech-Language-Hearing Association, St. Louis.

Mizuko, M. I., & Esser, J. M. (1990). Effects of array sizes and selection techniques on visual memory. Paper presented at the annual meeting of the American Speech-Language-Hearing Association, Seattle.

Mizuko, M. I., & Esser, J. M. (1991). The effect of direct selection and circular scanning on visual sequential recall. *Journal of Speech and Hearing Research, 34*, 43–48.

Mizuko, M. I., Esser, J. M., & Richardson, K. (1990). Visual sequential memory: Direct selection versus scanning. *Augmentative and Alternative Communication, 6*, 112–113.

Mizuko, M. I., & Hohnstadt, H. (1992a). The use of alternate input devices with Macintosh computers. Paper presented at the annual meeting of the American Speech-Language-Hearing Association, San Antonio.

Mizuko, M. I., & Hohnstadt, H. (1992b). Use of HyperCard utilities to crreate communication boards. Paper presented at the annual meeting of the American Speech-Language-Hearing Association, San Antonio.

Mizuko, M. I., & Reichle, J. (1988a). The effects of different training strategies on the learning of Blissymbols and Picsyms. *Augmentative and Alternative Communication*, 4, 147.

Mizuko, M. I., & Reichle, J. (1988b). Transparency and recall of symbols among intellectually handicapped adults. Paper presented at the annual meeting of the American Speech-Language-Hearing Association, Boston.

Mizuko, M. I., & Reichle, J. (1989). Transparency and recall of symbols among intellectually handicapped adults. *Journal of Speech and Hearing Disorders*, 54, 627–633.

Molidor, R. A., & Martin, M. (1981). Creative communicating: Easy alternatives for nonoral communicators. Paper presented at the annual meeting of the American Speech-Language-Hearing Association, Los Angeles.

Monfort, M., Rojo, A., & Juarez, A. (1982). *Programa Elemental de Comunicacion Bimodel* [Elementary Program of Bimodal Communication]. Madrid: Ciencias de la Educacion Preescolar y Especial.

Montgomery, J. K. (1977). Review of "The L Board"—A language board for nonoral communication. *Asha*, 19, 379–380.

Montgomery, J. K. (1979). Potential funding sources for the purchase of non-oral communication systems. In C. Cohen, J. K. Montgomery, & D. Yoder (Eds.), *Phonic Mirror Handivoice Seminar Manual*. Mill Valley, CA: H. C. Electronics, pp. 166–167.

Montgomery, J. K. (1980a). Measuring communication aid effectiveness. *Non-Oral Communication Center Newsletter*, 3, 1–3.

Montgomery, J. K. (Ed.) (1980b). *Non-oral Communication: A Training Guide for the Child Without Speech*. Fountain Valley, CA: Fountain Valley School District, Plavan School.

Montgomery, J. K. (Ed.) (1982). *The Assisted Communicator: A Monograph on the Use of the Phonic Mirror Handivoice*. Mill Valley, CA: Phonic Ear.

Montgomery, J. K. (1983). Communication systems for the child without speech. In William H. Perkins (Ed.), *Dysarthria and Apraxia*. New York: Thieme-Stratton, pp. 35–45.

Montgomery, J. K. (1984). Augmentative communication—An approach for the severely physically handicapped person without oral speech. *International Rehabilitation Medicine*, 6(3), 135-138.

Montgomery, J. K. (Ed.) (1987a). *Applications of Augmentative Communication in Schools and Clinics*. Seminars in Speech and Language, Vol. 8. New York: Thieme-Stratton.

Montgomery, J. K. (1987b). Augmentative communication: Selecting successful interventions. *Seminars in Speech and Hearing*, 8, 187–197.

Montgomery, J. K., Dashiell, S., Alvlis, V., Maxham, J., & Smith, M. (1988). Personal experiences of AAC users in a mainstreamed school environment. *Augmentative and Alternative Communication*, 4, 169.

Moody, E. J. (1982). Sign language acquisition by a global aphasic. *Journal of Nervous and Mental Diseases*, 170(2), 113–116.

Moogk-Soulis, C. A. (1977). An experimental evaluation of selected communication technical aids. Paper presented at the Fourth Annual Conference on Systems and Devices for the Disabled, Seattle, Washington. (Paper is published in the conference proceedings volume, available from Continuing Medical Education, University of Washington School of Medicine.)

Moore, E., Allen, D., Anderson, V., & Dunn, N. (1986). An outreach program: Addressing the augmentative communication needs of the physically handicapped in rural communities. *Augmentative and Alternative Communication*, 2, 105.

Moore, M. V. (1972). Binary communication for the severely handicapped. *Archives of Physical Medicine and Rehabilitation*, 53, 532–533.

Moores, D. F. (1980). Alternative communication modes: Visual-motor systems. In R. L. Schiefelbusch (Ed.), *Nonspeech Language and Communication: Analysis and Intervention*. Baltimore: University Park Press, pp. 27–47.

Moores, D. F. (1974). Nonvocal systems of verbal communication. In Richard L. Schiefelbusch & Lyle L. Lloyd (Eds.), *Language Perspectives—Acquisition, Retardation, and Intervention*. Baltimore: University Park Press, pp. 377–417.

Morasso, P., Penso, M., Suetta, G. P., & Tagliasco, V. (1979). Toward standardization of communication and control systems for motor impaired people. *Medical and Biological Engineering and Computing*, 17, 481–488.

Moratinos, G. S. (1992). A semiotic approach to AAC. *Augmentative and Alternative Communication*, 8, 155.

Moratinos, G. S., Schlosser, R. W., Haynes, C., & Belfiore, P. (1992). Teaching specific request behavior to a person with profound mental retardation: A comparative analysis of two communication modalities. *Augmentative and Alternative Communication*, 8, 155–156.

Morningstar, D. (1981). Blissymbol communication: Comparison of interaction with naive vs. experienced listeners. Unpublished manuscript, University of Toronto.

Morris, C., Newell, A. F., Booth, L., & Ricketts, I. W. (1992). Syntax PAL: A writing aid for language-impaired users. *Augmentative and Alternative Communication*, 8, 156.

Morris, L., & Belair, B. (1988). The client's role on the AAC assessment team. *Augmentative and Alternative Communication*, 4, 168–169.

Morris, S. E. (1981). Communication/interaction development at mealtimes for the multiply handicapped child: Implications for the use of augmentative communication systems. *Language, Speech, and Hearing Services in Schools*, 12, 216–232.

Morris-Manchester, E., & Shane, H. (1992). Maximizing AAC through the collaboration of two medical facilities. Paper presented at the annual meeting of the American Speech-Language-Hearing Association, San Antonio.

Morrow, D., Beukelman, D., & Mirenda, P. (1989). Augmentative and alternative communication: Three vocabulary selection techniques. Paper presented at the annual meeting of the American Speech-Language-Hearing Association, St. Louis.

Morrow, D., Beukelman, D., Mirenda, P., & Yorkston, K. (in press). Vocabulary selection for augmentative communication systems: A comparison of three techniques. *American Journal of Speech-Language Pathology*.

Moss, C. S. (1972). *Recovery from Aphasia: The Aftermath of My Stroke*. Urbana: University of Illinois Press.

Mount, M., & Shea, V. (1982). *How to Recognize and Assess Pre-language Skills in the Severely Handicapped*. Austin, TX: Pro-Ed.

Mountain, M. (1984). Signing with the visually and mentally handicapped noncommunicating child. *Bulletin of the College of Speech Therapists*, 386, 12.

Mountain, M. (1987). Working with Makaton. *Talking Sense*, 33, 10–11.

Mulholland, T., & Evans, C. R. (1965). An unexpected artifact in the human electroencephalogram concerning the alpha rhythm and the orientation of the eyes. *Nature*, 207, 36.

Munson, J. A., Nordquist, C., & Thuma-Rew, S. (1987). *Communication Systems for Persons with Severe Neuromotor Impairment.* Iowa City: University of Iowa.

Munson-Davis, J. A. (1989). Case coordination in AAC: A family model for success. Paper presented at the annual meeting of the American Speech-Language-Hearing Association, St. Louis.

Munson-Davis, J. A., Gilliland, V., Fried-Oken, M., & Mitch, J. L. (1990). Augmentative communication in Oregon. Paper presented at the annual meeting of the American Speech-Language-Hearing Association, Seattle.

Murdock, J. Y. (1978). A non-oral expressive communication program for a nonverbal retardate. *Journal of Childhood Communication Disorders*, 2, 18–25.

Murphy, C., Miller, L., & Eldridge, G. (1990). Service delivery: Assessment and follow-up in remote areas. *Augmentative and Alternative Communication*, 6, 121.

Murphy, J., Scott, J., Boa, S., & Markova, I. (1992). AAC systems used by people with cerebral palsy in Scotland. *Augmentative and Alternative Communication*, 8, 156.

Murray, P., Bedrosian, J., & Higginbotham, J. (1992a). Communicative characteristics of interactions between VOCA users: Effect of task. *Augmentative and Alternative Communication*, 8, 156–157.

Murray, P., Bedrosian, J., & Higginbotham, J. (1992b). Effect of task on communicative interactions between VOCA users. Paper presented at the annual convention of the American Speech-Language-Hearing Association, San Antonio.

Murray-Branch, J., Udavari-Solner, A., & Bailey, B. (1991). Textured communication systems for individuals with severe intellectual and dual sensory impairments. *Language, Speech, and Hearing Services in Schools*, 22, 260–268.

Musselwhite, C. R. (1982). A comparison of three symbolic communication systems. Unpublished doctoral dissertation, West Virginia University.

Musselwhite, C. R. (1984). Use of ideosyncratic signals by motorically impaired non-speakers. *Aug-Communique*, 3(4), 2.

Musselwhite, C. R. (1985). *Songbook: Signs and Symbols for Children.* Wauconda, IL: Don Johnson Developmental Equipment.

Musselwhite, C. R. (1986a). *Adaptive Play for Special Need Children: Strategies to Enhance Communication and Learning.* San Diego: Singular.

Musselwhite, C. R. (1986b). Barriers to interaction in augmented communicators: Early training strategies. *Augmentative and Alternative Communication*, 2, 105–106.

Musselwhite, C. R. (1986c). Introducing augmentative communication: Interactive training strategies. *NSSLHA Journal*, 14, 68–82.

Musselwhite, C. R. (1986d). Referential communication games as a training strategy for augmented communicators. *Augmentative and Alternative Communication*, 2, 106.

Musselwhite, C. R. (1987a). Augmentative communication. In E. McDonald (Ed.), *Treating Cerebral Palsy: For Clinicians by Clinicians*, Austin, TX: Pro-Ed., pp. 209–238.

Musselwhite, C. R. (1987b). Further comments on terminology. *Augmentative and Alternative Communication*, 3, 164–165.

Musselwhite, C. R. (1988). Singing augmentatively: Strategies for introducing aided and unaided music. *Augmentative and Alternative Communication*, 4, 145.

Musselwhite, C. R. (1990). Topic setting: Generic and specific strategies. *Augmentative and Alternative Communication*, 6, 87.

Musselwhite, C. R. (1992). Emerging literacy: Using devices to promote bookreading and early story writing. *Augmentative and Alternative Communication*, 8, 157.

Musselwhite, C. R., & Ruscello, D. M. (1984). Transparency of three communication symbol systems. *Journal of Speech and Hearing Research, 27,* 436–443.

Musselwhite, C. R., & St. Louis, K. (1982). *Communication Programming for the Severely Handicapped: Vocal and Nonvocal Strategies.* San Diego: College-Hill.

Musselwhite, C. R., & St. Louis, K. W. (1988). *Communication Programming for Persons with Severe Handicapps: Vocal and Augmentative Strategies.* Boston: College-Hill Press.

Musson, N. (1987). Application of Minspeak with geriatric rehabilitation patient population. Paper presented at the Second Annual Minspeak Conference, New Orleans.

Mustonen, T., Locke, P., Reichle, J., Solbrack, M., & Lindgren, A. (1991). An overview of augmentative and alternative communication systems. In J. Reichle, J. Y. York, & J. Sigafoos, *Implementing Augmentative and Alternative Communication: Strategies for Learners with Severe Disabilities.* Baltimore: Paul H. Brookes, pp. 1–37.

Myklebust, H. (1954). *Auditory Disorders in Children.* New York: Grune & Stratton.

Nail, B. J., Lloyd, L. L., & Francis, W. C. (1990). Comparative iconicity of pictographic symbols with two adult groups. *Augmentative and Alternative Communication, 6,* 93.

Nantais, T., Shein, F., Treviranus, J., & Apkarian, J. (1992). Predictive direct selection using pattern recognition. *Augmentative and Alternative Communication, 8,* 157.

Napper, S. A., Robey, B. L., & McAfee, P. H. (1989). An expert system for use in the prescription of electronic augmentative and alternative communication devices. *Augmentative and Alternative Communication, 5,* 128–136.

National Joint Committee for the Communicative Needs of Persons with Severe Disabilities (1992). Guidelines for meeting the communication needs for persons with severe disabilities. *Asha,* 34 (March, Supp. 7), 1–8.

Nelms, G., & Fuller, P. (1990). A service for children with communication impairments. *Augmentative and Alternative Communication, 6,* 143.

Nelms, G., Fuller, P., & Colven, D. (1990). Aids to communication in education. *Augmentative and Alternative Communication, 6,* 143.

Nelms, G., & Lysley, A. (1992). A communication system for David. *Augmentative and Alternative Communication, 8,* 157–158.

Nelms, G. M. (1986). A grammatical analysis of Blissymbol utterances of twenty cerebral palsied children. *Augmentative and Alternative Communication, 2,* 106–107.

Nelson, N. W. (1992). Performance is the prize: Language competence and performance among AAC users. *Augmentative and Alternative Communication, 8,* 3–18.

Nelson, P. J. (1977). Speech synthesis for non-verbal children—A progress report. Paper presented at the Fourth Annual Conference on Systems and Devices for the Disabled, Seattle, Washington. (Paper is published in the conference proceedings volume, available from Continuing Medical Education, University of Washington Medical School.)

Nelson, P. J. (Ed.) (1978). *Proceedings of Workshop on Communication Aids.* Ottawa: Canadian Medical and Biological Engineering Society, National Research Council.

Nelson, V. S., Leonard, J. A., Jr., Fisher, S. V., Esquenazi, A., & Hicks, J. E. (1989). Prosthetics, orthotics, and assistive devices. 2. Specialized seating and assistive devices. *Archives of Physical Medicine and Rehabilitation, 70* (5-1S), S202–S205.

Nenonen, T. (1990). How does an aphasia patient learn Blissymbol communication? *Augmentative and Alternative Communication, 6,* 88.

Newell, A. F. (1974). Morse code and voice control for the disabled (VOTEM). In Keith Copeland (Ed.), *Aids for the Severely Handicapped.* New York: Grune & Stratton, pp. 54–58.

Newell, A. F. (1987). How can we develop better communication aids? *Augmentative and Alternative Communication*, 3(1), 36–40.

Newell, A. F. (1992). Today's dream—Tomorrow's reality. *Augmentative and Alternative Communication*, 8, 81–88.

Newell, A. F., Arnott, J. L., & Alm, N. (1990). An integrated development of computer-based alternative communication systems. *Augmentative and Alternative Communication*, 6, 97–98.

Newell, A. F., Arnott, J. L., Booth, L., Beattie, W., Brophy, B., & Ricketts, I. W. (1992). Effect of the "PAL" word prediction system on the quality and quantity of text generation. *Augmentative and Alternative Communication*, 8, 304–311.

Newell, A. F., Arnott, J. L., & Waller, A. (1992). On the validity of user-modeling in AAC: Comments on Horstmann and Levine (1990). *Augmentative and Alternative Communication*, 8, 89–92.

Newell, A. F., Beynon, J. D. E., Brumfitt, P. J., & Hossain, K. S. (1975). An alphanumeric display as a communication aid for the dumb. *Medical and Biological Engineering*, 13, 84–88.

Newell, A. F., & Bour, J. S. (1971). Voice operated powered devices. *Biomechanics*, 4, 45–48.

Newell, A. F., & Brumfitt, P. J. (1974). "Talking brooch" communication aid. In Keith Copeland (Ed.), *Aids for the Severely Handicapped*. New York: Grune Stratton, pp. 204–208.

Newell, A. F., & Nabaui, C. D. (1969). VOTEM: The voice operated typewriter employing Morse Code. *Journal of Scientific Instruments*, Series 2, 2.

Newman, G. C., Sparrow, A. R., & Hospod, F. E. (1989). Two augmentative communication systems for speechless disabled patients. *American Journal of Occupational Therapy*, 43(8), 529–534.

Nicol, E. (1972). Breakthrough to communication. *Special Education*, 61(4), 25–28.

Nielson, H. R. C. (1983). Augmentative communication systems with aphasic patients: Direct nonvocal selection vs. synthesized voice. Unpublished Ph.D. dissertation, University of Utah.

Nietupski, J., & Hamre-Nietupski, S. (1979). Teaching auxillary communication skills to severely handicapped students. *AAESPH Review*, 4, 107–124.

Nietupski, J., & Williams, W. (1974). Teaching severely handicapped students to use the telephone to initiate recreational activities and to respond to telephone requests to engage in selected recreational activities. In L. Brown, W. Williams, & T. Crowner (Eds.), *A Collection of Papers and Programs Related to Public School Services for Severely Handicapped Students*. Vol. 4. Madison: Madison Metropolitan School District, pp. 507–560.

Nir, M. (1992). Augmentative communication with Inbal. *Augmentative and Alternative Communication*, 6, 125.

Nir, M. (1992). The process of six years' intervention with a patient with expressive aphasia. *Augmentative and Alternative Communication*, 8, 158.

Nisbet, P. D., & Odor, J. P. (1990). Integrating communication, learning, and mobility tools. *Augmentative and Alternative Communication*, 6, 135.

Nishikawa, S., Harada, H., Nakashima, K., Funamoto, J., & Takahashi, K. (1984). [Communication by patients with late amyotrophic lateral sclerosis: A document creating system by input of muscle action potentials.] *Rinsho-Shinkeigaku.*, 24(10), 963–967.

Nishimura, B., Watamaki, T., & Sato, M. (1987). The criteria for early use of nonvocal communication systems with nonspeaking autistic children. *Journal of Autism and Developmental Disorders*, 17(2), 243–253

Nolan, C. (1981). *Dam-Burst of Dreams.* New York: St. Martin's Press.

Nolan, C. (1987). *Under the Eye of the Clock.* New York: St. Martin's Press.

Nordquist, C., & Stepanek, S. (1992). Poets plus technology: Meeting AAC goals through an arts program. *Augmentative and Alternative Communication, 8,* 158.

Nordquist, C., & Thuma-Rew, S. (1990). Long term AAC users speak out. *Augmentative and Alternative Communication, 6,* 93.

Norris, L. (1985). Parent involvement in augmentative communication programs. *Communicating Together,* 3(2), 13.

Norris, L., & Belair, B. (1988). The client's role on the AAC assessment team. *Augmentative and Alternative Communication, 4,* 168–169.

Norris, L., Parnes, P., Boschen, K., & Schuller, R. (1992). Evaluation of a new approach to augmentative communication service delivery. *Augmentative and Alternative Communication, 8,* 158–159.

Norris, L., & Tamura, S. (1986). A model for supporting the use of the microcomputer for written communication. *Augmentative and Alternative Communication, 2,* 107.

Noyes, J. M., & Frankish, C. R. (1992). Speech recognition technology for individuals with disabilities. *Augmentative and Alternative Communication, 8,* 297–303.

Nozaki, K., Mochizuki, A., Yairo, C., & Tsunoda, T. (1991). Signing environment in an institution: Teaching sign vocabulary to residents with mental retardation for communication with deaf peers. *Behavioral Residental Treatment,* 6(2), 79–95.

Nuffer, P. S. (n.d.). *Communication Bracelet Manual.* Distributed by Ideas, Box 741, Tempe, AZ.

Nugent, C. L. (December 1977). Rehabilitative speech and language pathology and non-oral communication. *Resources* (Everest & Jennings, Inc., Los Angeles).

Nyberg, E. H., Demasco, P. W., Baker, B. R., McCoy, K., & Higgins, J. M. (1990). Intelligent parsing in AAC systems. *Augmentative and Alternative Communication, 6,* 104–105.

Oakander, S. (1980). *Language Board Instruction Kit.* Fountain Valley, CA: Non Oral Communication Center, Plavan School.

O'Connor, L., & Schery, S. (1986). A comparison of microcomputer-aided and traditional language therapy for developing communication skills in nonoral toddlers. *Journal of Speech and Hearing Disorders, 51,* 356–361.

Odell, S., & McNaughton, S. (1990). Teaching and learning—Blissymbol Component—Minspeak—Word Strategies. *Augmentative and Alternative Communication, 6,* 104.

Offir, C. W. (June 1976). Visual speech: Their fingers do the talking. *Psychology Today,* 10(1), 72–78.

Ogletree, B. T., & Schneeberger, M. (1992). Response sensitivity and consistency: Evaluation of an SMH preschool team. Paper presented at the annual meeting of the American Speech-Language-Hearing Association, San Antonio.

O'Keefe, B. M., & Camarata, S. M. (1988). Conversation control of communication board users during different response times. *Augmentative and Alternative Communication, 4,* 167.

O'Keefe, B. M., & Dattilo, J. (1990). Teaching the response-recode to adult AAC system users. *Augmentative and Alternative Communication, 6,* 136.

O'Keefe, B. M., & Dattilo, J. (1992). Teaching the response-recode form to adults with mental retardation using AAC systems. *Augmentative and Alternative Communication, 8,* 224–233.

O'Keefe, B. M., & Parnes, P. (1991). Effect of communication aid output on the attitudes of speakers. Paper presented at the annual meeting of the American Speech-Language-Hearing Association, Atlanta.

O'Keefe, B. M., & Parnes, P. (1992). Communication aid output effects on attitudes and preferences. *Augmentative and Alternative Communication*, 8, 159.

Oliver, C., & Halle, J. (1982). Language learning in the everyday environment: Teaching functional sign use to a retarded child. *Journal of the Association for the Severely Handicapped*, 8, 50–62.

Olofsson, Å. (1990). Can dyslexia be compensated for by computer-aided reading and synthetic speech? *Augmentative and Alternative Communication*, 6, 131.

Olson, T. (1976). Return of the nonverbal. *Asha*, 18, 823.

Olsson, C., Cain, S., Burcher, L., & Owen, S. (1990). Protocol for interviewing child abuse victims who use augmentative communication. *Augmentative and Alternative Communication*, 6, 124–125.

Olswang, L., Kriegsmann, E., & Mastergeorge, A. (1982). Facilitating functional requesting in pragmatically impaired children. *Language, Speech, and Hearing Services in Schools*, 13, 202–222.

Ontario Crippled Children's Centre Bliss Project Team (1973). *Ontario Crippled Children's Centre Symbol Communication Research Project 1972–1973*. Toronto.

Ontario Crippled Children's Centre Symbol Communication Programme Year End Report (1974). Distributed by the Ontario Crippled Children's Centre, 350 Rumsey Road, Toronto, Ont., Canada.

Oostinjen-Verschuur, E. (1990). Easy to make augmentative and alternative communication devices and techniques. *Augmentative and Alternative Communication*, 6, 113.

Orcutt, D. (1984a). Worldsign: A kinetic language. *Communicating Together*, 2 (3), 17–19.

Orcutt, D. (1984b). *The Worldsign Symbolbook*. Winlaw, B.C. Worldsign Communication Society.

Orcutt, D. (1985). Worldsign update. *Communicating Together*, 3(4), 24–25.

Oregon Research Institute (1989). *Bringing Out the Best: Encouraging Expressive Communication in Children with Multiple Handicaps* [videotape]. Champaign, IL: Research Press.

Osguthorpe, R. T., & Chang, L. L. (1987). Computerized symbol processors for individuals with severe communication disabilities. *Journal of Special Education Technology*, 8, 43–54.

Osguthorpe, R. T., & Chang, L. L. (1988). The effects of computerized symbol processor instruction on the communication skills of nonspeaking students. *Augmentative and Alternative Communication*, 4, 23–34.

Ostrander, D., & Barker, M. R. (1992a). A survey of scanning tools and strategies. *Augmentative and Alternative Communication*, 8, 159.

Ostrander, D., & Barker, M. R. (1992b). Transporting and positioning AAC devices. *Augmentative and Alternative Communication*, 8, 159.

Otos, M. (1983). *Nonverbal Prelinguistic Communication: A Guide to Communication Levels in Prelinguistic Handicapped Children*. Salem: Oregon Department of Education.

Ourand, P. R., Abrams, K., & Dix, C. (1990). Augmentative and alternative communication: Service delivery in Maryland. Paper presented at the annual meeting of the American Speech-Language-Hearing Association, Seattle.

Owens, M., & Harper, B. (1971). *Sign Language: A Teaching Manual for Cottage Parents of Non-verbal Retardates*. Pineville, LA: Pinecrest State School.

Owens, R. (1982). *Program for the Acquisition of Language with the Severely Impaired (PALS)*. Columbus, OH: Charles E. Merrill.

Owens, Jr., R. E., & House, L. I. (1984). Decision-making process in augmentative communication. *Journal of Speech and Hearing Disorders*, 49, 18–25.

Page, J. L. (1981). Comparisons of translucency ratings of manual signs representing nomination, action and attribution by preschool, school age, and adult subjects. Unpublished Ph.D. dissertation, Purdue University.

Palin, M., & Ray, S. (1992). Communication and instructional strategies for dynamic display devices. *Augmentative and Alternative Communication*, 8, 159–160.

Palmborg, J., Malmstedt, C., Lindin, A., & Wahlberg, K. (1990). THF—The Association for Speech Impaired: A presentation. *Augmentative and Alternative Communication*, 6, 115.

Parish, G. (1974). Prescription of remote-control devices for disabled adults. In Keith Copeland (Ed.), *Aids for the Severely Handicapped*. New York: Grune & Stratton, pp. 15–21.

Parish, J. G. (1979–1980). A study of the use of electronic environmental control systems by severely paralyzed patients. *Paraplegia*, 17, 147–152.

Park, K. (1986). Doing Makaton: A response. *British Journal of Special Education*, 13, 39.

Parkel, D. A., White, R. A., & Warner, H. (1977). Implications of the Yerkes technology for mentally retarded human subjects. In Duane M. Rumbaugh (Ed.), *Language Learning by a Chimpanzee: The LANA Project*. New York: Academic Press.

Parnes, P. (1989). Augmentative communication services: An organizational model. Paper presented at the annual meeting of the American Speech-Language-Hearing Association, St. Louis.

Parnes, P., Light, J., & Lee, K. (1990). Evolution of a service delivery model. *Augmentative and Alternative Communication*, 6, 121.

Pashek, G., & Jinks, A. (1992). Conversational use of communication books by persons with aphasia. *Augmentative and Alternative Communication*, 8, 160.

Peck, C. A. (1985). Increasing opportunities for social control by children with autism and severe handicaps: Effects on learner behavior and perceived classroom climate. *Journal of the Association for Persons with Severe Handicaps*, 10, 183–193.

Pecyna, P. M. (1988). Rebus symbol communication training with a severely handicapped preschool child: A case study. *Language, Speech, and Hearing Services in Schools*, 19, 128–143.

Pecyna-Rhyner, P. M., Lehr, D. H., & Pudlas, K. A. (1990). An analysis of teacher responsiveness to communication initiations of preschool children with handicaps. *Language, Speech, and Hearing Services in Schools*, 21, 91–97.

Peddie, H., Cairns, A. Y., Filz, G., Arnott, J. L., & Newell, A. F. (1992). A platform for extraordinary computer human operation (ECHO). *Augmentative and Alternative Communication*, 8, 160.

Pehringer, J. L. (1989). Assistive devices: Technology to improve communication. *Otolaryngologic Clinics of North America*, 22(1), 143–174.

Pei, M. (1965). *The Story of Language*. Philadelphia: Lippincott.

Peizer, E., Lorenze, E. J., & Dixon, M. (1982). Environmental controls to promote independence in severely disabled elderly persons. *Medical Instrumentation*, 16(3), 171–172.

Penfield, W., & Roberts, L. (1959). *Speech and Brain Mechanisms*. Princeton, NJ: Princeton University Press.

Penner, K. A., & Williams, W. N. (1982). Comparison of sign versus verbal symbol training in retarded adults. *Perceptual and Motor Skills*, 55, 395–401.

Pennington, L. (1992). "My turn to speak": An approach for schools. *Augmentative and Alternative Communication*, 8, 160–161.

Perron, J. V. (1965). Typewriter control for an aphasic quadriplegic patient. *Canadian Medical Association Journal*, 92, 557.

Perry, A. R., Gawel, M., & Rose, F. C. (1981). Communication aids for patients with motor neuron disease. *British Medical Journal*, 282, 1690–1692.

Peters, L. (1973). Sign language stimulus in vocabulary learning of a brain-injured child. *Sign Language Studies*, 3, 116–118.

Peters, N. A. (1986). The impact of augmentative and alternative communication systems on individual and family functioning: An update on the comparison of users of high and low tech systems. *Augmentative and Alternative Communication*, 2, 107–108.

Peters, S. J. (1990). Virginia Alternative Communication Association. Paper presented at the annual meeting of the American Speech-Language-Hearing Association, Seattle.

Peterson, L. N., & Kirshner, H. S. (1981). Gestural impairment and gestural ability in aphasia: A review. *Brain and Language*, 14, 333–348.

Petheran, B. (1986). Enabling stroke victims to interact with a microcomputer—A comparison of input devices. *Augmentative and Alternative Communication*, 2, 108.

Petheran, B. (1988). Towards adaptive communication aids—The possible impact of artifical intelligence concepts. *Augmentative and Alternative Communication*, 4, 157.

Phipps, D., & Soper, H. (1992). Augmentative communication program design in the public schools. Paper presented at the annual meeting of the American Speech-Language-Hearing Association, San Antonio.

Physically handicapped children learn to communicate (April 1973). *Science Dimension*, 8–13.

Piche, L., & Reichle, J. (1991). Teaching scanning techniques. In J. Reichle, J. Y. York, & J. Sigafoos, *Implementing Augmentative and Alternative Communication: Strategies for Learners with Severe Disabilities*. Baltimore: Paul H. Brookes, pp. 257–274.

Piche, L. M., Windsor, J., & Locke, P. A. (1992). Reinforcer preference testing: A comparison of two presentation strategies. *Augmentative and Alternative Communication*, 8, 161.

Pickering, G. A., & Bristow, D. C. (1990). The impact of functional visual deficits in augmentative communication. *Augmentative and Alternative Communication*, 6, 96.

PIC-MAN (1984). Toronto: Blissymbolics Communication Institute.

Pictogrammer (1989). Olso, Norway: Aventura forlag.

Pierce, P. L., & Kublin, K. (1993). *Access to Employability and Independence: The Case of Terry Lee*. Chapel Hill: Carolina Literacy Center, University of North Carolina.

Pierce, P. L., & McWilliams, P. J. (1993). Emerging literacy and children with SSPI: Issues and possible intervention strategies. *Topics in Language Disorders*, 13(2), 47–57.

Pierson, B. (1982). Help-Mate: Computer communication for the handicapped. *Colorado Medicine*, 79(1), 31.

Pigache, G., & Nieuwesteeg, Y. (1992). Laptops: The keys to integration. *Augmentative and Alternative Communication*, 8, 161.

Pischke, M., & Rossdeutscher, W. (1990). A programmable communication aid with Blissymbolics—A video tape presentation. *Augmentative and Alternative Communication*, 6, 129.

Plotnik, C., Lenhart, N., & Miano, L. (1992). Whole language and augmentative and alternative communication (AAC). *Augmentative and Alternative Communication*, 8, 161–162.

Pollak, I. V. (1982). Microprocessor-based communication system for the non-verbal person with serious motor handicaps: A preliminary report. *Bulletin of Prosthetics Research*, 19(1), 7–17.

Pollak, V. A., Gallagher, B. (1989). A fast communication aid for non-verbal subjects with severe motor handicaps. *Journal of Medical Engineering and Technology*, 13(1–2), 23–27.

Poock, G. K. (1990). Know your speech recognizer's "personality" when recognizing dysarthric speech! *Augmentative and Alternative Communication*, 6, 109.

Poock, G. K., & Blackstone, S. W. (1992). Using information theory to measure effectiveness of an augmentative and alternative communication display. *Augmentative and Alternative Communication*, 8, 287–296.

Poock, G. K., Blackstone, S. W., & Berg, M. H. (1992). Measuring the effectiveness of communication displays: Information theory and multiattribute analysis. *Augmentative and Alternative Communication*, 8, 162.

Poon, P. (1986). A team approach to the design and development of educational software. *Augmentative and Alternative Communication*, 2, 108.

Porch, B. (1971). *Porch Index of Communicative Ability*. Palo Alto, CA: Consulting Psychologists Press.

Porter, P. B. (198?). Augmentative communication: Selection of an initial vocabulary. *Journal of Occupational and Physical Therapy in Pediatrics*.

Porter, P. B. (1986). Communication systems for the dying patient. *Augmentative and Alternative Communication*, 2, 108.

Porter, P. B. (1989). Intervention in end stage of multiple sclerosis: A case study. *Augmentative and Alternative Communication*, 5, 125–127.

Porter, P. B. (1990). Are all prerequisites presumptuous? *Augmentative and Alternative Communication*, 6, 92.

Porter, P. B., Carter, S., Goolsby, E., Martin, N., Reed, M., Stowers, S., & Wurth, B. (1985). *Prerequisites to the Use of Augmentative Communication*. Chapel Hill, NC: University of North Carolina, Division for Disorders of Development and Learning.

Porter, P. B., & Schroeder, S. R. (1980). Generalization and maintenance of skills acquired in non-speech language initiation program training. *Applied Research in Mental Retardation*, 1, 71–84.

Position statement on nonspeech communication (1981). *Asha*, 23(10), 577–581.

Potter, R., Blackoe, V., Dymond, E., & McClemont, E. (1990). Software-based AAC for patients with acquired disorders: A system for life. *Augmentative and Alternative Communication*, 6, 143.

Potter, R., Dymond, E., Griffiths, P., McClemont, E. (1990). Design criteria for speech synthesis systems used with environmental controls. *Augmentative and Alternative Communication*, 6, 123–124.

Potter, R., Griffiths, P., Dymond, E. A., & Watts, P. (1988). Daily living at a glance. *Augmentative and Alternative Communication*, 4, 153–154.

Poulton, K. T., & Algozzine, B. (1980). Manual communication and mental retardation: A review of research and implications. *American Journal of Mental Deficiency*, 85(2), 145–152.

Premack, A. J., & Premack, D. (1972). Teaching language to an ape. *Scientific American*, 277, 92–99.

Premack, D. (1970). A functional analysis of language. *Journal of Experimental Analysis of Behavior*, 14, 107–125.

Premack, D. (1971a). Language in chimpanzee? *Science*, 172, 808–822.

Premack, D. (1971b). On the assessment of language competence in the chimpanzee. *Behavior of Non-human Primates*, 4, 198–228.

Premack, D., & Premack, A. J. (1974). Teaching visual language to apes and language-deficient persons. In Richard L. Schiefelbusch & Lyle L. Lloyd (Eds.), *Language Perspec-*

tives—Acquisition, Retardation, and Intervention. Baltimore: University Park Press, pp. 347–376.

Prentke-Romich Funding Packet (1986). Wooster, OH: Prentke-Romich Co.

Presley, S. (October 1980). When it comes to communicating without words . . . Cyrus was an expert. *Nursing*, 82–85.

Pressman, D. E., Whalen, T., & Pressman, I. S. (1986). The Technology Adjusted Functionality Score: New developments and case studies. *Augmentative and Alternative Communication*, 2, 109.

Pressman, E., & Heah, L. H. (1988). Augmentative and alternative communication use in Malaysia and the Pacific: Status and relevance. *Augmentative and Alternative Communication*, 4, 139.

Prevost, P. I. (1983). Using the Makaton vocabulary in early language learning with a Down's baby. *Mental Handicap*, 11, 28–29.

Price, K., McConachie, H., & Jolleff, N. (1992). "What's in the box?" Assessing children's communication skills. *Augmentative and Alternative Communication*, 8, 162.

Priest, L. W., & Cecconi, C. P. (1987). A case study: Augmentative communication with an autistic child. Paper presented at the annual meeting of the American Speech-Language-Hearing Association, New Orleans.

Prince, S. (1976). Something new. *Asha*, 18, 880.

Prinz, P. M., Nelson, K. E., Arford, L. M., & Mugg, S. E. (1988). "Recasting" during microcomputer-aided language intervention with multihandicapped children. Paper presented at the annual meeting of the American Speech-Language-Hearing Association, Boston.

Prinz, P. M., & Shaw, N. (1981). Communication development by speech and sign in mentally retarded individuals. Paper presented at the annual meeting of the American Speech-Language-Hearing Association, Los Angeles.

Prior, M. R. (1977). Psycholinguistic disabilities of autistic and retarded children. *Journal of Mental Deficiency Research*, 21, 37–45.

Prior, M., & Cummins, R. (1992). Questions about facilitated communication and autism. *Journal of Autism and Developmental Disorders*, 22(3), 331–338.

Prizant, B. (1983). Language and communication behavior in autism: Toward an understanding of the "whole" of it. *Journal of Speech and Hearing Disorders*, 46, 241–249.

Prizant, B., & Schuler, A. (1987). Facilitating communication: Theoretical foundations. In D. J. Cohen & A. M. Donnellan (Eds.), *Handbook of Autism and Pervasive Developmental Disorders*. New York: John Wiley & Sons.

Prizant, B., & Wetherby, A. (1988). Providing services to children with autism (ages 0 to 2 years) and their families. *Topics in Language Disorders*, 9(1), 1–23.

Provisional Dictionary (Blissymbolics) (1976). Toronto: Blissymbolics Communication Institute.

Puig de la Bellacasa, R. (1980). Telecommunications, computers and other complementary communication means on behalf of the disabled. *International Journal of Rehabilitation Research*, 3(2), 191–204.

Puig de la Bellacasa, R., & Lopez, J. (1981). *Comunicaciones y Discapacidad* [Communication and Handicaps]. Madrid: Tecnos.

Pulli, T., & Jaroma, M. (1990). Exploring novel solutions for motivating simplified signing, pictorializing, and vocalizing. *Augmentative and Alternative Communication*, 6, 103.

Purdy, M. H., Duffy, R. J., & Coelho, C. A. (1992). Functional communication in aphasic adults following multimodality training. Paper presented at the annual meeting of the American Speech-Language-Hearing Association, San Antonio.

Quist, R. W., & Blischak, D. M. (1992). Assistive communication devices: Call for specifications. *Augmentative and Alternative Communication*, 8, 312–317.

Quist, R. W., & Lloyd, L. L. (1988). Sequence effects of high vs. low translucency on learning Blissymbols. *Augmentative and Alternative Communication*, 4, 143.

Quist, R. W., Lloyd, L. L., Forde, B., Gordon, D., Romich, B., Weis, L., & Woltosz. W. (1990). Electronic communication devices: What specifications are needed? *Augmentative and Alternative Communication*, 6, 128.

Rabush, D. R., Lloyd, L. L., & Gerdes, M. (1982, 1983). Aided nonspeech communication: An extensive bibliography (Parts I, II, and III). *Communication Outlook*, 3(4) and 4(1 and 2).

Radwin, R. G., Vanderheiden, G. C., & Lin, M. L. (1990). A method for evaluating head-controlled computer input devices using Fitts' law. *Human Factors*, 32(4), 423–438.

Raghavendra, P., & Fristoe, M. W. (1987). What three-year-olds see in standard and enhanced Blissymbols. Paper presented at the annual meeting of the American Speech-Language-Hearing Association, New Orleans.

Raghavendra, P., & Fristoe, M. W. (1988). Standard and enhanced Blissymbols: Responses by Indian and U.S. children. *Augmentative and Alternative Communication*, 4, 146.

Raghavendra, P., & Fristoe, M. W. (1990a). "A spinach with a V on it": What 3-year-olds see in standard and enhanced Blissymbolics. *Journal of Speech and Hearing Disorders*, 55, 149–159.

Raghavendra, P., & Fristoe, M. W. (1990b). Standard and enhanced Blissymbols: Learning and use by preschool children. Paper presented at the annual meeting of the American Speech-Language-Hearing Association, Seattle.

Raghavendra, P., Rosengren, E., & Hunnicutt, S. (1992). Multi-Talk II: An evaluation of the updated VOCA from Sweden. *Augmentative and Alternative Communication*, 8, 162.

Rahimi, M. A., & Eulenberg, J. B. (1973). A computer terminal with synthetic speech output. Paper presented at the National Conference on the Use of On-Line Computers in Psychology, St. Louis.

Rahimi, M. A., & Eylenberg, J. B. (1974). A computing environment for the blind. Paper presented at the AFIPS National Computer Conference. (Paper is published in conference proceedings volume.)

Raitzer, G. A., Vanderheiden, G. C., & Holt, C. S. (1976). Interfacing computers for the physically handicapped—A review of international approaches. Paper presented at the AFIPS National Computer Conference. (Paper is published in conference proceedings volume, pp. 209–216.)

Ralston, A., & Meek, C. L. (Eds.) (1976). *Encyclopedia of Computer Science*. New York: Petrocelli/Charter.

Rambo Jr., R. R. (1992). Expanding the concept of telecommunication through advocacy. *Augmentative and Alternative Communication*, 8, 163.

Randall, C., & Stevens, L. (1988). Breaking the barriers to communication: Physical, behavioral, emotional. *Augmentative and Alternative Communication*, 4, 168.

Raney, C., & Silverman, F. H. (1992). Attitudes toward nonspeaking individuals who use communication boards. *Journal of Speech and Hearing Research*, 35, 1269–1271.

Ransay, D. A., Snapper, A. G., & Kop, P. F. M. (1972). A foot-operated typewriter. *Archives of Physical Medicine and Rehabilitation*, 53, 190.

Rao, P. R. (1986). The use of Amer-Ind code with aphasic adults. In R.Chapey (Ed.), *Language Intervention Strategies in Adult Aphasia*. Baltimore: Williams & Wilkins, pp. 360–367.

Rao, P. R., Basili, A. G., Koller, J. J., Fullerton, B., Diener, S., & Burton, P. L. (1979). The use of Amer-Ind code by severe aphasic adults. Paper presented at the annual meeting of the American Speech-Language-Hearing Association, Atlanta.

Rao, P. R., & Horner, J. (1980). Nonverbal strategies for functional communication in aphasic persons. In M. Burns & J. Andrews (Eds.), *Neuropathologies of Speech and Language Diagnosis and Treatment Selected Papers*. Evanston, IL: Institute for Continuing Professional Education.

Ratcliff, A. E. (1987). A comparison of two message selection techniques used in augmentative communication systems by normal children with differing cognitive styles. Unpublished dissertation, University of Wisconsin, Madison.

Ratcliff, A. E. (1988a). Can user cognitive style predict augmentative and alternative communication use? *Augmentative and Alternative Communication*, 4, 157–158.

Ratcliff, A. E. (1988b). Differences between scanning and direct selection: Information from normal children. Paper presented at the annual meeting of the American Speech-Language-Hearing Association, Boston.

Ratusnik, C. M., & Ratusnik, D. L. (1974). A comprehensive communication approach for a ten-year-old nonverbal autistic child. *American Journal of Orthopsychiatry*, 44, 396–403.

Ratusnik, C. M., & Ratusnik, D. L. (1976). A comprehensive communication approach for a ten-year-old autistic child. Paper presented at the annual meeting of the American Speech-Language-Hearing Association, Houston.

Ray, S., & Palin, M. W. (1992). Linguistically-based acceleration strategies for AAC: Function words/units, Minspeak, VoisShapes. Paper presented at the annual meeting of the American Speech-Language-Hearing Association, San Antonio.

Record-player "voice" for mutes (Spring 1977). *NASA Tech Briefs*, 97–98.

Reich, P. A., & Shein, F. (1990). VOCI: A Voice Output Intelligent Communication Interface. *Augmentative and Alternative Communication*, 6, 104.

Reichle, J. (1988). Stimulus control applictions in the establishment of an initial communicative repertoire. Unpublished manuscript, University of Minnesota, Minneapolis.

Reichle, J. (1991a). Defining the decisions involved in designing and implementing augmentative and alternative communication systems. In J. Reichle, J. Y. York, & J. Sigafoos, *Implementing Augmentative and Alternative Communication: Strategies for Learners with Severe Disabilities*. Baltimore: Paul H. Brookes, pp. 39–60.

Reichle, J. (1991b). Describing initial communicative intents. In J. Reichle, J. Y. York, & J. Sigafoos, *Implementing Augmentative and Alternative Communication: Strategies for Learners with Severe Disabilities*. Baltimore: Paul H. Brookes, pp. 71–88.

Reichle, J. (1991c). Developing communicative exchanges. In J. Reichle, J. Y. York, & J. Sigafoos, *Implementing Augmentative and Alternative Communication: Strategies for Learners with Severe Disabilities*. Baltimore: Paul H. Brookes, pp. 133–156.

Reichle, J., Anderson, H., & Schermer, G. (1986). Establishing the discrimination between requesting objects, requesting assistance, and "helping yourself." Unpublished manuscript, University of Minnesota.

Reichle, J., Barrett, C., Tetlie, R. R., & McQuarter, R. J. (1987). The effect of prior intervention to establish generalized requesting on the acquisition of object labels. *Augmentative and Alternative Communication*, 3(1), 3–11.

Reichle, J., & Brown, L. (1986). Teaching the use of a multipage direct selection communication board to an adult with autism. *Journal of the Association for Persons with Severe Handicaps.* 11, 68–73.

Reichle, J., Feeley, K., & Johnston, S. (1993). Communicative intervention for persons with severe and profound disabilities. *Clinics in Communication Disorders*, 3(2), 7–30.

Reichle, J., & Karlan, G. (1985). The selection of an augmentative communication system in communication intervention: A critique of decision rules. *Journal of the Association for Persons with Severe Handicaps*, 10, 146–156.

Reichle, J., & Karlan, G. (1988). Selecting augmentative communication interventions: A critique of candidacy criteria and a proposed alternative. In R. L. Schiefelbusch & L. L. Lloyd (Eds.), *Language Perspectives: Acquisition, Retardation, and Intervention*, 2nd ed. Austin, TX: Pro-Ed, pp. 321–339.

Reichle, J., & Koegh, W. (1985). Communication intervention: A selective review of what, when, and how to teach. In S. Warren & A. Rogers-Warren (Eds.), *Teaching Functional Language.* Austin, TX: Pro-Ed, pp. 25–59.

Reichle, J., & Koegh, W. (1986). Communication instruction for learners with severe handicaps: Some unresolved issues. In R. Horner, L. Meyer, & H. Fredericks (Eds.), *Education of Learners with Severe Handicaps: Exemplary Service Strategies.* Baltimore: Paul H. Brookes.

Reichle, J., Rogers, N., & Barrett, C. (1984). Establishing pragmatic discrimination among the communicative functions of requesting, rejecting, and commenting in an adolescent. *Journal of the Association for Persons with Severe Handicaps*, 9, 31–36.

Reichle, J., & Sigafoos, J. (1991a). Bringing communication behavior under the control of the appropriate stimuli. In J. Reichle, J. Y. York, & J. Sigafoos, *Implementing Augmentative and Alternative Communication: Strategies for Learners with Severe Disabilities.* Baltimore: Paul H. Brookes, pp. 193–213.

Reichle, J., & Sigafoos, J. (1991b). Establishing an initial repertoire of requesting. In J. Reichle, J. Y. York, & J. Sigafoos, *Implementing Augmentative and Alternative Communication: Strategies for Learners with Severe Disabilities.* Baltimore: Paul H. Brookes, pp. 89–114.

Reichle, J., & Sigafoos, J. (1991c). Establishing spontaneity and generalization. In J. Reichle, J. Y. York, & J. Sigafoos, *Implementing Augmentative and Alternative Communication: Strategies for Learners with Severe Disabilities.* Baltimore: Paul H. Brookes, pp. 157–171.

Reichle, J., & Ward, M. (1985). Teaching the descriminative use of an encoding electronic communication device and signing exact English to a moderately handicapped child. *Language, Speech, and Hearing Services in Schools*, 16, 58–63.

Reichle, J., Williams, W., & Ryan, S. (1981). Selecting signs for the formulation of an augmentative communication modality. *Journal of the Association for the Severely Handicapped*, 6, 48–56.

Reichle, J., & Yoder, D. (1979). Assessment and early stimulation of communication in the severely and profoundly mentally retarded. In R. York & E. Edgar (Eds.), *Teaching the Severely Handicapped.* Vol. 4. Columbus, OH: Special Press, pp. 155–179.

Reichle, J., & Yoder, D. (1985). Communication board use in severely handicapped learners. *Language, Speech, and Hearing Services in Schools*, 16, 146–157.

Reichle, J., York, J., & Eynon, D. (1989). Influence of indicating preferences for initiating, maintaining, and terminating interactions. In F. Brown & D. H. Lehr (Eds.), *Persons with Profound Disabilities: Issues and Practices.* Baltimore: Paul H. Brookes, pp. 191–211.

Reichle, J., York, J., & Sigafoos, J. (1991). *Implementing Augmentative and Alternative Communication: Strategies for Learners with Severe Disabilities.* Baltimore: Paul H. Brooks.

Reid, B., & Kiernan, C. (1979). Spoken words and manual signs as encoding categories in short-term memory for mentally retarded children. *American Journal of Mental Deficiency,* 84, 200–203.

Reid, B., & McNaughton, S. (1988). Graphics: Reviewing the literature. *Augmentative and Alternative Communication,* 4, 169–170.

Reid, D. H., & Hurlbut, B. (1977). Teaching nonvocal communication skills to multihandicapped retarded adults. *Journal of Applied Behavioral Analysis,* 10, 591–603.

Reisfeld, M. D. (1992). "Picture-in-pocket" symbol selection method. *Augmentative and Alternative Communication,* 8, 163.

Remington, B., & Clarke, S. (1983). Acquisition of expressive signing by autistic children: An evaluation of the relative effects of simultaneous communication and sign-alone training. *Journal of Applied Behavior Analysis,* 16, 315–327.

Remington, B., & Clarke, S. (1993a). Acquisition of expressive signing: Comparison of reinforcement strategies. *Augmentative and Alternative Communication,* 9, 26–35.

Remington, B., & Clarke, S. (1993b). Simulaneous communication and speech comprehension. Part I: Comparison of two methods of teaching expressive signing and speech comprehension skills. *Augmentative and Alternative Communication,* 9, 36–48.

Remington, B., & Clarke, S. (1993c). Simultaneous communication and speech comprehension. Part II: Comparison of two methods of overcoming selective attention during expressive sign training. *Augmentative and Alternative Communication,* 9, 49–60.

Remington, B., & Light, P. (1983). Some problems in the evaluation of research on non-oral communication systems. *Advances in Mental Handicaps,* 2, 69–94.

Remington, B., Watson, J., & Light, P. (1990). Beyond the single sign: A matrix approach to teaching productive sign combinations. *Mental Handicap Research,* 3(1), 33–50.

Remington-Gurney, J., Crossley, R., & Batt, M. (1990). Facilitated communication in mainstream schools. *Augmentative and Alternative Communication,* 6, 127.

Rentschler, G. J. (1985). Computer synthesized speech: Intelligibility and the language-impaired child. Paper presented at the annual meeting of the American Speech-Language-Hearing Association, Washington, DC.

Renuk, J. (1990). Upgrading a VOCA. *Augmentative and Alternative Communication,* 6, 126.

Resch, R. C., Pizzuti, S., & Woods, A. (1988). The later creation of a transitional object. *Psychoanalytic Psychology,* 5(4), 369–387.

Reuter, D. B. (1974). Speech synthesis under APL. *Proceedings of the Sixth International APL Users Conference,* pp. 585–596.

Rice, O. M., & Combs, R. G. (1972). Practical aids for non-verbal handicapped. *Proceedings of the 1972 Carnahan Conference on Electronic Prosthetics.*

Richardson, T. (1975). Sign language for SMR and PMR. *Mental Retardation,* 13(3), 17.

Ricketts, I. W., & Booth, L. (1993). PAL—A predictive word processing system. *International Journal of Computers in Adult Education and Training,* 3(1), 6–11.

Ricks, D. M., & Wing, L. (1975). Language, communication, and use of symbols in normal and autistic children. *Journal of Autism and Childhood Schizophrenia,* 5, 191–221.

Ridgway, L., Nixon, C., McKears, S., Pulsford, J. F., Gallagher, J., & Gallagher, C. (1986).

COMPAID: Computer aid for speech impaired and disabled people. *Augmentative and Alternative Communication*, 2, 109.

Riley, J. K. (1992). An augmentative telephone booth: Observations of first year of service. *Augmentative and Alternative Communication*, 8, 163.

Riley, J. K., & Moes, S. C. (1990a). Innovations in augmentative telecommunications: An augmentative telephone booth. *Augmentative and Alternative Communication*, 6, 88–89.

Riley, J. K., & Moes, S. C. (1990b). Technology for augmentative telecommunications: An augmentative telephone booth. *Augmentative and Alternative Communication*, 6, 113.

Rimac, R. T. (1991) How to make "talking" communication boards on the Macintosh computer. Paper presented at the annual meeting of the American Speech-Language-Hearing Association, Atlanta.

Rimland, B. (1992). Facilitated communication: Now the bad news. *Autism Research Review International*, 6(1), 3.

Rinard, G. A. (1978). An ocular-controlled video terminal. In P. Nelson (Ed.), *Proceedings of Workship on Communication Aids*. Ottawa: Canadian Medical and Biological Engineering Society, National Research Council.

Rinard, G. A., Matteson, R. W., Quine, R. W., & Tegtmeyer, R. S. (1980). An infrared system for determining ocular position. *ISA Transactions*, 19(4), 3–6.

Rinard, G. A., & Rugg, D. (1978). Application of the ocular transducer to the Etran (1) communicator. *Proceedings of the Fifth Annual Conference on Systems and Devices for the Disabled*. Houston: Baylor College of Medicine, Texas Institute for Rehabilitation and Research, pp. 164–166.

Ring, N. (1974). Possum typewriter—Consumer experience. In Keith Copeland (Ed.), *Aids for the Severely Handicapped*. New York: Grune & Stratton, pp. 124–128.

Ring, N. (1978). Specification of interfaces for communication aid. In P. Nelson (Ed.), *Proceedings of Workshop on Communication Aids*. Ottawa: Canadian Medical and Biological Engineering Society, National Research Council.

Ripich, D. N., & Lewis, B. A. (1983). Discourse analysis of vocal/nonvocal cerebral palsied adult group interaction. Paper presented at the annual meeting of the American Speech-Language-Hearing Association, Cincinnati.

Rivarola, A., Panzera, S., Schiaffino, A., & Fronticellia, G. (1990). Analysis of the development of augmentative and alternative communication in Italy. *Augmentative and Alternative Communication*, 6, 106.

Rivarola, A., & Risatti, F. (1990). Including Blissymbols in the communication system of a nonverbal aphasic individual. *Augmentative and Alternative Communication*, 6, 88.

Rivarola, A., Vallini, S., & Gava, L. (1986). "Mainstreaming" children with communication problems in normal Italian schools. *Augmentative and Alternative Communication*, 2, 109–110.

Robbins, N. (1976). Selected sign systems for multi-handicapped students. Paper presented at the annual meeting of the American Speech-Language-Hearing Association, Houston.

Robenault, I. P. (1973). *Functional Aids for the Multiply Handicapped*. Evanston, IL: Harper & Row.

Roberts, M. L., Donoghue, K. A., & Parker, E. K. (1990). Augmenting oral communication in the nonspeaking traumatic brain injured. Paper presented at the annual meeting of the American Speech-Language-Hearing Association, Seattle.

Robinson, B. F., Wilkinson, K. M., Sevcik, R. A., & Romski, M. A. (1990). Integrating AAC systems into the classroom: Strategies and applications. Paper presented at the annual meeting of the American Speech-Language-Hearing Association, Seattle.

Robinson, C., Bataillon, K., Fieber, N., Jackson, B., & Rasmussen, J. (1985). *Sensorimotor Assessment Form*. Omaha, NE: Meyer Rehabilitation Center.

Robison, A. (1986). An open letter to my daughter's teacher. *Communicating Together*, 4, 8–9.

Robison, G., & Robison, A. (1985). Obtaining insurance funding for your handicapped dependent's needs. *Communication Outlook*, 7(3), 7–8.

Rodgers, B. L. (1984). The holistic application of high technology for conversation, writing, and computer access aid system. In Christopher Smith (Ed.), *Discovery '84: Technology for Disabled Persons Conference Papers*. Menomonie, WI: Materials Development Center, Stout Vocational Rehabilitation Institute, University of Wisconsin-Stout.

Rodgers, B. L., Kelso, D. P., Vanderheiden, G. C., & Schauer, J. (1987). *Simple Electronic Transducer (SET) Compatibility Standard Proposal*. Madison: Trace Research and Development Center for the Severely Communicatively Handicapped, University of Wisconsin.

Rodgers, B. L., Schauer, J., Kelso, D. P., Vanderheiden, G. C., & Lee, C. C. (1987). *Keyboard Emulating Interface (KEI) Compatibility Standard Proposal*. Madison: Trace Research and Development Center for the Severely Communicatively Handicapped, University of Wisconsin.

Roland, C. (1990). Communication in the classroom for children with dual sensory impairments: Studies of teacher and child behavior. *Augmentative and Alternative Communication*, 6, 262–274.

Romich, B. A., & Bruno, J. (1990a). Current issues in AAC: A survey of ASHA membership. *Augmentative and Alternative Communication*, 6, 106.

Romich, B. A., & Bruno, J. (1990b). Identifying and addressing ethical dilemmas in AAC. *Augmentative and Alternative Communication*, 6, 152–153.

Romich, B. A., & Zangari, C. (1989). Augmentative and alternative communication; Ethics and authenticity in clinical practice. *Augmentative and Alternative Communication*, 5, 199–202.

Romski, M. A. (1984). Effects of speech and speech and sign instruction on oral language learning and generalization of action + object combinations by Down's syndrome children. *Journal of Speech and Hearing Disorders*, 49, 293–302.

Romski, M. A. (May 1989). Two decades of language research with great apes. *Asha*, 31, 81–82.

Romski, M. A., Lloyd, L. L., & Sevcik, R. A. (198?). Augmentative and alternative communication issues. In R. L. Schiefelbusch & L. L. Lloyd (Eds.), *Language Perspectives*. Vol. II. San Diego: College-Hill.

Romski, M. A., & Ruder, K. (1984). Effects of speech and speech and sign instruction on oral language learning and generalization of action + object combinations by Down's syndrome children. *Journal of Speech and Hearing Disorders*, 49, 293–302.

Romski, M. A., & Savage-Rumbaugh, E. S. (1986). A nonhuman primate model: Implications for language intervention research. In E. S. Savage-Rumbaugh (Ed.), *Ape Language: From Conditioning Response to Symbol*. New York: Columbia University Press.

Romski, M. A., & Sevcik, R. A. (1984). Symbol meaning boundaries in severely retarded adults: Three case profiles. Paper presented at the annual meeting of the American Speech-Language-Hearing Association, San Francisco.

Romski, M. A., & Sevcik, R. A. (1988a). Augmentative and alternative communication systems: Considerations for individuals with severe intellectual disabilities. *Augmentative and Alternative Communication*, 4, 83–93.

Romski, M. A., & Sevcik, R. A. (1988b). Augmentative communication system acquisition and use: A model for teaching and assessing progress. *NSSLHA Journal*, 16, 61–75.

Romski, M. A., & Sevcik, R. A. (1988c). Speech-output communication systems: Acquisition/ use by youngsters with retardation. *Augmentative and Alternative Communication*, 4, 167.

Romski, M. A., & Sevcik, R. A. (1989). An analysis of visual-graphic symbol meanings for two nonspeaking adults with severe mental retardation. *Augmentative and Alternative Communication*, 5, 109–114.

Romski, M. A., & Sevcik, R. A. (1991). Patterns of language learning by instruction: Evidence from nonspeaking persons with mental retardation. In N. Krasnegor, D. Rumbaugh, R. Schiefelbusch, & M. Studdert-Kennedy (Eds.), *Biological and Behavioral Determinants of Language Development*. Hillsdale, NJ: Lawrence Erlbaum Associates, 429–445.

Romski, M. A., & Sevcik, R. A. (1992). Augmented language development in children with severe mental retardation. In S. Warren & J. Reichle (Eds.), *Causes and Effects in Communication and Language Intervention*. Baltimore: Paul H. Brookes, pp. 113–130.

Romski, M. A., Sevcik, R. A., Collier, V., & Hartsell, K. (1992). Project FACTT: From research to practice in augmentative communication. *Augmentative and Alternative Communication*, 8, 163.

Romski, M. A., Sevcik, R. A., & Joyner, S. E. (1984). Nonspeech communication systems: Implications for language intervention with mentally retarded children. *Topics in Language Disorders*, 5, 66–81.

Romski, M. A., Sevcik, R. A., & Pate, J. L. (1988). Establishment of symbolic communication in persons with severe retardation. *Journal of Speech and Hearing Disorders*, 53, 94–107.

Romski, M. A., Sevcik, R. A., Pate, J. L., & Rumbaugh, D. M. (1985). Discrimination of lexigrams and traditional orthography by nonspeaking severely mentally retarded persons. *American Journal of Mental Deficiency*, 90(2), 185–189.

Romski, M. A., Sevcik, R. A., Reumann, R., & Pate, J. L. (1989). Youngsters with moderate or severe mental retardation and severe spoken language impairments I: Extant communicative patterns. *Journal of Speech and Hearing Disorders*, 54, 366–373.

Romski, M. A., Sevcik, R. A., Robinson, B., & Bakeman, R. (1994). Adult-directed communication of youth with mental retardation using the System for Augmenting Language. *Journal of Speech and Hearing Research*, 37, 617–628.

Romski, M. A., Sevcik, R. A., Robinson, B., & Wilkinson, K. (1990). Intelligibility and form changes in the vocalizations of augmented communicators. Paper presented at the annual meeting of the American Speech-Language-Hearing Association, Seattle.

Romski, M. A., Sevcik, R. A., & Rumbaugh, D. M. (1985). Retention of symbolic communication skills by severely mentally retarded persons. *American Journal of Mental Deficiency*, 89(4), 441–444.

Romski, M. A., Watkins, R., & Sevcik, R. A. (1989). Augmented linguistic input to nonspeaking children with mental retardation. Paper presented at the annual meeting of the American Speech-Language-Hearing Association, St. Louis.

Romski, M. A., White, R. A., Millen, C. E., & Rumbaugh, D. M. (1984). Effects of computer keyboard teaching on the symbolic communication of severely retarded persons: Five case studies. *Psychological Record*, 34, 39–54.

Roodenburg, N. (1988). Speech therapy in intensive-and medium-care settings. *Augmentative and Alternative Communication*, 4, 154.

Roper, I., & Kalbe, U. (1984). [Aid for physically handicapped children: Five year experience with a collection facility]. *Rehabilitation (Stuttgart)*, 23(3), 117–119.

Rosen, M., Drinker, P., & Dalrymple, G. (1976). *A Display Board for Non-verbal Communication Encoded as Eye Movement*. Cambridge, MA: Department of Mechanical Engineering, Massachusetts Institute of Technology.

Rosen, M., & Goodenough-Trepagnier, C. (1981). Factors affecting communication rate in non-vocal communication systems. *Proceedings of the Fourth Annual Conference on Rehabilitation Engineering*. Washington, DC: Rehabilitation Engineering Society of North America, pp. 194–195.

Rosen, M., & Goodenough-Trepagnier, C. (1983). Development of a computer-aided system for prescription of non-vocal communication devices: A progress report. *Proceedings of the RESNA [Research Engineering Society of North America] 6th Annual Conference on Rehabilitation Engineering*, pp. 191–193.

Rosenberg, G. (1968). *Assistive Devices for the Handicapped*. Atlanta: American Rehabilitation Foundation.

Rosengren, E., & Hunnicutt, S. (1990). A speech recognition-controlled predicting word processor. *Augmentative and Alternative Communication*, 6, 109.

Ross, A., & Flanagan, K. (1977). Communication system using Morse code to printed English translation. Paper presented at the Fourth Annual Conference on Systems and Devices for the Disabled, Seattle. (Paper is published in the conference proceedings volume, available from Continuing Medical Education, University of Washington School of Medicine.)

Ross, A. J. (1979). A study of the application of Blissymbolics as a means of communication for a young brain damaged adult. *British Journal of Disorders of Communication*, 14, 103–109.

Ross, L. L., Butt, D. S., & Williams, J. K. (1991). Learning and recalling symbol sequences in augmentative communication using computers. Paper presented at the annual meeting of the American Speech-Language-Hearing Association, Atlanta.

Rossdeutscher, W., & Pischke, M. (1990). A programmable communication aid with Blissymbolics. *Augmentative and Alternative Communication*, 6, 129.

Roth, F. P., & Cassatt-James, E. L. (1989). The language assessment process: Clinical implications for individuals with severe speech impairments. *Augmentative and Alternative Communication*, 5, 165–172.

Rothchild, N., & Collier, B. (1986). Some issues regarding the clinical application of Minspeak. Paper presented at the First Annual Minspeak Conference, Detroit.

Rotholz, D. A., Berkowitz, S. F., & Burberry, J. (1989). Functionality of two modes of communication in the community by students with developmental disabilities: A comparison of signing and communication books. *Journal of the Association for Persons with Severe Handicaps*, 14, 227–233.

Rothschild, N. (1992). Centralized equipment pool project (CEPP): A new system of service delivery. *Augmentative and Alternative Communication*, 8, 163.

Rothschild, N., Parnes, P. H., Poss, J., Treviranus, J. E., Fulford, E. N., & Manji, S. (1990). Custom database development to support augmentative and alternative communication. Paper presented at the annual meeting of the American Speech-Language-Hearing Association, Seattle.

Rothschild, N. (1984). Sharing ideas with Nora. *Communicating Together*, 2(3), 15.

Rothschild, N. (1985). Sharing ideas with Nora. *Communicating Together*, 3(4), 17–18.

Rothschild, N. (1986). Partner assisted scanning. *Communicating Together*, 4(3), 22–23.

Roustan, A., Glazer, S., & Burbidge, N. (1986). Sign language: Communicating with developmentally delayed children under three years of age. *Augmentative and Alternative Communication*, 2, 110.

Rowe, J. A., & Rapp, D. L. (1980). Tantrums: Remediation through communication. *Child: Care, Health, and Development*, 6, 197–208.

Rowland, C. (1988). Opportunities to communicate for multisensory impaired versus communication-disordered students. *Augmentative and Alternative Communication*, 4, 162–163.

Rowland, C. (1990). Communication in the classroom for children with dual sensory impairments: Studies of teacher and child behavior. *Augmentative and Alternative Communication*, 6, 262–274.

Rowland, C., & Schweigert, P. D. (1989). Tangible symbols: Symbolic communication for individuals with multisensory impairments. *Augmentative and Alternative Communication*, 5, 226–234.

Rowland, C., & Schweigert, P. D. (1990). *Tangible Symbol Systems: Symbolic Communication for Individuals with Multisensory Impairments*. Tucson, AZ: Communication Skill Builders.

Rowland, C., & Schweigert, P. D. (1992). Structuring functional activities to encourage communication in children without speech. *Augmentative and Alternative Communication*, 8, 164.

Rowland, C., Schweigert, P. D., & Brummett, B. (1988). Tangible symbol communication systems for individuals with multiple sensory impairments. *Augmentative and Alternative Communication*, 4, 146.

Roy, D. M. (1992). Computer recognition of movement for people with athetoid cerebral palsy. *Augmentative and Alternative Communication*, 8, 164.

Roy, O. Z. (1965). A communication system for the handicapped. *Medical Electronics and Biological Engineering*, 3, 427.

Roy, O. Z. (1982). I. Y. D. P. in retrospect: Technology for the disabled. *Dimensions of Health Services*, 59(1), 9.

Roy, O. Z., & Charbonneau, J. R. (1974). A communication system for the handicapped (COMHANDI). In Keith Copeland (Ed.), *Aids for the Severely Handicapped*. New York: Grune & Stratton, pp. 89–98.

Roy, S. (1986). Computer-assisted nonspeech communication. *Augmentative and Alternative Communication*, 2, 110.

Rubin, R. B., & Stark, L. (1984). A preliminary investigation of the information carrying potential of voluntary eye movements. *Computers in Biology and Medicine*, 14(3), 303–313.

Ruder, K. F., & Sims, M. B. (1987). Smiling: An effective interaction maintenance strategy for multiply handicapped individuals? Paper presented at the annual meeting of the American Speech-Language-Hearing Association, New Orleans.

Ruggles, V. (1979). *Funding of Non-vocal Communication Aids: Current Issues and Strategies*. New York: Muscular Dystrophy Association.

Rumbaugh, D. M. (Ed.) (1977). *Language Learning by a Chimpanzee: The LANA Project*. New York: Academic Press.

Rush, W. (1986). *Journey out of Silence*. Lincoln, NE: Media Publishing and Marketing.

Rygaard, K., Norup, B., Kirkegaard, C., Riis, J., Nesgaard, V., & Knudsen, A. B. (1992).

Semantically structured communication Mac-program for aphasic people. *Augmentative and Alternative Communication*, 8, 164.

Saarnio, I. (1974). Typewriter control by dental palate key. In Keith Copeland (Ed.), *Aids for the Severely Handicapped*. New York: Grune & Stratton, pp. 59–62.

Sack, S., Etter, R., & Simmons, S. (1992). Using picture symbol reading to adapt curriculum for augmentative communicators. Paper presented at the annual meeting of the American Speech-Language-Hearing Association, San Antonio.

Sadare, A. D. (1986). Transferred technology vs. appropriate technology: Providing a communication aids service for the handicapped in the third world. *Augmentative and Alternative Communication*, 2, 110–111.

Salciccia, C. E., Christopher, F., Parathyras, A., Uellendahl, B., Van Sant, K., Zaretsky, H., Kerman-Lerner, P., & Lipton, J. (1986). Augmentative communication intervention in long-term care: A multidisciplinary approach. *Augmentative and Alternative Communication*, 2, 111.

Salonen, L. (1990). A systems approach and computer assisted rehabilitation for language disorders. *Augmentative and Alternative Communication*, 6, 90.

Salvin, A., Routh, D. K., Foster, R. E., & Lovejoy, K. M. (1977). Acquisition of Modified American Sign Language by a mute autistic child. *Journal of Autism and Childhood Schizophrenia*, 7, 359–371.

Samanski, M. D. (1977). Singing, signing, and smiling: Total communication for nonverbal hearing children. *Canadian Nurse*, 73(2), 28–29.

Sampson, D. (1970). A communication device for patients unable to speak. *Medical and Biological Engineering*, 8, 99–101.

Samworth, K. T. (1992). Using a diphone inventory with parallel formant synthesis. *Augmentative and Alternative Communication*, 8, 164–165.

Sanders, D. A. (1976). A model of communication. In Lyle L. Lloyd (Ed.), *Communication Assessment and Intervention Strategies*. Baltimore: University Park Press, pp. 1–32.

Sappington, J., Reedy, S., Welch, R., & Hamilton, J. (1989). Validity of messages from quadriplegic persons with cerebral palsy. *American Journal on Mental Retardation*, 94(1), 49–52.

Sarno, J., Swisher, L., & Sarno, M. (1969). Aphasia in a congenitally deaf man. *Cortex*, 5, 398–414.

Sauer, M. (1989). The mobile outreach program—The first year. Paper presented at the annual meeting of the American Speech-Language-Hearing Association, St. Louis.

Sauer, M., Albanese, M. K., & Jarrell, N. (1992). Communication system for cognitively intact, physically disabled, deaf-blind user. Paper presented at the annual meeting of the American Speech-Language-Hearing Association, San Antonio.

Sauer, M., Brown, C., & Wyatt, C. (1990). Research findings for a voice-activated communication system with graphics. Paper presented at the annual meeting of the American Speech-Language-Hearing Association, Seattle.

Sauer, M., Brown, C., Wyatt, C., & Cavalier, A. (1992). Research findings for a voice-activated communication system with graphics. Paper presented at the annual meeting of the American Speech-Language-Hearing Association, San Antonio.

Sauer, M., McLetchie, B., & Postma, S. (1988). Effective use of computers by low functioning severely handicapped persons. *Augmentative and Alternative Communication*, 4, 160.

Sawyer, C. A., & Uebel, J. M. (1990). Listener perceptions: Severely dysarthric speech versus electronic augmentative communication system. Paper presented at the annual meeting of the American Speech-Language-Hearing Association, Seattle.

Sawyer-Woods, L. (1992). The facilitating role of Blissymbolics in aphasia rehabilitation. *Augmentative and Alternative Communication*, 6, 88.

Saya, M. (1979). Adult aphasics and Bliss symbol language. Paper presented at the annual meeting of the American Speech-Language-Hearing Association, Atlanta.

Saya, M. J., & Burrows, J. (1990). Bending Paradox to your augmentative communication service. *Augmentative and Alternative Communication*, 6, 143–144.

Sayre, J. M. (November/December 1963). Communication for the non-verbal cerebral palsied. *CP Review*, 24, 3–8.

Schaeffer, B. (1980). Simultaneous language through signed speech. In R. L. Schiefelbusch (Ed.), *Nonspeech Language and Communication: Analysis and Intervention*. Baltimore: University Park Press, pp. 421–446.

Schaeffer, B., Kollinzas, G., Musil, A., & McDowell, P. (1975). Signed speech: A new treatment for autism. Paper presented at the annual meeting of the National Society for Autistic Children, San Diego.

Schaeffer, B., McDowell, P., Musil, A., & Kollinzas, G. (1976). Spontaneous verbal language for autistic children through signed speech. *Research Relating to Children* (ERIC Clearinghouse for Early Childhood Education), Bulletin 37, 98–99.

Schaeffer, B., Musil, A., & Kollinzas, G. (1980). *Total Communication*. Champaign, IL: Research Press.

Schaffer, T. R., & Goehl, H. (1974). The alinguistic child. *Mental Retardation*, 12(2), 3–6.

Schauer, J., & Rodgers, B. L. (1987). *Highlights of the Current Standards Proposals*. Madison: Trace Research and Development Center for the Severely Communicatively Handicapped, University of Wisconsin.

Schepis, M. M., Reid, D. H., Fitzgerald, J. R., Faw, G. D., Van Den Pol, R. A., & Welty, P. A. (1982). A program for increasing manual signing by autistic and profoundly retarded youth within the daily environment. *Journal of Applied Behavior Analysis*, 15, 363–379.

Scherer, M. J. (1992). AAC users in the workplace: What employers want to know. *Augmentative and Alternative Communication*, 8, 165.

Scherer, M. J., & McKee, B. J. (1990). High-tech communication devices: What separates users from nonusers? *Augmentative and Alternative Communication*, 6, 99.

Schery, T. K., & O'Connor, L. C. (1989). Assessing effectiveness of computer language intervention with severely handicapped students. Paper presented at the annual meeting of the American Speech-Language-Hearing Association, St. Louis.

Schery, T. K., & Wilcoxen, A. (1982). *Initial Communication Processes*. Monterey, CA: Publishers Test Service.

Scheuerman, N., Baumgart, D., Sipsma, K., & Brown, L. (1976). Toward the development of a curriculum for teaching nonverbal communication skills to severely handicapped students: Teaching basic tracking, scanning, and selection skills. In L. Brown, N. Scheuerman, & T. Crowner (Eds.), *Madison's Alternative for Zero Exclusion: Toward an Integrated Therapy Model for Teaching Motor, Tracking, and Scanning Skills to Severely Handicapped Students*. Vol. 6, P. 3. Madison, WI: Department of Specialized Educational Services, Madison Metropolitan School District.

Schiaffino, A., Costa, G., Bertolami, A., & Giannoni, P. (1990). Approach to synthesized speech for communication: An experience in Italy. *Augmentative and Alternative Communication*, 6, 129.

Schiefelbusch, R. L. (Ed.) (1979). *Nonspeech Language Intervention.* Baltimore: University Park Press.

Schlanger, P. H. (1976). Training the adult aphasic to pantomime. Paper presented at the annual meeting of the American Speech-Language-Hearing Association, Houston.

Schlanger, P. H., & Schlanger, B. B. (1970). Adapting role-playing activities with aphasic patients. *Journal of Speech and Hearing Disorders,* 35, 229–235.

Schlanger, P. H., Geffner, D. S., & DiCarrado, C. (1974). A comparison of gestural communication with aphasics: Pre- and post-therapy. Paper presented at the annual meeting of the American Speech-Language-Hearing Association, Las Vegas.

Schlosser, R. W., & Karlan, G. R. (1992a). AAC and aberrant behavior: Solution and problem. *Augmentative and Alternative Communication,* 8, 165.

Schlosser, R. W., & Karlan, G. R. (1992b). Effects of functional communication training on self-injurious behavior. *Augmentative and Alternative Communication,* 8, 165–166.

Schlosser, R. W., & Lloyd, L. L. (1991). Augmentative and alternative communication: An evolving field. *Augmentative and Alternative Communication,* 7, 154–160.

Schlosser, R. W., Lloyd, L. L., & Quist, R. W. (1991). Effects of initial element teaching on Blissymbol learning and generalization. Paper presented at the annual meeting of the American Speech-Language-Hearing Association, Atlanta.

Schmidt, M. J.., Carrier Jr., J. K., & Parsons, S. D. (1971). Use of a nonspeech mode in teaching language. Paper presented at the annual meeting of the American Speech-Language-Hearing Association, Chicago.

Schrader, B. K., & Mizuko, M. I. (1989). Interactive approach to training graphic systems among developmentally delayed adults. Paper presented at the annual meeting of the American Speech-Language-Hearing Association, St. Louis.

Schreiber, C. (March 1979). To communicate with Mrs. Savage, we put bells on her toes. *Nursing,* 47–49.

Schuler, A. (198?). Selecting augmentative communication systems on the basis of current communicative means and functions. *Australian Journal of Human Communication Disorders.*

Schuler, A., & Baldwin, M. (1981). Nonspeech communication and childhood autism. *Language, Speech, and Hearing Services in Schools,* 12, 246–257.

Schuler, A., & Prizant, B. (1987). Facilitating communication: Pre-language approaches. In D. Cohen & A. Donnellan (Eds.), *Handbook of Autism and Pervasive Developmental Disorders.* New York: John Wiley, pp. 301–315.

Schultz-Muehling, L. D., & Beukelman, D. R. (1990). An augmentative and alternative writing system for a college student with fibrositis: A case study. *Augmentative and Alternative Communication,* 6, 250–255.

Schurman, J. A. (1974). Custom designing communication board frames: The role of the occupational therapist. In Beverly Vicker (Ed.), *Nonoral Communication System Project 1964/1973.* Iowa City: Campus Stores, University of Iowa, pp. 177–211.

Schwab, E., Nusbaum, H., & Pisoni, D. (1985). Some effects of training on the perception of synthetic speech. *Human Factors,* 27, 395–408.

Schwartz, P. J. (1988). A comparative study of two augmentative communication methods: Words strategy and traditional orthography. Unpublished master's thesis, Ohio University.

Schweigert, P. D. (1988). Social contingencies to intentional communication through microswitch technology: Case study. *Augmentative and Alternative Communication,* 4, 165.

Schweigert, P. D. (1989). Use of microswitch technology to facilitate social contingency awareness as a basic for early communication skills. *Augmentative and Alternative Communication*, 5, 192–198.

Schweigert, P. D., & Rowland, C. M. (1992a). Early communication and microtechnology: Instructional sequence and case studies of children with severe multiple disabilities. *Augmentative and Alternative Communication*, 8, 273–286.

Schweigert, P. D., & Rowland, C. M. (1992b). Social contingencies and the early communication process using microswitch technology. *Augmentative and Alternative Communication*, 8, 166.

Schweigert, P. D., Rowland, C. M., & Brummett, B. (1988). New CONCEPT videodisk: Communication training program. *Augmentative and Alternative Communication*, 4, 150–151.

Schweitzer, M. T., & Carney, K. A. (1992). Towards communication competence: Performance of an adult with mental retardation. *Augmentative and Alternative Communication*, 8, 166.

Schwejda, P. (1984). *Motor Training Games*. Seattle: Washington Research Foundation. [Apple II computer switch training program.]

Scull, J., & Hill, L. (1988). A computerized communication message preparation program that "learns" the user's vocabulary. *Augmentative and Alternative Communication*, 4, 40–44.

Seamone, W. (1982). A new communication technique for the nonvocal person, using the Apple II computer. *Bulletin of Prosthetics Research*, 19(1), 28–33.

Sedey, A. L., Rosin, M., & Miller, J. F. (1991). A survey of sign use among children with Down syndrome. Paper presented at the annual meeting of the American Speech-Language-Hearing Association, Atlanta.

Seery, J. (1985). *Eye Gaze Communication Systems, Games, Activities, Interactions*. Spring Valley, NY: Author.

Segalman, R. (1992). Communication, perceptions, and interaction: Part 1. Speech interpreters for dysarthric speakers. *Augmentative and Alternative Communication*, 8, 166.

Seidel, A. L., Alsup, J., & Prestigiacomo, G. (1988). A model service delivery program for a rural/urban area. *Augmentative and Alternative Communication*, 4, 138.

Selders, G., Prentice, J., Barry, R., Kent, P. A., & Baker, B. (1992). Employment of individuals with severe physical and speech impairments. *Augmentative and Alternative Communication*, 8, 167.

Seligman, J., & Gannon, R. (1972). A new approach to communication for the severely physically handicapped child. Paper presented at the annual meeting of the American Speech-Language-Hearing Association, San Francisco.

Seligman-Wine, J. (1988). A Blissymbol bar mitzvah. *Communicating Together*, 6(2), 16–17.

Seligman-Wine, J. (1990). A national model for inservice training in AAC. *Augmentative and Alternative Communication*, 6, 102–103.

Seligman-Wine, J., & Amir, N. (1986). The use of Blissymbols with preschool children with severe nondysarthric speech and language disorders. *Augmentative and Alternative Communication*, 2, 111.

Seligman-Wine, J., & Amir, N. (1990). AAC in the rehabilitation process of a postencephalitic child. *Augmentative and Alternative Communication*, 6, 146.

Seligman-Wine, J., & Jaimovich, M. (1990). Integrating AAC in a dynamic-language-oriented classroom program. *Augmentative and Alternative Communication*, 6, 117–118.

Seligman-Wine, J., Yaniv, K., & Carmeli, S. (1992). Parental perceptions within the pragmatics of AAC. *Augmentative and Alternative Communication*, 8, 167.

Sensenig, L. D., Mazeika, E. J., & Topf, B. (1989). Sign language facilitation of reading with students classified as trainable mentally-handicapped. *Education and Training in Mental Retardation*, 24(2), 121–125.

Serenella, B., & Chinato, M. G. (1992). Cognitive development and interaction between systems: A Bliss user's decennial history. *Augmentative and Alternative Communication*, 8, 167.

Sevcik, R. A., Chabon, S. S., & Romski, M. A. (1988). Residental communicative interaction patterns of nonspeaking adults with severe retardation. Paper presented at the annual meeting of the American Speech-Language-Hearing Association, Boston.

Sevcik, R. A., Plenge, T. F., & Romski, M. A. (1987). Augmentative communication system acquisition and use: A model for assessing progress. Paper presented at the annual meeting of the American Speech-Language-Hearing Association, New Orleans.

Sevcik, R. A., & Romski, M. A. (1984). Group instruction: A viable communication approach to severely retarded persons. Paper presented at the annual meeting of the American Speech-Language-Hearing Association, San Francisco.

Sevcik, R. A., & Romski, M. A. (1985). Comprehension of synthesized speech by nonspeaking severely retarded persons. Paper presented at the annual meeting of the American Speech-Language-Hearing Association, Washington, DC.

Sevcik, R. A., & Romski, M. A. (1986). Representative matching skills of persons with severe retardation. *Augmentative and Alternative Communication*, 2(4), 160–164.

Sevcik, R. A., Romski, M. A., & Adamson, L. B. (1992). Augmentative communication development by a preschool child with severe disabilities. Paper presented at the annual meeting of the American Speech-Language-Hearing Association, San Antonio.

Sevcik, R. A., Romski, M. A., & Wilkinson, K. M. (1991). Roles of graphic symbols in the language acquisition process for persons with severe cognitive disabilities. *Augmentative and Alternative Communication*, 7, 161–170.

Shaeffer, B., Kollinzas, G., Musil, A., & McDowell, P. (1975). Signed speech: A new treatment for autism. Paper presented at the annual meeting of the National Society for Autistic Children, San Diego.

Shaffer, T. R., & Goehl, H. (1974). The alinguistic child. *Mental Retardation*, 12(2), 3–6.

Shahar, E., Nowaczyk, M., & Tervo, R. C. (1987). Rehabilitation of communication impairment in dystonia musculorum deformans. *Pediatric Neurology*, 3(2), 97–100.

Shalit, A., & Boonzaier, D. (1990). Macintosh-based semantographic technique with adaptive-predictive algorithm for Blissymbolics communication. *Augmentative and Alternative Communication*, 6, 122.

Shalit, A., & Boonzaier, D. (1992). Why should the "semantographic" method be used for teaching and retrieving of Blissymbols? *Augmentative and Alternative Communication*, 8, 167–168.

Shane, H. C. (1981a). Decision making in early augmentative communication. In R. L. Schiefelbusch & D. D. Bricker (Eds.), *Early Language: Acquisition and Intervention*. Baltimore: University Park Press, pp. 389–425.

Shane, H. C. (1981b). The value of toys. *Communication Outlook*, 3(1), 8.

Shane, H. C. (1986). Goals and Uses. In Sarah W. Blackstone (Ed.), *Augmentative Communication: An Introduction*. Rockville, MD: American Speech-Language-Hearing Association, pp. 29–47.

Shane, H. C., & Anastasio, V. C. (1989). Augmentative communication considerations in pediatric otolaryngology. *Otolaryngologic Clinics of North America*, 22(3), 501–517.

Shane, H. C., & Bashir, A. S. (1980). Election criteria for the adoption of an augmentative communication system: Preliminary considerations. *Journal of Speech and Hearing Disorders*, 45, 408–414.

Shane, H. C., & Cohen, C. (1981). A discussion of communicative strategies and patterns by nonspeaking persons. *Language, Speech, and Hearing Services in Schools*, 12, 205–210.

Shane, H. C., Lipshultz, S., & Shane, C. (1982). Facilitating the communication interaction of nonspeaking persons in large residential settings. *Topics in Language Disorders*, 2(2), 73–84.

Shane, H. C., & Melrose, J. (1975). An electronic conversation board and an accompaning training program for aphonic expressive communication. Paper presented at the annual meeting of the American Speech-Language-Hearing Association, Washington, DC.

Shane, H. C., & Sauer, M. (1986). *Augmentative and Alternative Communication*. Austin, TX: Pro-Ed.

Shane, H. C., Thompson, E. J., & Carpenter, C. (1990). The use of voice recognition in a competitive work environment. *Augmentative and Alternative Communication*, 6, 108–109.

Shane, H. C., & Wilbur, R. B. (1980). Potential for expressive signing based on motor control. *Sign Language Studies*, 29, 331–347.

Shane, H. C., & Wilbur, R. B. (1989). A conceptual framework for AAC strategy based on sign language parameters. Paper presented at the annual meeting of the American Speech-Language-Hearing Association, St. Louis.

Shane, H. C., & Wilbur, R. B. (1990). An introduction to the Vois Shapes system for language production. *Augmentative and Alternative Communication*, 6, 105.

Shane, H. C., & Wilson, M. S. (1977). Blissymbolics. *Asha*, 19, 223.

Shannon, C. E., & Weaver, W. (1963). *A Mathematical Theory of Communication*. Urbana: University of Illinois Press.

Shea, V., & Mount, M. (1982). *How to Arrange the Environment to Stimulate and Teach Prelanguage Skills in the Severely Retarded*. Lawrence, KS: H & H Enterprises.

Shell, D., Horn, C., & Bruning, R. (October–November 1989). Technologies for the information age: Enhancing disabled persons' access and use of text based information. *Closing the Gap*, 24–27.

Shenhav, H., & Gorfil, L. (1990). Integration of Blissymbols in a reading program with AAC users. *Augmentative and Alternative Communication*, 6, 131.

Shepherd, T. A., & Haaf, R. G. (1992). Comparison of two training methods of Blissymbols. *Augmentative and Alternative Communication*, 8, 168.

Shevin, M., & Klein, N. (1984). The importance of choice-making skills for students with severe disabilities. *Journal of the Association for Persons with Severe Handicaps*, 9, 159–166.

Shewan, C. M., & Blake, A. (May 1991). Augmentative and alternative communication. *Asha*, 33, 46.

Shimizu, N. (1988). Sign language training for children with developmental retardation in speech. *Tokushu Kyoiku Kenkyu Shisetsu Hokoku/RIEEC Report*, 37, 73–78.

Shipley, K. G., & Jarrow, J. E. (1976). An experimental university clinic training program for a non-language child. *Journal of the National Student Speech and Hearing Association*, 4, 9–16.

Shook, E. S. (1992). Integrating teaching and technology: AAC device-facilitating strategies. *Augmentative and Alternative Communication*, 8, 168.

Shrewsbury, R. G., Lass, M. J., & Joseph, L. S. (1985). A survey of special educators' awareness of, experience with, and attitudes toward nonverbal communication aids in the schools. *Language, Speech, and Hearing Services in Schools*, 16, 293–298.

Shvadron, Z. (1990). From a parent's point of view. *Augmentative and Alternative Communication*, 6, 87.

Shwedyk, E., & Gordon, J. (1977). Communication aids for nonvocal handicapped people. *Medical and Biological Engineering and Computing*, 15, 189–194.

Siegel-Causey, E., & Downing, J. (1987). Nonsymbolic communication development: Theoretical concepts and educational strategies. In L. Goetz, D. Guess, & K. Stremel-Campbell (Eds.), *Innovative Program Design for Individuals with Dual Sensory Impairments*. Baltimore: Paul H. Brookes, pp. 15–48.

Siegel-Causey, E., & Ernst, B. (1989). Theoretical orientation and research in non-symbolic development. In E. Siegel-Causey & D. Guess (Eds.), *Enhancing Nonsymbolic Communication Interactions Among Learners with Severe Disabilities*. Baltimore: Paul H. Brookes, pp. 17–51.

Siegel-Causey, E., & Guess, D. (1988). *Enhancing Interactions Between Service Providers and Individuals Who Are Severely Multiply Disabled: Strategies for Developing Nonsymbolic Communication*. Monmouth, OR: Teaching Research.

Siegel-Causey, E., & Guess, D. (Eds) (1989). *Enhancing Nonsymbolic Communication Interactions Among Learners with Severe Disabilities*. Baltimore: Paul H. Brookes.

Sienkiewicz-Mercer, R., & Costello, J. (1992). Becoming independent and an effective communicator: One consumer's experience. *Augmentative and Alternative Communication*, 8, 168.

Sigafoos, J., Doss, S., & Reichle, J. (1989). Developing mand and tact repertoires in persons with severe developmental disabilities using graphic symbols. *Research in Developmental Disabilities*, 10, 183–200.

Sigafoos, J., Mustonen, T., DePaepe, P., Reichle, J., & York, J. (1991). Defining the array of instructional prompts for teaching communication skills. In J. Reichle, J. Y. York, & J. Sigafoos, *Implementing Augmentative and Alternative Communication: Strategies for Learners with Severe Disabilities*. Baltimore: Paul H. Brookes, pp. 173–192.

Sigafoos, J., & Reichle, J. (1991). Establishing an initial repertoire of rejecting. In J. Reichle, J. Y. York, & J. Sigafoos, *Implementing Augmentative and Alternative Communication: Strategies for Learners with Severe Disabilities*. Baltimore: Paul H. Brookes, pp. 115–132.

Sigafoos, J., & Reichle, J. (1992). Comparing explicit to generalized requesting in an augmentative communication mode. *Journal of Developmental and Physical Disabilities*, 4(2), 167–188.

Sigafoos, J., & York, J. (1991). Using ecological inventories to promote functional communication. In J. Reichle, J. Y. York, & J. Sigafoos, *Implementing Augmentative and Alternative Communication: Strategies for Learners with Severe Disabilities*. Baltimore: Paul H. Brookes, pp. 61–70.

Sigelman, C., Vengroff, L., & Spanhel, C. (1984). Disability and the concept of life functions. In R. Marinelli & A. Dell Orto (Eds.), *The Psychological and Social Impact of Physical Disability*. 2nd ed. New York: Springer.

Silliphant, D. L., & Bedrosian, J. L. (1990). Communication initiations by an AAC user in a mainstreamed classroom. Paper presented at the annual meeting of the American Speech-Language-Hearing Association, Seattle.

Silverman, E.-M., & Silverman, F. H. (1979). Attitudes toward the adoption of an international language. In William C. McCormack & Stephen A. Wurm (Eds.), *Language and Society: Anthropological Issues*. The Hague and Paris: Mouton.

Silverman, F. H. (1977a). A bibliography of literature relevant to nonspeech communication modes for the speechless. *Ohio Journal of Speech and Hearing*, 12, 83–102.

Silverman, F. H. (1977b). Why not Amerind. *Asha*, 19, 463.

Silverman, F. H. (1977c). Criteria for assessing therapy outcome in speech pathology and audiology. *Journal of Speech and Hearing Research*, 20, 5–20.

Silverman, F. H. (1978). Non-vocal communication systems: Implications for the neurosciences. *Trends in Neurosciences*, 1, 147–148.

Silverman, F. H. (1980). *Communication for the Speechless*. Englewood Cliffs, NJ: Prentice Hall.

Silverman, F. H. (1983). Dysarthria: Communication augmentation systems for adults without speech. In William H. Perkins (Ed.), *Dysarthria and Apraxia*. New York: Thieme-Stratton, pp. 115–121.

Silverman, F. H. (1985). La communicazione per il privo di parola ieri, oggi e domani. In Oskar Schindler (Ed.), *Foniatria e Logopedia Oggi*. Torino, Italy: Edizioni Omega.

Silverman, F. H. (1986). *Why Is It Being Recommended That My Child Learn Sign Language?* [Apple II program for use with parents of mentally retarded children]. Greendale, WI: CODI Publications, 5918 Currant Lane.

Silverman, F. H. (1987a). *La Communicazione per il Privo di Parola*. Torino, Italy: Edizioni Omega.

Silverman, F. H. (1987b). *Microcomputers in Speech-Language Pathology and Audiology: A Primer*. Englewood Cliffs, NJ: Prentice Hall.

Silverman, F. H. (1987c). T-shirt communication board. *The Clinical Connection*, 1(2), 2.

Silverman, F. H. (1989a). Augmenting the residual communication skills of severely-communicatively-impaired adults who are aphasic. Paper presented at the National Symposium on Rehabilitation of Patients with Aphasia, Krakow, Poland.

Silverman, F. H. (1989b). *Communication for the Speechless*. 2nd ed. Englewood Cliffs, NJ: Prentice Hall.

Silverman, F. H. (1989c). Communication for the speechless: State of the art. Paper presented at the All-Union Symposium on Treatment and Rehabilitation of Patients with Speech Disorders, Moscow.

Silverman, F. H. (1989d). Manual communication for people with mental retardation: Why? and Why not? Paper presented at the annual meeting of the American Association for Mental Retardation, Chicago.

Silverman, F. H. (1990). Augmenting the residual communication skills of severely-communicatively-impaired persons, particularly those who are aphasic. Paper presented at the Sixteenth Congress of European Phoniatricians, Salsomaggiori, Italy.

Silverman, F. H. (1992a). Augmentative communication strategies for speechless children. Paper presented at the First Conference of the Saudi Benevolent Association for Disabled Children, Riyadh, Saudi Arabia.

Silverman, F. H. (1992b). *Legal-Ethical Considerations, Restrictions, and Obligations for Clinicians Who Treat Communicative Disorders*. Springfield, IL: Charles C. Thomas.

Silverman, F. H. (1993a). *Research Design and Evaluation in Speech-Language Pathology and Audiology*. 3rd ed. Englewood Cliffs, NJ: Prentice Hall.

Silverman, F. H. (1993b). Telecommunication relay services: An option for persons who are severely speech impaired. *Augmentative and Alternative Communication*.

Silverman, F. H., and Bady, J. (1978). Need for including coursework on nonvocal communication systems: A survey. *Asha*, 20, 1023.

Silverman, F. H., & Bhatnagar, S. (1992). Development of Hindi language communication boards. Unpublished manuscript, Marquette University.

Silverman, F. H., & Kazmarek, D. (1992). Development of a Polish language communication device for severely-communicatively-impaired children and adults. Paper presented at the First European Congress of Speech and Language Pathology, Athens.

Silverman, F. H., & Meagher, M. (1980). The speechless population: How large is it? *Perceptual and Motor Skills*, 51, 1178.

Silverman, F. H., & Merz-Johnson, G. (1990). Development of a German language communication board. Unpublished manuscript, Marquette University.

Silverman, F. H., & Rivilis, G. (1990). Development of a Russian language communication board. Unpublished manuscript, Marquette University.

Silverman, F. H., & Schorsch, J. C. (November 1992). Augmentative communication coursework needed. *Asha*, 34, 66.

Silverman, F. H., & Schuyler, H. J. (1994). Can AAC help person with dementia? *Augmentative and Alternative Communication*, 10, 60.

Silverman, H., & Kelso, D. (1977). The Bliss-Com: A portable symbol printing communication aid. Paper presented at the Fourth Annual Conference on Systems and Devices for the Disabled, Seattle. (Paper is published in the conference proceedings volume, available from Continuing Medical Education, University of Washington School of Medicine.)

Silverman, H., McNaughton, S., & Kates, B. (1978). *Handbook of Blissymbolics for Instructors, Users, Parents, and Administrators*. Toronto: Blissymbolics Communication Institute.

Simon, B. M. (1985). Illustration of augmentative communication modifications in two ventilator-dependent children. Paper presented at the annual meeting of the American Speech-Language-Hearing Association, Washington, DC.

Simpson, K. O., Cumley, G. D., Novak, B., & Tegtmeier, J. (1992). Issues related to instruction of technology in AAC. Paper presented at the annual meeting of the American Speech-Language-Hearing Association, San Antonio.

Simpson, M. (1979). A total communication approach in an interdisciplinary infant development program. Paper presented at the annual meeting of the American Speech-Language-Hearing Association, Atlanta.

Simpson, S. (1988). If only I could tell them . . . !! *Communication Outlook*, 9(4), 9–11.

Single-Input Control Assessment (1983). Lake Zurich, IL: Don Johnson Developmental Equipment. [Computer program.]

Sisson, L. A., & Barrett, R. P. (1984). An alternating treatment comparison of oral and total communication training with minimally verbal retarded children. *Journal of Applied Behavior Analysis*, 17(4), 559–566.

Sitver, M., & Kraat, A. (1982). Augmentative communication for the person with amyotrophic lateral sclerosis (ALS). *Asha*, 24, 783.

Skelly, M. (1977). Amerind clarified. *Asha*, 19, 746–747.

Skelly, M. (1979). *Amer-Ind Gestural Code*. New York: Elsevier (1979).

Skelly, M., Donaldson, R. C., & Fust, R. S. (1973). *Glossectomee Speech Rehabilitation*. Springfield, IL: Charles C. Thomas.

Skelly, M., Schinsky, L., Smith, R. W., Donaldson, R., & Griffin, J. (1975). American Indian Sign: A gestural communication system for the speechless. *Archives of Physical Medicine and Rehabilitation*, 56, 156–160.

Skelly, M., Schinsky, L., Smith, R. W., & Fust, R. S. (1974). American Indian Sign (AMER-IND) as a facilitator of verbalization for the oral verbal apraxic. *Journal of Speech and Hearing Disorders*, 39, 445–456.

Sklar, M., & Bennett, D. N. (1956). Initial communication chart for aphasics. *Journal of the Association of Physical and Mental Rehabilitation*, 10, 43–53.

Small-Morris, S. (1986). Transparency of two representational systems: Picsyms and picture communication symbols. Unpublished master's thesis, Western Carolina University.

Smebye, H. (1986). A new method for teaching communication through technology on child-initiative to multiply handicapped children. *Augmentative and Alternative Communication*, 2, 111–112.

Smebye, H. (1990). A theoretical basis for early communication intervention. *Augmentative and Alternative Communication*, 6, 148.

Smith, A. K., & Lageer, N. (1988). Introducing literacy to children who use augmentative and alternative communication systems. *Augmentative and Alternative Communication*, 4, 140.

Smith, A. K., Thurston, S., Light, J., Parnes, P., & O'Keefe, B. (1989). The form and use of written communication produced by physically disabled individuals using microcomputers. *Augmentative and Alternative Communication*, 5, 115–124.

Smith, C. H. (1975). Total communication utilizing the simultaneous method. In M. P. Creedon (Ed.), *Appropriate Behavior Through Communication: A New Program in Simultaneous Language*. Chicago: Dysfunctioning Child Center, pp. 45–74.

Smith, L. (1986a). A measure of natural nonverbal behavior in aphasia. *Augmentative and Alternative Communication*, 2, 112.

Smith, L. (1986b). Natural nonverbal behavior in aphasic and nonaphasic adults. *Augmentative and Alternative Communication*, 2, 112–113.

Smith, L., & von Tetzchner, S. (1986). Communicative, sensorimotor, and language skills of young children with Down syndrome. *American Journal of Mental Deficiency*, 91, 57–66.

Smith, M. D., & Belcher, R. G. (1993). Brief report: Facilitated communication with adults with autism. *Journal of Autism and Developmental Disorders*, 23(1), 175–183.

Smith, M. M. (1989). Reading without speech: A study of children with cerebral palsy. *Irish Journal of Psychology*, 10(4), 601–614.

Smith, M. M. (1990). Reading achievement in nonspeaking children: A comparative study. *Augmentative and Alternative Communication*, 6, 132.

Smith, M. M. (1991). Assessment of interaction patterns and AAC use: A case study. *Journal of Clinical Speech and Language Studies*, 1, 76–102.

Smith, M. M. (1992a). Reading abilities of nonspeaking students: Two case studies. *Augmentative and Alternative Communication*, 8, 57–66.

Smith, M. M. (1992b). Spelling abilities of nonspeaking students. *Augmentative and Alternative Communication*, 8, 168–169.

Smith, R. O., Christiaansen, R., Borden, B., Lindberg, D., Gunderson, J., & Vanderheiden, G. C. (1989). Effectiveness of a writing system using a computerized long-range optical pointer and 10-branch abbreviation expansion. *Journal of Rehabilitation Research and Development*, 26(1), 51–62.

Smith, R. O., Cress, C. J., Murray-Branch, J., & Vanderheiden, G. C. (1992). InterACT: Interdisciplinary augmentative communication and technology training program. *Augmentative and Alternative Communication*, 8, 169.

Smith-Lewis, M. R. (1992). Culturally diverse nonspeakers: Comparison of home/school communication interactions. *Augmentative and Alternative Communication*, 8, 169.

Smith-Lewis, M. R., & Ford, A. (1987). A user's perspective on augmentative communication. *Augmentative and Alternative Communication*, 3(1), 12–17.

Smorto, M. P., & Basmajian, J. V. (1977). *Electrodiagnosis: A Handbook for Neurologists.* New York: Harper & Row.

Smullen, J., & Watts, P. (1986). Classroom experience with "MIKE": A flexible keyboard emulator. *Augmentative and Alternative Communication*, 2, 113.

Snyder, M. P., Crockett, K. E., & Kesnecka, C. T. (1990). Switch selection and wheelchair mounting considerations with augmentative systems. Paper presented at the annual meeting of the American Speech-Language-Hearing Association, Seattle.

Snyder-McLean, L. (1978a). Functional stimulus and response variables in sign training with retarded subjects. Paper presented at the annual meeting of the American Speech-Language-Hearing Association, San Francisco.

Snyder-McLean, L. (1978b). Language training procedures for non-verbal severely retarded clients: Functional stimulus and response variables. Paper presented at the annual meeting of the American Association for the Education of the Severely/Profoundly Handicapped, Baltimore.

Sobsey, R., & Bieniek, B. (1983). A family approach to functional sign language. *Behavior Modification*, 7, 488–502.

Soede, M., & Foulds, R. A. (1986). Prediction (P)reviewed. *Augmentative and Alternative Communication*, 2, 113–114.

Soede, M., van Balkon, H. L., Deroost, G., van Knippenberg, F. H., & Kamphuis, H. (1989). New possibilities for enhanced keyboard input for the handicapped. *Journal of Medical Engineering and Technology*, 13(1–2), 34–36.

Soede, M., & Stassen, H. G. (1973). A light spot operated typewriter for severely disabled patients. *Medical and Biological Engineering*, 11, 641–644.

Soede, M., Stassen, H. G., Lunteren, A. V., & Luitse, W. J. (1974). A lightspot-operated typewriter (LOT). In Keith Copeland (Ed.), *Aids for the Severely Handicapped.* New York: Grune & Stratton, pp. 42–53.

Solon, E. M. (1992). Smooth transitions: From low technology to high technology AAC systems. *Augmentative and Alternative Communication*, 8, 169.

Sommer, K. S., Whitman, T. L., & Keogh, D. A. (1988). Teaching severely retarded persons to sign interactively through the use of a behavioral script. *Research in Developmental Disabilities*, 9(3), 291–304.

Song, A. (1979). Acquisition and use of Blissymbols by severely mentally retarded adolescents. *Mental Retardation*, 17, 253–255.

Sontag, E. Smith, J., & Certo, N. (Eds.) (1977). *Educational Programming for the Severely and Profoundly Handicapped.* Reston, VA: Council for Exceptional Children.

Soper, H., L., & Phipps, D. C. (1992). Augmentative communication: Program design in the public schools. Paper presented at the annual meeting of the American Speech-Language-Hearing Association, San Antonio.

Soro, E., Basil, C., & von Tetzchner, S. (1992). Teaching initial communication and language skills to AAC users. *Augmentative and Alternative Communication*, 8, 169–170.

Sparker, A. W. (Fall/Winter 1989). Communication alternatives for intubated, trached, and/or ventilator dependent patients. *Tejas*, 15(2), 25–26.

Spiegel, B. B. (1987). Pragmatic considerations in augmentative communication use. Paper presented at the annual meeting of the American Speech-Language-Hearing Association, New Orleans.

Spradlin, J. (1963). Assessment of speech and language of retarded children: The Parsons Language Sample. *Journal of Speech and Hearing Disorders*, Monograph Supplement 10, 8–31.

Spragale, D. M., & Micucci, D. (1989). Functional sign language training for staff: Signs of the week. Paper presented at the annual meeting of the American Speech-Language-Hearing Association, St. Louis.

Spragale, D. M., & Micucci, D. (1990). Signs of the week: A functional approach to manual sign training. *Augmentative and Alternative Communication*, 6, 29–37.

Sprague, L. G. (1983). Equipment-free communication. *Communication Outlook*, 4(4), 6–7.

Starch, S. A. (1990). Increasing children's understanding of aphasia: An educational approach. Paper presented at the annual meeting of the American Speech-Language-Hearing Association, Seattle.

Stassen, H. G., Soede, M., & Bakker, H. (1982). The lightspot operated typewriter: A communication aid for severely bodily handicapped patients. *Scandinavian Journal of Rehabilitation*, 14, 159–161.

Staudenbauer, T. (1985). An on-line analysis of communicative intention displayed by young children with severe physical handicaps while interacting with various partners. Unpublished master's thesis, University of Wisconsin, Madison.

Steadman, J. W., Ferris, C. D., & Rhodine, C. N. (1980). Prosthetic communication device. *Archives of Physical Medicine and Rehabilitation*, 61, 93–97.

Steele, D. (1974). Visual effect from muscular movement (Systems 7 and 9). In Keith Copeland (Ed.), *Aids for the Severely Handicapped*. New York: Grune & Stratton, pp. 63–71.

Steele, R. D., Newell, A. F., Soede, M., Fagerberg, G., Bernstein, J., & Parnes, P. (1988). International forum on current issues in AAC research. *Augmentative and Alternative Communication*, 4, 157.

Steele, R. D., Weinrich, M., Wertz, R. T., Kleczewska, M. K., and Carlson, G. S. (1989). Computer-based visual communication in aphasia. *Neuropsychologia*, 27(4), 409–426.

Steelman, J. D. (1992a). *High Tech Literacy Learning: We've Only Just Begun*. Chapel Hill: Carolina Literacy Center, University of North Carolina.

Steelman, J. D. (1992b). TILLT: Technology, interaction, literacy, learning, and teaching. *Augmentative and Alternative Communication*, 8, 170.

Steelman, J. D., Coleman, P. P., & Koppenhaver, D. A. (1992). Minspeak: A tool for developing literacy. Paper presented at the Seventh Annual Minspeak Conference.

Steelman, J. D., Pierce, P. L., Alger, M. J., Shannon, J., Koppenhaver, D. A., & Yoder, D. E. (1993). *Developing an Emergent Literacy Curriculum for Children with Developmental Disabilities*. Chapel Hill: Carolina Literacy Center, University of North Carolina.

Steelman, J. D., Pierce, P. L., & Koppenhaver, D. A. (1993). The role of computers in promoting literacy in children with severe speech and physical impairment. *Topics in Language Disorders*, 13(2), 76–91.

Steiner, S., & Larson, V. (1991). Integrating microcomputers into language intervention with children. *Topics in Language Disorders*, 11(2), 18–30.

Stemach, G., & Williams, W. (1988). *Word Express: The First 2,500 Words of Spoken English.* Novato, CA: Academic Therapy Publications.

Stephens, R., & Lauro, C. (1988). Development of communication centre in Lisbon and case studies. *Augmentative and Alternative Communication*, 4, 137.

Stephens, R. M. (1986). Voice recognition, computing, and the disabled. *Augmentative and Alternative Communication*, 2, 114–115.

Stephens, R. M., & Cottle, M. (1988). Voice activated workstation for disabled people. *Augmentative and Alternative Communication*, 4, 153.

Stephenson-Wright, B. (1990). The educator's role in integrating the augmentative and alternative communication user. *Augmentative and Alternative Communication*, 6, 107.

Sterling, L. R., & Kluppel-Vetter, D. (1990). Measuring the ASL translucency continuum: Magnitude estimation vs. interval scaling. Paper presented at the annual meeting of the American Speech-Language-Hearing Association, Seattle.

Sternberg, L., McNerney, C. D., & Pegnatore, L. (1987). Developing primitive signalling behavior of students with profound mental retardation. *Mental Retardation*, 25(1), 13–20.

Stevenson-Wright, B., Todaro, M. P., & Morrison, C. (1992). Integrating AAC into the classroom: A panel discussion. *Augmentative and Alternative Communication*, 8, 170.

Stewart, K. P. (1989). Facilitating the success for an augmentative communication system. Paper presented at the annual meeting of the American Speech-Language-Hearing Association, St. Louis.

Stillman, R. D., & Battle, C. (1984). Developing prelanguage communication in the severely handicapped: An interpretation of the Van Dijk method. *Seminars in Speech and Language*, 5, 159–170.

Stillman, R. D., & Battle, C. (1985). *The Callier-Azusa Scales for the Assessment of Communicative Abilities.* Dallas: Callier Center, University of Texas.

Stillman, R. D., & Williams, C. (1990). Severely handicapped children's responsiveness to verbal and nonverbal communication. Paper presented at the annual meeting of the American Speech-Language-Hearing Association, Seattle.

St. Louis, K. W. (1988). Development of vocabularies for three voice output communication aids. *Augmentative and Alternative Communication*, 4, 143–144.

St. Louis, K. W. (1990). Devices as teaching and speaking aids in a public school. *Augmentative and Alternative Communication*, 6, 126.

St. Louis, K. W., Mattingly, S., & Esposito, A. (1986). Receptive language curriculum for the moderately, severely, and profoundly handicapped. In J. D. Cone (Ed.), *Pyramid System Curriculum.* Morgantown, WV: Pyramid Press.

St. Louis, K. W., & Rejzer, R. (1986). Expressive language curriculum for the moderately, severely, and profoundly handicapped. In J. D. Cone (Ed.), *Pyramid System Curriculum.* Morgantown, WV: Pyramid Press.

Stovsky, B., Rudy, E., & Dragonette, P. (1988). Comparison of two types of communication methods used after cardiac surgery with patients with endotracheal tubes. *Heart and Lung*, 17(3), 281–289.

Stowers, S., Altheide, M. R., & Shea, V. (1987). Motor assessment for unaided and aided augmentative communication. *Physical and Occupational Therapy in Pediatrics*, 7, 61–77.

Stratil, M., & Burkhardt, D. (1986). Spanish speech synthesis used with CAL language laboratory. *Augmentative and Alternative Communication*, 2, 115.

Strauss, K. P. (June/July 1992). Nationwide relay services. *Asha*, 34, 48–49.

Stremel-Campbell, K., Cantrell, D., & Halle, J. (1977). Manual signing as a language system and as a speech initiator for the non-verbal severely handicapped student. In E. Sontag (Ed.), *Educational Programming for the Severely and Profoundly Handicapped*. Reston, VA: Council for Exceptional Children.

Strong, G. W. (1992). Usability evaluation of the PRC Touchtalker with Minspeak. *Augmentative and Alternative Communication*, 8, 170.

Stuart, S., Gordon, D., Hofman, A., Romich, B., Weis, L., & Woltosz, W. (1988). Insights related to manufacturing augmentative and alternative communication equipment—Panel discussion. *Augmentative and Alternative Communication*, 4, 155.

Stuart, S. L. (1986). Expanding sequencing, turntaking, and timing skills through play acting. In Sarah W. Blackstone (Ed.), *Augmentative Communication: An Introduction*. Rockville, MD: American Speech-Language-Hearing Association, pp. 389–395.

Stuart, S. L. (1988). Expanding sequencing, turn-taking and timing skills through play acting. In S. Blackstone, E. Cassatt-James, & D. Bruskin (Eds.), *Augmentative Communication: Implementation Strategies*. Rockville, MD: American Speech-Language-Hearing Association, pp. 5.8-21–5.8-26.

Stuart, S. L. (1991a). Differences in words/topics used by elderly men and women. Paper presented at the annual meeting of the American Speech-Language-Hearing Association, Atlanta.

Stuart, S. L. (1991b). Topic and vocabulary use patterns of elderly men and women in two age cohorts. Unpublished doctoral dissertation, University of Nebraska, Lincoln.

Stuart, S. L., Jones, R. S., & Beukelman, D. R. (1992). Vocabulary by topic analysis in the speech of elderly persons. *Augmentative and Alternative Communication*, 8, 170–171.

Stuart, S. L., Jones, R. S., & Harrington, L. L. (1992). Analyzing repetitive storytelling narratives for vocabulary selection in AAC systems. Paper presented at the annual meeting of the American Speech-Language-Hearing Association, San Antonio.

Stum, G. M., Demasco, P., & McCoy, K. F. (1992). Flexible abbreviation expansion. *Augmentative and Alternative Communication*, 8, 171.

Stump, R. (1986). Large scale vocabulary selection technique. Paper presented at the First Annual Minspeak Conference, Detroit.

Stump, R. T. (1988). Implementing augmentative and alternative communication: A vocational rehabilitation counselor's perspective. *Augmentative and Alternative Communication*, 4, 146.

Stump, R. T. (1990). Successful augmentative and alternative communicators in vocational rehabilitation programs. *Augmentative and Alternative Communication*, 6, 139.

Stump, R. T. (1992). Transitional technology: Opening to independence, opening to the world. *Augmentative and Alternative Communication*, 8, 171.

Stump, R. T., Weinberg, W., & Baker, B. (1987). *Vocabulary Development for Augmentative Communication*. Pittsburgh: Authors.

Such, P. (1988). New software and hardware for motor disabled people. *Augmentative and Alternative Communication*, 4, 161.

Sutherland, D., & Kates, B. (1975). *Considerations in Assessing a Child's Communication Needs*. Toronto: Blissymbolics Communication Institute.

Sutherland, G. F., & Beckett, J. W. (1969). Teaching the mentally retarded sign language. *Journal of Rehabilitation of the Deaf*, 2, 56–60.

Sutherland, L., & Joss, A. (1990). Training materials for teachers/therapists/caregivers involved in assessment. *Augmentative and Alternative Communication*, 6, 144.

Sutter, E. (1983). An oculo-encephalographic communication system. *Proceedings of the Sixth Annual Conference on Rehabilitation Engineering*. Rehabilitation Engineering Society of North America, pp. 242–244.

Sutton, A. C. (1988). The Expressive One-Word Vocabulary Test via Blissymbols. *Augmentative and Alternative Communication*, 4, 145.

Sutton, A. C. (1989). The social-verbal competence of AAC users. *Augmentative and Alternative Communication*, 5, 150–164.

Sutton, A. C., & Gallagher, T. (1992). Linguistic comprehension of past time references in AAC system users. *Augmentative and Alternative Communication*, 8, 171.

Svanfeldt, I. (1992). TALTJANST—A new communication service for speech impaired in Uppsala. *Augmentative and Alternative Communication*, 6, 107.

Swartz, S. (1984). Blissymbols go to India. *Communicating Together*, 2(1), 4–6.

Sweda, J. P., & Coleman, L. G. (1983). Communicative interaction between nonverbal, severely handicapped children and their mothers. Paper presented at the annual meeting of the American Speech-Language-Hearing Association, Cincinnati.

Sweeney, L. A. (1980). Simultaneous communication versus vocal training with severely language-impaired adults. Paper presented at the annual meeting of the American Speech-Language-Hearing Association, Detroit.

Sweeney, L. A. (1990). A protocol for assessment of early manual communication skills. *Augmentative and Alternative Communication*, 6, 109–110.

Sweeney, L. A. (1992). Assessment of learned dependency among potential users of AAC. *Augmentative and Alternative Communication*, 8, 171–172.

Sweeney, L. A., & Finkley, E. (1989). Early manual communication skills assessment. In S. Blackstone, E. Cassatt-James, & D. Bruskin (Eds.), *Augmentative Communication: Implementation Strategies*. Rockville, MD: American Speech-Language-Hearing Association, pp. 3-159–3-168.

Sweeney, L. A., & Jones, J. (1988). Speech-language pathologists and equipment distributors: Cooperative problem solving. *Augmentative and Alternative Communication*, 4, 173.

Sweeney, L. A., & Mathy-Laikko, P. (1992). Management and supervision issues in AAC. *Augmentative and Alternative Communication*, 8, 172.

Sweeney, L. A., & Neal, A. E. (1986). Sign language notation: Analysis and application. *Augmentative and Alternative Communication*, 2, 115.

Swerissen, H. (1990). Alternative communication strategies for people with intellectual disability. *Australian Journal of Human Communication Disorders*, 18(1), 63–77.

Swiffin, A. L., Arnott, J. L., Pickering, J. A., & Newell, A. F. (1987). Adaptive and predictive techniques in a communication prosthesis. *Augmentative and Alternative Communication*, 3(4), 181–191.

Swiffin, A. L., Newell, A. F., & Arnott, J. L. (1986). Linguistic prediction in a portable communication system for the physically handicapped. *Augmentative and Alternative Communication*, 2, 115–116.

Sy, B. K., & Deller Jr., J. R. (1989). An AI-based communication system for motor and speech disabled persons: Design methodology and prototype testing. *IEEE Transactions on Biomedical Engineering*, 36(5), 565–571.

Symbols are Bliss (1977). *Asha*, 19, 104.

Syntax Supplement No. 1 [for Blissymbols] (n.d.). Toronto: Blissymbolics Communication Institute.

Szeto, A. Y. J., Allen, E. J., & Littrell, M. C. (1993). Comparison of speed and accuracy for selected electronic communication devices and imput methods. *Augmentative and Alternative Communication*, 9, 229–242.

Tallman, T. M. (1986). Making the most of what you have: Adapting available materials for developing interactive skills in augmentative communication users. *Augmentative and Alternative Communication*, 2, 116.

Tallman, T. M., & Favin, D. L. (1986). Audible prompting to the handicapped for communication and environmental control. *Augmentative and Alternative Communication*, 2, 116–117.

Tamura, S., Webber, S., Richard, A., & Mahoney, P. (1992). Sexual abuse: Issues for adult users of AAC. *Augmentative and Alternative Communication*, 8, 172–173.

Tangerud, H., Rustoy, F., & Brande, E. (1990). Computers in special education in Norway—Strategies and product development. *Augmentative and Alternative Communication*, 6, 92.

Tanner, D. C. (1980). Loss and grief: Implications for the speech-language pathologist and audiologist. *Asha*, 22, 916–928.

Tapajna, M., & Blau, A. (1985). *The Choice Board: Perspectives on Training and Use.* Lake Zurich, IL: Don Johnson Developmental Equipment.

Tatman, T., & Webster, C. D. (1973). *Teaching Autistic-Retarded Children Through Simultaneous (Gestural and Verbal) Communications* (15-minute black and white film). Distributed by Clarke Institute of Psychiatry, Toronto.

Taylor, L., Hook, S., & Phoenix, R. (1990). Speaking, reading, writing—Mainstreaming the technology dependent student. *Augmentative and Alternative Communication*, 6, 152.

Teaching Aids for Children with Cerebral Palsy (1966). Albany: New York State Department of Education.

Teaching Guidelines [for Blissymbols] (n.d.). Toronto: Blissymbolics Communication Institute.

Teller, D. Y., McDonald, M. A., Preston, K., Sebris, S. L., & Dobson, V. (1986). Assessment of visual acuity in infants and children: The acuity card procedure. *Developmental Medicine and Child Neurology*, 28, 779–789.

Tenenbaum, D., & Schlanger, B. B. (1968). Gestural communication by aphasics in dyadic situations. Paper presented at the annual meeting of the American Speech-Language-Hearing Association, Denver.

ten Kate, J. H., & Hepp, B. (1989). Optical and eye-controlled communication aids. *Journal of Medical Engineering and Technology*, 13(1–2), 63–67.

ten Kate, J. H., & van Nifterick, W. (1988). The design of a saccade-size predictor for eye communication. *Medical Progress through Technology*, 13(4), 179–193.

ten Kate, J. H., Verbeek, D. G., Hogerworst, R., & Donker, D. J. (1985). Discrete eye-position recording for alternative communication. *Medical Progress and Technology*, 10(4), 201–211.

Tennell, B. (1986). Talking with Tina. *Proceedings, Minspeak Conference.* Wooster, OH: Prentke Romich Co., pp. 44–49.

Tetlie, R., & Reichle, J. (1986). The match between signed requests and objects selection in four learners with severe handicaps. Unpublished master's thesis, University of Minnesota.

Thal, D. J., & Tobias, S. (1992). Communicative gestures in children with delayed onset of oral expressive vocabulary. *Journal of Speech and Hearing Research*, 35, 1281–1289.

Theriault, P. A. (1993). *Mike's Story*. Ridgetown, Ont., Canada: The Bliss Book Foundation, P.O. Box 354.

Thomas, L., Hope, M., & Odor, P. (1986). Compatibility standards for communication aids in the EEC. *Augmentative and Alternative Communication*, 2, 117.

Thorley, B., Ward, J., Binepal, T., & Dolan, K. (1991). Communicating with printed words to augment signing: Case study of a severely disabled deaf-blind child. *Augmentative and Alternative Communication*, 7, 80–87.

Thornett, C. E. E., Langer, M. C., Billington, G. D., Dymond, E. A., & Bracey, D. I. (1986). The technology is here—Can we use it? *Augmentative and Alternative Communication*, 2, 117.

Thornett, C. E. E., Langner, M. C., & Brown, A. W. (1990). Disabled access to information technology—a portable adaptable multipurpose device. *Journal of Biomedical Engineering*, 12(3), 205–208.

Three new groups work for people with communication disorders (May 1989). *Asha*, 31, 89,

Thurlow, W. R. (1980a). Studies on hand-held visual communication device for the deaf and speech-impaired: 1. Visual display window size. *Ear and Hearing*, 1(3), 137–140.

Thurlow, W. R. (1980b). Studies on hand-held communication device for deaf and speech-impaired: 2. Keyboard design. *Ear and Hearing*, 1(3), 140–147.

Thursfield, C. D., Robinson, K., & Ryan, M. (1986). The use of portable computers in the field of alternative and augmentative communication. *Augmentative and Alternative Communication*, 2, 117–118.

Thurston, S., & Deegan, S. (1990). "Hooked on groups": Expansion of VOCA vocabularies through group intervention. *Augmentative and Alternative Communication*, 6, 148.

Thurston, S., Tressel, J., & Brawn, R. (1992). Is 20 too late to learn to read and write? *Augmentative and Alternative Communication*, 8, 173.

Tolstrup, I. M. (1975). VIDIALOG: TV-based communication system for the motor handicapped. Paper presented at the Third Nordic Meeting on Medical and Biological Engineering, Tampere, Finland. (Paper is published in the conference proceedings volume.)

Tomkins, W. (1969). *Indian Sign Language*. New York: Dover Publications.

Topper, S. T. (1975). Gestural language for a non-verbal severely retarded male. *Mental Retardation*, 13(1), 30–31.

Topper-Zweibwan, S. (1977). Indicators of success in learning a manual communication mode. *Mental Retardation*, 15, 47–49.

Torok, Z. (1974). A typewriter operated by electromyographic potentials (GMMI). In Keith Copeland (Ed.), *Aids for the Severely Handicapped*, New York: Grune & Stratton, pp. 77–82.

Torok, Z., & Hammond, P. H. (1971). On the performance of single motor units as sources of control signals. Paper presented at the Conference of Human Locomotor Engineering, University of Sussex. (Paper is published in conference proceedings volume, pp. 35–40.)

Toulotte, J., Baudel-Cantgrit, B., & Trehou, G. (1990). Acceleration method using a dictionary access in a Blissymbolics communicator. *Augmentative and Alternative Communication*, 6, 122.

Trace Research and Development Center (1991). *HyperABLEDATA*. 4th ed. [computer compact disk]. Madison, WI: Author.

Tracy, W. F., & Bevans, D. (1984). Switch rules and considerations for communicator use. *Communication Outlook*, 5(3), 7.

Traub, D. A. (1977). Training teachers to use communication boards with the mentally retarded. Paper presented at the annual meeting of the American Speech-Language-Hearing Association, Chicago.

Traynor, C. D. (1977). A breath-controlled computer data system. Paper presented at the Fourth Annual Conference on Systems and Devices for the Disabled, Seattle. (Paper is published in conference proceedings volume, available from Continuing Medical Education, University of Washington School of Medicine.)

Trefler, E. (Ed.) (1984). *Seating for Children with Cerebral Palsy: A Resource Manual.* Memphis: University of Tennessee, Rehabilitation Engineering Program.

Trefler, E., & Crislip, D. (1985). No aid, an Etran, a Minspeak: A comparison of efficiency and effectiveness during structured use. *Augmentative and Alternative Communication*, 1(4), 151–155.

Trefler, E., Nickey, J., & Hobson, D. A. (1983). Technology in the education of multiply-handicapped children. *American Journal of Occupational Therapy*, 37, 381–387.

Trevinarus, J., & Drynan, D. (1990). Indirect selection techniques: A comparison. *Augmentative and Alternative Communication*, 6, 124.

Trevinarus, J., Shein, F., Parnes, P., & Milner, M. (1992). Speech recognition to enhance computer access for AAC users. *Augmentative and Alternative Communication*, 8, 173.

Trevinarus, J., & Tannock, R. (1987). A scanning computer access system for children with severe physical disabilities. *American Journal of Occupational Therapy*, 41, 733–738.

Treviranus, J., & McFadden, G. (1986). Auditory scanning: A case study. *Augmentative and Alternative Communication*, 2, 118.

Treviranus, J., & Tamura, S. (1986). The Elementary MOD keyboard: Scan access to children's software. *Augmentative and Alternative Communication*, 2, 118.

Treviranus, J., & Tannock, R. (1987). A scanning computer access system for children with severe physical disabilities. *American Journal of Occupational Therapy*, 41, 733–738.

Trittin, P. J., & Foulds, R. (1992). Automatic intonation application to synthesized Spanish speech. *Augmentative and Alternative Communication*, 8, 173–174.

Tronconi, A. (1990). Blissymbolics-based telecommunications. *Communication Outlook*, 11(2), 8–11.

Tronconi, A., Billi, M., Boscaleri, A., Graziani, P., & Susini, C. (1988). Some approaches to computerized graphics for disabled people. *Augmentative and Alternative Communication*, 4, 151.

Tsuchiya, K. (1984). [Review of the environmental control system for the severely handicapped.] *Iyodenshi-To-Seitai-Kogaku.*, 22(5), 305–310.

Turner, G. (1981). Eliciting spontaneous speech and peer group interaction. *Communication Outlook*, 3(1), 6–7.

Turner, G. A. (1988). The WOLF Pack: Inexpensive VOCA's from Wayne County schools, Michigan. *Augmentative and Alternative Communication*, 4, 153.

Turner, G. A. (1992). Synthesis of foreign language vocabularies at ADAMLAB. *Augmentative and Alternative Communication*, 8, 174.

Tyvand, S., Nilsson, K. B., & von Tetzchner, S. (1992). Evaluation of linguistic prediction techniques. *Augmentative and Alternative Communication*, 8, 174.

Vaccari, P., Fronticelli, G., & Sarti, P. (1990). Communication aids customization for disabled mainstreamed children in normal schools. *Augmentative and Alternative Communication*, 6, 134.

Vagnini, C. (1984). Critical questions to consider in selecting a communication aid. *Communicating Together*, 2(3), 16–17.

Vail, J. L., & Spas, D. L. (1974). *A Manual Communication Program for Non-Verbal Retardates*. DeKalb, IL: MWSEARCH-Title 1, 145 Fisk Avenue.

Valentic, V. (1991). Successful integration from a student's perspective. *Communicating Together*, 9(2), 9.

Valentine, M. (1988). An augmentative and alternative communication classroom project—Does it really work? *Augmentative and Alternative Communication*, 4, 140.

van Balkom, L. J. M. (1986). Is communication assessable? Perspectives for communicative interaction analysis. *Augmentative and Alternative Communication*, 2, 119.

van Balkom, H., & Donker-Gimbrere, M. (1988). *Kiezen vor Communicatie* [Choosing for Communication]. Nijerk, Netherlands: Intro.

van Balkom, H., van Blom, K., Donker, M. W., Lloyd, L., Nail, B. J., & Quist, R. W. (1990a). Graphic symbol communication. *Augmentative and Alternative Communication*, 6, 98–99.

van Balkom, H., van Blom, K., Donker, M. W., Lloyd, L., Nail, B. J., & Quist, R. W. (1990b). Research concerning description and comparison of graphic symbols. *Augmentative and Alternative Communication*, 6, 151.

VanBiervliet, A. (1977). Establishing words and objects as functionally equivalent through manual sign training. *American Journal of Mental Deficiency*, 82, 178–186.

VanBiervliet, A. (1986). Talking stripes: Utilization of bar code technology for augmentative communication. *Augmentative and Alternative Communication*, 2, 119.

VanBiervliet, A. (1988). Development of a multipurpose communication aid using compact disk technology. *Augmentative and Alternative Communication*, 4, 151.

VanBiervliet, A., & Paratte, H. P. (1992). Preliminary examination of rate enhancement techniques for graphic-based AAC aids. *Augmentative and Alternative Communication*, 8, 174.

VanBiervliet, A., & Wilson, L. (1988). Evaluation of the Magic Wand Speaking Reader as an augmentative and alternative communication aid. *Augmentative and Alternative Communication*, 4, 151.

van Blom, K. (1990). Computer-aided cognitive training in aphasia. *Augmentative and Alternative Communication*, 6, 96–97.

van Blom, K., & van Balkom, H. (1990). Follow-up service and training for aphasic patients. *Augmentative and Alternative Communication*, 6, 121.

van Coile, B., & Martens, P. (1990). Development and evaluation of two speech aids which are based on Dutch text-to-speech synthesis. *Augmentative and Alternative Communication*, 6, 123.

van den Hoven, M., & Mariotti, J. (1990). Increasing sociocommunication for augmentative and alternative communication users. *Augmentative and Alternative Communication*, 6, 144.

Vanderheiden, D. H., Brown, W. P., MacKenzie, P., Reinen, S., & Scheibel, C. (1975). Symbol communication for mentally handicapped. *Mental Retardation*, 13, 34–37.

Vanderheiden, G. C. (1975). *Evaluation and Further Development of the Automonitoring Communication Board as an Educational Aid for Severely Handicapped Children: Summary Final Report*. Madison: Trace Research and Development Center for the Severely Communicatively Handicapped, University of Wisconsin.

Vanderheiden, G. C. (1976a). Providing the child with a means to indicate. In Gregg C. Vanderheiden & Kate Grilley (Eds.), *Non-vocal Communication Techniques and Aids for the Severely Physically Handicapped*. Baltimore: University Park Press.

Vanderheiden, G. C. (1976b). *Synthesized Speech as a Communication Mode for Non-vocal Severely Handicapped Individuals*. Madison: Trace Research and Development Center for the Severely Communicatively Handicapped, University of Wisconsin.

Vanderheiden, G. C. (1977). *Design and Construction of a Laptray: Preliminary Notes*. Madison: Trace Research and Development Center for the Severely Communicatively Handicapped, University of Wisconsin.

Vanderheiden, G. C. (Ed.) (1978). *Non-vocal Communication Resourcebook*. Baltimore: University Park Press.

Vanderheiden, G. C. (1982a). Hybrid optical headpointing technique. *Proceedings of the Fifth Annual Conference on Rehabilitation Engineering*. Houston: Rehabilitation Engineering Society of North America, p. 24.

Vanderheiden, G. C. (1982b). Lightbeam headpointer research. *Communication Outlook*, 3(4), 11.

Vanderheiden, G. C. (1982c). Trace-hybrid lightbeam/sensor technique. *Communication Outlook*, 3(3), 6–7.

Vanderheiden, G. C. (1984a). A high efficiency flexible keyboard input acceleration technique: SPEEDKEY. *Proceedings of the Second International Conference on Rehabilitation Engineering*. Research Engineering Society of North America, pp. 353–354.

Vanderheiden, G. C. (1984b). A unified quantitative modeling approach for selection-based augmentative communication systems. Unpublished Ph.D. dissertation, University of Wisconsin, Madison.

Vanderheiden, G. C. (1987a). Advanced technology aids for communication, education, and employment. In E. McDonald (Ed.), *Treating Cerebral Palsy: For Clinicians by Clinicians*. Austin, TX: Pro-Ed, pp. 257–273.

Vanderheiden, G. C. (1987b). Service delivery mechanisms in rehabilitation technology. *American Journal of Occupational Therapy*, 41, 703–710.

Vanderheiden, G. C. (1988). Overview of basic selection techniques for augmentative communication: Present and future. In L. E. Bernstein (Ed.), *The Vocally Impaired: Clinical Practice and Research*. New York: Academic Press.

Vanderheiden, G. C. (1990a). Temporal relationship of the components of the selection act. *Augmentative and Alternative Communication*, 6, 94.

Vanderheiden, G. C. (1990b). Use of Hyper-text to create user-accessible databases. *Augmentative and Alternative Communication*, 6, 116.

Vanderheiden, G. C., Brandenburg, S., Brown, B., & Bottorf, C. (1987). *Toy Modification Note*. Madison: Trace Research and Development Center for the Severely Communicatively Handicapped, University of Wisconsin.

Vanderheiden, G. C., Brown, W. P., & Fothergill, J. (1978). Master chart of communication aids. In Gregg C. Vanderheiden (Ed.), *Non-vocal Communication Resourcebook*. Baltimore: University Park Press.

Vanderheiden, G. C., & Grilley, K. (Eds.) (1976). *Non-vocal Communication Techniques and Aids for the Severely Physically Handicapped*. Baltimore: University Park Press.

Vanderheiden, G. C., & Harris-Vanderheiden, D. (1976a). Communication techniques and aids for the nonvocal severely handicapped. In Lyle L. Lloyd (Ed.), *Communication Assessment and Intervention Strategies*. Baltimore: University Park Press.

Vanderheiden, G. C., & Harris-Vanderheiden, D. (1976b). Field evaluation of the Auto-Com, an auto-monitoring communication board. *Research Relating to Children* (ERIC Clearinghouse for Early Childhood Education), Bulletin 37, 86–87.

Vanderheiden, G. C., & Harris-Vanderheiden, D (1977). Developing effective modes of response and expression in nonvocal severely handicapped children. In P. Mittler (Ed.), *Research in Practice in Mental Retardation.* Baltimore: University Park Press.

Vanderheiden, G. C., & Kelso, D. (1982). *The Talking Blissapple.* Madison: Trace Research and Development Center for the Severely Communicatively Handicapped, University of Wisconsin.

Vanderheiden, G. C., & Kelso, D. (1987). Comparative analysis of fixed-vocabulary communication acceleration techniques. *Augmentative and Alternative Communication*, 3(4), 196–206.

Vanderheiden, G. C., Kelso, D. P., Holt, C. S., & Raitzer, G. A. (1976). *A Teacher Modifiable Portable Microprocessor Based Aid for Nonvocal Severely Physically Handicapped Individuals.* Madison: Trace Research and Development Center for the Severely Communicatively Handicapped, University of Wisconsin.

Vanderheiden, G. C., Kelso, D. P., Holt, C. S., & Raitzer, G. A. (1978). Cost reduction in the development of new communication aids through use of a common control system: A case example, the Blisscom. In P. Nelson (Ed.), *Proceedings of Workshop on Communication Aids.* Ottawa: Medical and Biological Engineering Society, National Research Council.

Vanderheiden, G. C., Lamers, D. F., Volk, A. M., & Geisler, C. D. (1975). *A Portable Nonvocal Communication Prosthesis for the Severely Physically Handicapped.* Distributed by the Trace Research and Development Center for the Severely Communicatively Handicapped, University of Wisconsin, Madison.

Vanderheiden, G. C., & Lloyd, L. L. (1986). Communication systems and their components. In Sarah W. Blackstone (Ed.), *Augmentative Communication: An Introduction.* Rockville, MD: American Speech-Language-Hearing Association, pp. 49–161.

Vanderheiden, G. C., & Luster, M. J. (1976). *Communication Techniques and Aids to Assist in the Education of Non-vocal Physically Handicapped Children: A State-of-the-Art Review.* Madison: Trace Research and Development Center for the Severely Communicatively Handicapped, University of Wisconsin.

Vanderheiden, G. C., Raitzer, G. A., & Kelso, D. P. (1976). *The Portable Auto-Com/Wordmaster: A Portable Non-vocal Communication Prosthesis for the Severely Physically Handicapped.* Madison: Trace Research and Development Center for the Severely Communicatively Handicapped, University of Wisconsin.

Vanderheiden, G. C., Raitzer, G. A., Kelso, D. P., & Geisler, C. D. (1974). *An Automated Technique for the Interpretation of Erratic Pointing Motions of Severely Cerebral Palsied Individuals.* Madison: Trace Research and Development Center for the Severely Communicatively Handicapped, University of Wisconsin.

Vanderheiden, G. C., & Smith, R. O. (1989). Application of communication technologies to an adult with a high spinal cord injury. *Augmentative and Alternative Communication*, 5, 62–66.

Vanderheiden, G. C., Snyder, T., & Kelso, D. (1992). Development of a user-friendly directly consumer accessible database service. *Augmentative and Alternative Communication*, 8, 175.

Vanderheiden, G. C., Volk, A. M., & Geisler, C. D. (1973). The auto-monitoring technique and its application in the automonitoring communication board. A new communication technique for the severely handicapped. Paper presented at the Carnahan Conference on Electronic Prostheses, Lexington, KY. (Paper is published in conference proceedings volume, pp. 47–51.)

Vanderheiden, G. C., Volk, A. M., & Geisler, C. D. (1974). An alternative interface to computers for the physically handicapped. Paper presented at the AFIPS National Computer Conference. (Paper is published in the conference proceedings volume, pp. 47–51.)

Vanderheiden, G. C., & Yoder, D. (1986). Overview. In S. Blackstone (Ed.), *Augmentative Communication: An Introduction*. Rockville, MD: American Speech-Language-Hearing Association, pp. 1–28.

Vandervelden, M. C. (1990). AAC users and development of word recognition and spelling. *Augmentative and Alternative Communication*, 6, 133.

Vandyke, J., McCoy, K. F., & Demasco, P. (1992). Using syntactic knowledge for word prediction. *Augmentative and Alternative Communication*, 8, 175.

van Dyck, M. C., Allaire, J. H., & Gressard, R. P. (1989). Decision making protocol used in augmentative/alternative communication. Paper presented at the annual meeting of the American Speech-Language-Hearing Association, St. Louis.

van Geel, R. C. (1986). Communication aid centers in the Netherlands? *Augmentative and Alternative Communication*, 2, 119–120.

van Hook, K. E., & Stohr, P. G. (1973). The development of manual communication in a profoundly retarded hearing population. Paper presented at the annual meeting of the American Speech-Language-Hearing Association, Detroit.

van Oosterom, J., & Devereux, K. (1982). REBUS at Rees Thomas School. *Special Education: Forward Trends*, 9(1), 31–33.

van Oosterom, J., & Devereux, K. (1984). *Rebus Glossary*. Blackhill, England: EARD.

van Oosterom, J., & Devereux, K. (1985). *Learning with Rebuses*. Cambridgeshire, England: EARO, The Resource Centre.

Van Tatenhove, G. M. (1978). Augmentative communication board development: A response training protocol. Paper presented at the annual meeting of the American Speech-Language-Hearing Association, Atlanta.

Van Tatenhove, G. M. (1986a). Transition through graphic symbol systems. *Communication Outlook*, 6(3), 27–29.

Van Tatenhove, G. M. (1986b). Vocabulary versatility for the person who is nonspeaking. *Communicating Together*, 4(3), 19–20.

Van Tatenhove, G. M. (1986c). Development of a location, color-coded ETRAN. In Sarah W. Blackwell (Ed.), *Augmentative Communication: An Introduction*. Rockville, MD: American Speech-Language-Hearing Association, pp. 397–409.

Van Tatenhove, G. M. (1987a). Assessing oral and speech motor abilities: Prognosis and student perspective. Intervention strategy developed under Contract No. 300-85-0139 (*Implementation Strategies for Improving the Use of Communication Aids in Schools Serving Handicapped Children*) from the U.S. Department of Education distributed by the American Speech-Language-Hearing Association.

Van Tatenhove, G. M. (1987b). Training caregivers and facilitators to select vocabulary. Intervention strategy developed under Contract No. 300-85-0139 (*Implementation Strategies for Improving the Use of Communication Aids in Schools Serving Handicapped Children*) from the U.S. Department of Education distributed by the American Speech-Language-Hearing Association.

Van Tatenhove, G. M. (1989). *Power in Play*. Wooster, OH: Prentke Romich Co.

Van Tatenhove, G. M., & Brothers, S. (1992). Using competent AAC users as peer trainers. *Augmentative and Alternative Communication*, 8, 175.

Van Tatenhove, G. M., & Osborn, S. (1987). Setting up and marketing an augmentative communication inservice for teachers/clinicians. Intervention strategy developed under Contract No. 300-85-0139 (*Implementation Strategies for Improving the Use of Com-*

munication Aids in Schools Serving Handicapped Children) from the U.S. Department of Education distributed by the American Speech-Language-Hearing Association.

Vasa, J. J. (1982). Electronic aids for the disabled and the elderly. *Medical Instrumentation*, 16(5), 261–262.

Vasa, J. J., & Lywood, D. W. (1972). A typing aid for the severely handicapped. Paper presented at the Canadian Medical and Biological Engineering Conference. (Paper is published in the conference digest volume, available from the Canadian Medical and Biological Engineering Society, National Research Council, Ottawa.)

Vasa, J. J., and Lywood, D. W. (1976). High-speed communication aid for quadriplegics. *Medical and Biological Engineering*, 14, 445–450.

Vasa, J. J., & Mansell, M. (1974). Queen's communication aids. Paper presented at the Seminar on Electronic Controls for the Severely Disabled, Vancouver, BC. (Paper is published in seminar proceedings volume, pp. 37–39.)

Venkatagiri, H. S. (1990). The effect of rate and pitch on Echo-II produced speech. Paper presented at the annual meeting of the American Speech-Language-Hearing Association, Seattle.

Venkatagiri, H. S. (1991). Effects of rate and pitch variations on the intelligibility of synthesized speech. *Augmentative and Alternative Communication*, 7, 284–289.

Venkatagiri, H. S. (1992). The Messenger: An assistive communication program. Paper presented at the annual meeting of the American Speech-Language-Hearing Association, San Antonio.

Venkatagiri, H. S. (1994). Effect of sentence length and exposure on the intelligibility of synthesized speech. *Augmentative and Alternative Communication*, 10, 96–104.

Verburg, G. (1986). A holistic model of symbol learning. *Augmentative and Alternative Communication*, 2, 120.

Vicker, B. (1974a). Advances in nonoral communication system programming: Project Summary No. 2, August 1973. In Beverly Vicker (Ed.), *Nonoral Communication System Project 1964/1973*. Iowa City: Campus Stores, University of Iowa, pp. 105–175.

Vicker, B. (1974b). Communication board programming with a four-year-old child: A case report. In Beverly Vicker (Ed.), *Nonoral Communication System Project 1964/1973*. Iowa City: Campus Stores, University of Iowa, pp. 213–261.

Vicker, B. (1974c). The communication process using a nonoral means. In Beverly Vicker (Ed.), *Nonoral Communication System Project 1964/1973*. Iowa City: Campus Stores, University of Iowa, pp. 15–56.

Vicker, B. (Ed.) (1974d). *Nonoral Communication System Project 1964/1973*. Distributed by Campus Stores, University of Iowa, Iowa City.

Vicker, B. (1992). AAC encounters of the first kind. *Augmentative and Alternative Communication*, 8, 175–176.

Vicker, B., & Mecca, A. (1988). Teaching nontraditional AAC behaviors to individuals with autism. *Augmentative and Alternative Communication*, 4, 170.

Vicker, B., & Quist, R. (1988). Upgrading the skills of professionals about augmentative and alternative communication. *Augmentative and Alternative Communication*, 4, 140.

Vicker, B., & Williams, D. L. (1990). AAC: Getting the word out in Indiana. Paper presented at the annual meeting of the American Speech-Language-Hearing Association, Seattle.

Viggiano, J. (1981). Ignorance as handicap. *Asha*, 23, 551–552.

Viggiano, J. (1982). Don't patronize me—Communicate with me. *Communication Outlook*, 3(4), 13.

Villarruel, F., Mathy-Laikko, P., Ratcliff, A., & Yoder, D. (1987). *Augmentative and Alterna-*

tive Communication Bibliography. Madison: Trace Research and Development Center for the Severely Communicatively Handicapped, University of Wisconsin.

Villiers, J. G. D., & McNaughton, J. M. (1974). Teaching a symbol language to autistic children. *Journal of Consulting and Clinical Psychology*, 42, 111–117.

Voda, J. A., Leibowitz, L., & Wu, Y. (1988). Unlocking locked-in syndrome: A unique solution. *Augmentative and Alternative Communication*, 4, 144.

von Glaserfeld, E. (1977). The Yerkish Language and its automatic parser. In Duane M. Rambaugh (Ed.), *Language Learning in a Chimpanzee: The LANA Project.* New York: Academic Press, pp. 91–130.

von Tetzchner, S. (1984). Facilitation of early speech development in a dysphatic child by use of signed Norwegian. *Scandinavian Journal of Psychology*, 25, 265–275.

von Tetzchner, S. (1988). Becoming an aided speaker. *Augmentative and Alternative Communication*, 4, 171.

von Tetzchner, S. (1990). First words. *Augmentative and Alternative Communication*, 6, 118.

von Tetzchner, S. (1992). Conversational aid for a girl with Spielmeyer-Vogt's disease. *Augmentative and Alternative Communication*, 8, 176.

von Tetzchner, S., & Basil, C. (1992). Prototype theories and language teaching. *Augmentative and Alternative Communication*, 8, 176.

von Tetzchner, S., & Berntzen, J. (1990). A conversational text telephone program for IBM-compatible computers. *Augmentative and Alternative Communication*, 6, 113.

von Tetzchner, S., & Martinsen, H. (1992). *Introduction to Symbolic and Augmentative Communication.* San Diego: Singular Publishing Group.

von Tetzchner, S., & Øien, I. (1990). Rett syndrome—Development and intervention. *Augmentative and Alternative Communication*, 6, 106–107.

Wachtmeister, H., & Hunnicut, S. (1992). Use of word prediction with speech recognition: A case study. *Augmentative and Alternative Communication*, 8, 176.

Wacker, D. P., Wiggins, B., Fowler, M., & Berg, W. K. (1988). Training students with profound or multiple handicaps to make requests via microswitches. *Journal of Applied Behavior Analysis*, 21(4), 331–343.

Wald, M. (1986). Speech synthesisers and special schools. *Augmentative and Alternative Communication*, 2, 120.

Waldman, S., Miudosar, D., Nebenzahi, I., & Chen, D. (1992). Decision support expert system for adopting AAC to disabled children. *Augmentative and Alternative Communication*, 8, 176.

Waldo, L. J. (1977). Functional communication board training for the severely handicapped. Paper presented at the annual meeting of the American Speech-Language-Hearing Association, Chicago.

Walejko, M., & Price, R. (1986). Computers as an instructional tool—Not a panacea. *Augmentative and Alternative Communication*, 2, 120–121.

Walker, M. (1986). *The Revised Makaton Vocabulary.* Camberley, Surrey, England: Makaton Vocabulary Development Project.

Walker, M. (1987). The Makaton Vocabulary: Uses and effectiveness. Paper presented at the first international AFASIC symposium, University of Reading, Reading, England.

Walker, M., & Grove, N. (1986). Communicating through Makaton: A symposium on aspects of the work of the Makaton Vocabulary Development Project. *Augmentative and Alternative Communication*, 2, 121–122.

Walker, M., Parsons, F., Cousins, S., Henderson, R., & Carpenter, B. (1985). *Symbols for Makaton.* Camberly, England: Makaton Vocabulary Development Project.

Waller, A., & Alm, N. (1990). Semantic help in a text database communication system for nonspeaking people. *Augmentative and Alternative Communication,* 6, 89.

Waller, A., Beattie, W., & Newell, A. F. (1990). Using a predictive word processor—A case study. *Augmentative and Alternative Communication,* 6, 138.

Waller, A., Broumley, L., & Newell, A. F. (1992). Incorporating conversational narratives in an AAC device. *Augmentative and Alternative Communication,* 8, 177.

Waller, A., & Van Der Walt, R. (1988). "Interface"—The first five years. *Augmentative and Alternative Communication,* 4, 150.

Ward, D. (1986). *Positioning the Handicapped Child for Function.* Chicago: Phoenix Press.

Wardell, R. (1978). Development of the eyewriter. In P. Nelson (Ed.), *Proceedings of Workshop on Communication Aids.* Ottawa: Canadian Medical and Biological Engineering Society, National Research Council.

Warner, H., Bell, C. L., & Brown, J. V. (1977). The conversation board. In Duane M. Rumbaugh (Ed.), *Language Learning in a Chimpanzee: The LANA Project.* New York: Academic Press, pp. 263–271.

Warren, S., & Rogers-Warren, A. (Eds.) (1985). *Teaching Functional Language.* Austin, TX: Pro-Ed.

Warrick, A. (1982). *Blissymbolics for Preschool Children.* 2nd ed. Toronto: Blissymbolics Communication Institute.

Warrick, A. (1984). Worldsign: A kinetic language. *Communicating Together,* 2(3), 17–19.

Warrick, A. (1985). Picture your Blissymbols. *Aug-Communique,* 3(1), 5–6.

Warrick, A. (1986). A socio-developmental model relating to graphic communication within augmentative communication. *Augmentative and Alternative Communication,* 2, 122.

Warrick, A. (1987). Can we play a game tonight? *Communicating Together,* 5(3), 15–16.

Warrick, A. (1988). Sociocommunicative considerations within augmentative and alternative communication. *Augmentative and Alternative Communication,* 4, 45–51.

Warrick, A., et al. (1978). Synthesized speech as an aid in communication and learning for the non-verbal. In P. Nelson (Ed.), *Proceedings of Workshop on Communication Aids.* Ottawa: Canadian Medical and Biological Engineering Society, National Research Council.

Warrick, A., & Woodall, S. (1990). Facilitator training: One component of AAC service delivery. *Augmentative and Alternative Communication,* 6, 144–145.

Wasson, P. (1986). Messaging and reporting. In Sarah W. Blackstone (Ed.), *Augmentative Communication: An Introduction.* Rockville, MD: American Speech-Language-Hearing Association, pp. 411–421.

Wasson, P., Tynan, T., & Gardiner, P. (1982). *Test Adaptations for the Handicapped.* San Antonio: Education Service Center Region 20.

Watkins, C. W. (1988). Communication considerations for quadriplegic patients with high spinal cord injury. *Augmentative and Alternative Communication,* 4, 144.

Watkins, C. W. (1990). Spinal cord injury: Communication needs. *Augmentative and Alternative Communication,* 6, 130.

Watkins, C. W., & Berryman, J. D. (1988a). Effects of cognitive level on augmentative and alternative communication learning. *Augmentative and Alternative Communication,* 4, 157.

Watkins, C. W., & Berryman, J. D. (1988b). Effects of selected stimulus variables on augmentative communication learning. Paper presented at the annual meeting of the American Speech-Language-Hearing Association, Boston.

Watkins., L. T., Sprafkin, J. N., & Krolikowski, D. M. (1990). Effects of video based training on spoken and signed language acquisition by students with mental retardation. *Research in Developmental Disabilities*, 11(3), 273–288.

Watters, R. G., Wheeler, L. J., & Watters, W. E. (1981). The relative efficiency of two orders for training autistic children in the expressive and receptive use of manual sign. *Journal of Communication Disorders*, 14, 273–285.

Watts, P. (1986). Keyboard emulation for the BBC Micro using a parallel interface. *Augmentative and Alternative Communication*, 2, 122–123.

Weatherill, M. M., & Haak, N. J. (1992). Attitudes toward dysarthric speech and an augmentative communication device. Paper presented at the annual meeting of the American Speech-Language-Hearing Association, San Antonio.

Webb, A. (1984). Dustin—3: Augmented communication for a preschool child. *Communication Outlook*, 6(2), 4–5.

Weber, S. C. (1972). Preliminary norms pertaining to the inner language construct in children. Unpublished manuscript, Marquette University.

Webster, C. D., McPherson, H., Sloman, L., Evans, M. A., & Kuchar, E. (1973). Communicating with an autistic boy with gestures. *Journal of Autism and Childhood Schizophrenia*, 3, 337–346.

Webster, J. G., Cook, A. M., Tompkins, W. J., & Vanderheiden, G. C. (1985). *Electronic Devices for Rehabilitation*. New York: John Wiley.

Weintraub, M. J. (1982). Computer assisted communication. *Archives of Neurology*, 39, 740.

Weiss, L., Thatch, D., & Thatch, J. (1987). *I Wasn't Finished with Life*. Dallas: E-Heart Press.

Welle Donker-Gimbrere, M., & van Balkom, H. (1992). Use of graphic symbols in communication in the Netherlands. *Augmentative and Alternative Communication*, 8, 177.

Weller, D. R. (1990). Voice interface access for persons with disabilities. *Augmentative and Alternative Communication*, 6, 88.

Wells, M. E. (1981). The effects of total communication training versus traditional speech training on word articulation in several retarded individuals. *Applied Research in Mental Retardation*, 2, 323–333.

Wender, D. (January 1990). Quality: A personal perspective. *Asha*, 32, 41–44.

Wendt, E., Sprague, M. J., & Marquis, J. (Fall 1975). Communication without speech. *Teaching Exceptional Children*, 38–42.

Westman, C., Bowen, K., & Crary, M. A. (1987). Touch-Talker intelligibility. Paper presented at the annual meeting of the American Speech-Language-Hearing Association, New Orleans.

Wetherby, A. (1989). Language intervention for autistic children: A look at where we have come in the past 25 years. *Revue d'orthophonie et d'audiologie* [Journal of Speech-Language Pathology and Audiology]. 13(4), 15–28.

Wetherby, A., & Prizant, B. (1990). *Communication and Symbolic Behavior Scales (CSBS)*. Tucson, AZ: Communication Skill Builders.

Wexler, K., Blau, A., Leslie, S., & Dore, J. (1983). *Conversational Interaction of Nonspeaking Cerebral Palsied Individuals and Their Speaking Partners with and without Augmentative Communication Aids*. Final Report R-313–80. New York: United Cerebral Palsy Research and Education Foundation.

Wherry, J. N., & Edwards, R. P. (1983). A comparison of verbal, sign, and simultaneous systems for the acquisition of receptive language by an autistic boy. *Journal of Communication Disorders*, 16, 201–216.

Whitley, K. (1985). Picture Communication Symbols (PCS): A review. *Aug-Communique*, 3(1), 3.

White, L. C., & Dobres, R. (1992). Carryover in the work setting: Where is the TouchTalker? Paper presented at the Seventh Annual Minspeak™ Conference.

White, L. C., Dobres, R., Haight, P. L., & Lee, N. (1990). Communicating in a community setting: Comparison of interactions with and without Minspeak™. Paper presented at the Fifth Annual Minspeak™ Conference, Seattle.

White, M. J., & Chambers, R. D. (1985). Practical modifications of communication boards to increase transmission rate. Paper presented at the annual meeting of the American Speech-Language-Hearing Association, Washington, DC.

White, S. C., Cornett, B. S., & Madak, T. W. (1988). A new procedure to facilitate payment for augmentative communication systems. *Augmentative and Alternative Communication*, 4, 146.

White, S. C., Madak, T. W., & Cornett, B. S. (1988). A new procedure to facilitate payment for augmentative communication systems. Paper presented at the annual meeting of the American Speech-Language-Hearing Association, Boston.

White, S. D. (1974). A modular communication device for paralyzed patients. *Archives of Physical Medicine and Rehabilitation*, 55, 94–95.

Wilber, R. B. (1976). The linguistics of manual language and manual systems. In Lyle L. Lloyd (Ed.), *Communication Assessment and Intervention Strategies*. Baltimore: University Park Press.

Wilber, R. B. (1980). Nonspeech symbol systems. In R. L. Schiefelbusch (Ed.), *Nonspeech Language and Communication: Analysis and Intervention*. Baltimore: University Park Press, pp. 325–356.

Wilbert, K. M. (1986). Communicative interaction. *Augmentative and Alternative Communication*, 2, 123.

Wilkinson, K. M., & Romski, M. A. (1989). Emerging symbol combinations in nonspeaking children with mental retardation. Paper presented at the annual meeting of the American Speech-Language-Hearing Association, St. Louis.

Wilkinson, K. M., Romski, M. A., & Sevcik, R. A. (1990a). Children with disabilities: Peer social competence and augmentative communication. Paper presented at the annual meeting of the American Speech-Language-Hearing Association, Seattle.

Wilkinson, K. M., Romski, M. A., & Sevcik, R. A. (1990b). Patterns of multi-symbol augmented input to youngsters with retardation. *Augmentative and Alternative Communication*, 6, 118.

Williams, B., Williams, M. B., & Broehl, D. (1992). Hear our voices. *Augmentative and Alternative Communication*, 8, 178.

Williams, B., Williams, M. B., Mata, E., & Richmond, G. (1992). Empowerment: The ultimate vehicle for change. *Augmentative and Alternative Communication*, 8, 178.

Williams, G. O. (1990). Augmentative communication in North Carolina. Paper presented at the annual meeting of the American Speech-Language-Hearing Association, Seattle.

Williams, J., Csongradi, J., & LeBlanc, M. (1982). *A Guide to Controls: Selecting, Mounting, Applications*. Palo Alto, CA: Rehabilitation Engineering Center, Children's Hospital at Stanford.

Williams, M. B. (1991). Message encoding: Comment on Light et al. (1990). *Augmentative and Alternative Communication, 7*, 133–134.

Williams, M. B., & Berg, M. H. (1992). Local consumer support groups: A pilot study. *Augmentative and Alternative Communication, 8*, 177.

Williams, M. B., & Krezman, C. (1992). Integration of an electronic communication system into daily life. *Augmentative and Alternative Communication, 8*, 177–178.

Williams, M. L. (1992). An algorithm for selecting a communication technique with intubated patients. *Dimensions of Critical Care Nursing, 11*(4), 222–233.

Williams, R. (1989). *In a Struggling Voice.* Seattle: TASH, The Association for Persons with Severe Handicaps.

Wills, K. E. (1981). Manual communication training for nonspeaking hearing children. *Journal of Pediatric Psychology, 6*(1), 15–27.

Wilson, P. S. (1974a). A manual language dialect for the retarded. Paper presented at the annual meeting of the American Speech-Language-Hearing Association, Las Vegas.

Wilson, P. S. (1974b). Sign language as a means of communication for the mentally retarded. Paper presented at the April meeting of the Eastern Psychological Association.

Wilson, P. S., Goodman, L., & Wood, R. K. (1975). *Manual Language for the Child Without Language.* Distributed by Paula Starks Wilson, Department of Mental Retardation Developmental Team, 79 Elm Street, Hartford, CT.

Wilson, W. R. (1982). Uses of a portable microprocessor-based communication system and personal computers in the instruction of persons with severe physical disabilities. *Journal of Special Education Technology, 5*(4), 40–41.

Windsor, J. (1991). Core references on augmentative and alternative communication: Core reference list 1991. *Augmentative and Alternative Communication, 7*, 224–228.

Windsor, J., & Fristoe, M. (1988). Can listeners hear singing? Some effects of signing on speech. Paper presented at the annual meeting of the American Speech-Language-Hearing Association, Boston.

Windsor, J., & Lloyd, L. L. (1987). Core (or basic) references on AAC. *Augmentative and Alternative Communication, 3*, 103–111.

Wint, G. (1965). *The Third Killer: Meditations on a Stroke.* New York: Abelard-Schuman.

Wisocki, P. A., & Mosher, P. M. (1980). Peer-facilitated sign language training for a geriatric stroke victim with chronic brain damage. *Journal of Geriatric Psychiatry, 13*(1), 89–102.

Wolf, S., & Mizuko, M. (1992). The intelligibility of synthesized speech: Monosyllabic words versus bissyllabic words. Paper presented at the annual meeting of the American Speech-Language-Hearing Association, San Antonio.

Woltosz, W. S. (1984). Personal computers as augmentative communication aids. *Communication Outlook, 5*(4), 4–7.

Woltosz, W. S. (1988a). Integrated or dedicated?;t.;t.;t. The new choice in augmentative and alternative communication systems. *Augmentative and Alternative Communication, 4*, 151–152.

Woltosz, W. S. (1988b). A proposed model for augmentative and alternative communication evaluation and system selection. *Augmentative and Alternative Communication, 4*, 233–235.

Woltosz, W. S. (1988c). When is scanning or encoding better than direct selection? *Augmentative and Alternative Communication, 4*, 161–162.

Woltosz, W. S., Dahlen, J. A., & Palin, M. W. (1988). State-of-the-art strategies for novel communication by literate augmentative and alternative communicators. *Augmentative and Alternative Communication*, 4, 151.

Woltosz, W. S., & Palin, M. W. (1988). Computerized evaluation and assessment for augmentative and alternative communication. *Augmentative and Alternative Communication*, 4, 158.

Wolverton, R., Beukelman, D., Haynes, R., & Sesow, D. (1992). Strategies in augmented literacy using microcomputer-based approaches. *Seminars in Speech and Language*, 13(2).

Wong, L., & MacKinnon, E. (1990). Mediator training: Overcoming inherent difficulties in the process. *Augmentative and Alternative Communication*, 6, 103.

Wood, C. (1990a). Blissymbol talk: New Blissymbols for teaching human sexuality. *Communicating Together*, 8(3), 12–13.

Wood, C. (1990b). Ignorance is not Bliss—Blissymbolics for learning about human sexuality. *Augmentative and Alternative Communication*, 6, 118.

Wood, C., & Storr, J. (1986). Blissymbolics: Interactive, interdisciplinary, international. *Augmentative and Alternative Communication*, 2, 123.

Wood, M. W. (1992). "Language, Learning, and Living" software: Two case studies. *Augmentative and Alternative Communication*, 8, 178.

Woodcock, R. W. (1958). An experimental test for remedial readers. *Journal of Educational Psychology*, 49, 23–27.

Woodcock, R. W. (Ed.) (1965). *The Rebus Reading Series*. Nashville, TN: Institute on Mental Retardation and Intellectual Development, George Peabody College.

Woodcock, R. W. (1968). Rebuses as a medium in beginning reading instruction. *IMRID Papers and Reports*, 5(4).

Woodcock, R. W., Clark, C. R., & Davies, C. O. (1968). *The Peabody Rebus Reading Program*. Minneapolis: American Guidance Service.

Woodcock, R. W., Clark, C. R., & Davies, C. O. (1969). *The Peabody Rebus Reading Program—Teacher's Guide*. Circle Pines, MN: American Guidance Service.

Woodfin, S. T., & Larson, J. (1988). Training staff members as effective partners of AAC users. *Augmentative and Alternative Communication*, 4, 165.

Woodfin, S. T., & Larson, J. (1992). Development levels framework: A continuum in AAC assessment and intervention. *Augmentative and Alternative Communication*, 8, 178–179.

Woolman, D. H. (1980). A presymbolic training program. In R. L. Schiefelbusch (Ed.), *Nonspeech Language and Communication: Analysis and Intervention*. Baltimore: University Park Press, pp. 325–356.

Wormnaes, S. (1987). *Bevegelsesvansker, Talevansker og Ny Teknologi* [Motor Handicap, Speech Handicap, and New Technology]. Statens Speciallaererhogskole, 1347 Hosle Norway.

Wright, C., & Nomura, M. (1987). *From Toys to Computers: Access for the Physically Disabled Child*. Wauconda, IL: Don Johnson Developmental Equipment.

Writing made possible for cerebral palsy victim (February, 1976). *Pacific Review*, 10(4), 3.

Wu, Y. C., & Voda, J. A. (1985). User-friendly communication board for nonverbal, severely physically handicapped individuals. *Archives of Physical Medicine and Rehabilitation*, 66(12), 827–828.

Wyper, D. J., Cunningham, E., Keating, D., & Evans, A. L. (1986). The art of conversation prompting. *Augmentative and Alternative Communication*, 2, 124.

Wyper, D. J., Evans, A. L., Cunningham, E., & Keating, D. (1986). A communication aid for the nonvocal in the intensive care unit. *Augmentative and Alternative Communication, 2,* 123–124.

Yarrington, D. (1992). Refining a synthesized child's voice. *Augmentative and Alternative Communication,* 8, 179.

Yngvesson, Y., & Johnsen, B. (1990). PictoCom—A computer based graphic communication aid for persons with aphasia. *Augmentative and Alternative Communication,* 6, 107.

Yoder, D. E. (Ed.) (1982). Communication intervention strategies for the severely communicatively impaired. *Topics in Language Disorders,* 2(2).

Yoder, D. E., & Kraat, A. (1983). Intervention issues in nonspeech communication. In J. Miller, D. E. Yoder, & R. Schiefelbusch (Eds.), *Contemporary Issues in Language Intervention.* ASHA Report No. 12. Rockville, MD: American Speech-Language-Hearing Association, pp. 27–51.

Yoder, P. J., & Layton, T. L. (1988). Speech following sign language training in autistic children with minimal verbal language. *Journal of Autism and Developmental Disorders,* 18(2), 217–229.

York, J., Nietupski, J., & Hamre-Nietupski, S. (1985). A decision-making process for using microswitches. *Journal of the Association for Persons with Severe Handicaps,* 10, 214–223.

York, J., & Weimann, G. (1991). Accomodating severe physical disability. In J. Reichle, J. Y. York, & J. Sigafoos, *Implementing Augmentative and Alternative Communication: Strategies for Learners with Severe Disabilities.* Baltimore: Paul H. Brookes, pp. 239–255.

Yorkston, K. M. (1989). Early intervention in amyotrophic lateral sclerosis: A case presentation. *Augmentative and Alternative Communication,* 5, 67–70.

Yorkston, K. M., Beukelman, D. R., & Bell, K. (1988). *Clinical Management of Dysarthric Speakers.* San Diego: College-Hill.

Yorkston, K. M., Beukelman, D. R., Smith, K., & Tice, R. (1990). Extended communication samples of augmented communicators II: Analysis of multiword sequences. *Journal of Speech and Hearing Disorders,* 55, 225–230.

Yorkston, K. M., Dowden, P. A., & Honsinger, M. J. (1988). Natural speech as a component of augmentative and alternative communication systems. *Augmentative and Alternative Communication,* 4, 156.

Yorkston, K. M., Dowden, P. A., Honsinger, M. J., Marriner, N., & Smith, K. (1988). Comparison of standard and user vocabulary lists. *Augmentative and Alternative Communication,* 4, 189–210.

Yorkston, K. M., Fried-Oken, M., & Beukelman, D. (1988). Single word vocabulary needs: Studies from various nonspeaking populations. *Augmentative and Alternative Communication,* 4(3), 149.

Yorkston, K. M., Honsinger, M. J., Dowden, P. A., & Marriner, N. (1989). Vocabulary selection: A case report. *Augmentative and Alternative Communication,* 5, 101–108.

Yorkston, K. M., & Karlan, G. (1986). Assessment procedures. In Sarah W. Blackstone (Ed.), *Augmentative Communication: An Introduction.* Rockville, MD: American Speech-Language-Hearing Association, pp. 163–196.

Yorkston, K. M., Marriner, N., Smith, K., Dowden, P., & Honsinger, M. (1987). *Vocabulary Selection.* Seattle: Authors.

Yorkston, K. M., Smith, K., & Beukelman, D. (1990). Extended communication samples of augmented communicators I: A comparison of individualized versus standard single-word vocabularies. *Journal of Speech and Hearing Disorders*, 55, 217–224.

Yorkston, K. M., Smith, K., Miller, R., & Hillel, A. (1991). Augmentative and alternative communication in amyotrophic lateral sclerosis. Unpublished manuscript, University of Washington.

Young, C. M., & Hough, S. D. (1992). Can old dogs learn new tricks? Two case studies. *Augmentative and Alternative Communication*, 8, 179.

Yovetich, W. S. (1985). Cognitive processing of Blissymbols by normal adults. Unpublished doctoral dissertation, University of Western Ontario.

Yovetich, W. S. (1986). A dual coding model relating to the processing of graphic symbol systems. *Augmentative and Alternative Communication*, 2, 124–125.

Yovetich, W. S., Fagerberg, G., Porter, J., & Stewart, D. (1992). Noise and predictability effects on the intelligibility of synthesized speech. *Augmentative and Alternative Communication*, 8, 179–180.

Yovetich, W. S., & Paivio, A. (1980). Cognitive processing of Bliss-like symbols by normal populations: A report of four studies. Paper presented at the European Association for Special Education, Helsinki, Finland.

Yovetich, W. S., & Young, T. A. (1988). The effects of representativeness and concreteness on the "guessability" of Blissymbols. *Augmentative and Alternative Communication*, 4, 35–39.

Zangari, C. (1990). AAC users in integrated settings: Working with personal aides. Paper presented at the annual meeting of the American Speech-Language-Hearing Association, Seattle.

Zangari, C., Kangas, K. A., & Lloyd, L. L. (1988). Augmentative and alternative communication: A field in transition. *Augmentative and Alternative Communication*, 4, 60–65.

Zangari, C., Karlan, G. R., & Haynes, C. W. (1989). Providing technical assistance in AAC. Paper presented at the annual meeting of the American Speech-Language-Hearing Association, St. Louis.

Zangari, C., & Lloyd, L. L. (1987). Methodological issues in Blissymbol translucency research. Paper presented at the annual meeting of the American Speech-Language-Hearing Association, New Orleans.

Zangari, C., & Lloyd, L. L. (1989). A continuing look at methodological issues in Blissymbol translucency research. Paper presented at the annual meeting of the American Speech-Language-Hearing Association, St. Louis.

Zangari, C., Lloyd, L. L., & Vicker, B. (1994). Augmentative and alternative communication: An historical pespective. *Augmentative and Alternative Communication*, 10, 27–59.

Zavalani, T. S. (1984). *Jet Era Glphs: A Utilitarian Graphic Sign System*. Van Nuys, CA: Tomor S. Zavalani, 14803 Friar Street, No. 8.

Zeitlin, D. (1990). Unlocking potential in a brainstem injured patient. *Augmentative and Alternative Communication*, 6, 124.

Zeitlin, D. (1992). How functional is technology without strong support mechanisms? *Augmentative and Alternative Communication*, 8, 180.

Zellhofer, C. M., & Beukelman, D. R. (1992). Service delivery in augmentative communication. *Clinics in Communication Disorders*, 2(2), 7–18.

Zielinski, K., & Thompson, D. K. (1992). Developing communicative competence for persons with severe cognitive impairments. *Augmentative and Alternative Communication*, 8, 180.

Zimmer, C. A., Devlin, P. M., Werner, J. L., Stamp, C. V., Bellian, K.T., Powell, D. M., & Edlich, R. F. (1991). Adaptive communication systems for patients with mobility disorders. *Journal of Burn Care and Rehabilitation*, 12(4), 354–360.

Ziskind, A., & Ziskind, R. (1959). Remote control typewriter for paraplegics. *Journal of the American Medical Association*, 169, 459–460.

Zweiben, S. T. (1977). Indicators of success in learning a manual communication mode. *Mental Retardation*, 15(2), 47–49.

Author Index

Subject Index